A Surgical Temptation

T0138346

A Surgical Temptation

*The Demonization of the Foreskin and
the Rise of Circumcision in Britain*

ROBERT DARBY

The University of Chicago Press   CHICAGO & LONDON

The University of Chicago Press, Chicago 60637
The University of Chicago Press, Ltd., London
© 2005 by The University of Chicago
All rights reserved. Published 2005.
Printed in the United States of America

22 21 20 19 18 17 16 15 14 13   2 3 4 5 6

ISBN-13: 978-0-226-13645-5 (cloth)
ISBN-13 978-0-226-10110-1 (paperback)
ISBN-10: 978-0-226-10978-7 (ebook)
DOI: 10.7208/chicago/ 9780226109787.001.0001

An earlier version of chapter 12 was published as "Where Doctors Differ: The Debate on
Circumcision as a Protection against Syphilis," *Social History of Medicine* 16 (2003): 57–78.

Library of Congress Cataloging-in-Publication Data

Darby, Robert (Robert J. L.)
    A surgical temptation: the demonization of the foreskin and the rise of circumcision in
Britain / Robert Darby.
        p.   cm.
    Includes bibliographical references and index.
    ISBN: 0-226-13645-0 (alk. paper)
    Circumcision—History. 2. Circumcision—Social aspects. I. Title.

GN484.D37 2005
392.1'09—dc22

                                                                                    2004027996

♾ This paper meets the requirements of ANSI/NISO Z39.48-1992 (Permanence of Paper).

In all cases [of masturbation] circumcision is undoubtedly the physician's closest friend and ally, offering as it does a certain means of alleviation and pronounced benefit. . . . Those cases in which the glans presents a moist, semi-oily appearance . . . long thickened foreskin, pliant and giving, large and often tortuous dorsal veins, go to make up a picture that is exceedingly tempting to the surgeon's scissors.

DR. EDGAR SPRATLING, "Masturbation in the Adult," 1895

They didn't have to think, only to endure. If you look at history you will see that men have always preferred suffering to thinking.

M. BARNARD ELDERSHAW, *Tomorrow and Tomorrow and Tomorrow,* 1947

CONTENTS

ACKNOWLEDGMENTS

Over the years it has taken me to complete this book, my greatest debt has been to the National Library of Australia, and particularly the staff of the Petherick reading room, who provide congenial conditions for research and have always made every effort to find the scarce items I have sought. The NLA's facilities for interlibrary loans and obtaining copies of journal articles are indispensable resources for independent scholars. I am also grateful to the staff of the Chifley and Hancock libraries at the Australian National University, and especially to Paul Quilty, for facilitating access to nineteenth-century medical periodicals at a time when they were stored in the basement. No medical historian in Australia would get far without the History of Medicine Library at the Royal Australasian College of Physicians in Sydney, and I am grateful to the former librarian there, Brenda Heagney, for her friendly assistance, enthusiasm, and kindness on many occasions; I know of nowhere else where a sudden whim to see the extant works of Aretaeus the Cappadocian could be gratified within five minutes. Librarians at Sydney and Melbourne universities have also been very helpful. At the Wellcome Library and as the founder and maintainer of the Hist-Sex (now H-Histsex) List for historians of sexuality, Dr. Lesley Hall replied to my many questions with detailed answers and kindly sent me an advance copy of her *Dictionary of National Biography* entry on William Acton, as well as providing much other material from her own research and commenting helpfully on several draft chapters. Dr. Ivan Crozier provided useful leads and advice in relation to Acton, Havelock Ellis, and male sexuality in the nineteenth century generally. Through the Hist-Sex List I was able to find a translator for the passage in Latin quoted in chapter 7, and I thank Chris Cudabec from the Classics Department, University of North Carolina, for his fluent rendering. Friends and colleagues overseas have also provided vital assistance by sending me photocopies of books and articles not available locally. I particularly thank Eddie Marcus for copying relevant pages from Isaac Baker Brown's infamous book in the British Library. This study would not have been possible without the trailblazing research of Dr. Frederick Hodges, whose meticulous investigations into the history of spermatorrhea and circumcision, and principled ethical stance on genital mutilation, have been a constant source of inspiration. His vast knowledge of the medical literature has guided me to many essential sources and helped me over numerous hurdles. Special and profound thanks are also due to the publisher's anonymous reader, whose relentless criticism of successive drafts and irrepressible suggestions for further reading and improvement have enabled me to produce a text far less imperfect than it would otherwise have been; and to Douglas Mitchell of the University of Chicago Press for his initial encouragement, his faith in the book, and his unfailing kindness and support. As my book neared completion I was invited to be a visiting fellow in the School of Social Sciences, Australian National University, and I thank the dean, Professor Frank Lewins, and Dr. Christopher Forth for their hospitality. Finally, it is a pleasure to thank my friends in Australia for their own contribution. To name them all would hold us up for too long, but I would particularly mention Peter Cochrane, Suzanne Rickard, Michael Johnson, and John Trevivian, who tolerated my obsession and provided congenial hospitality on my trips to Sydney and Melbourne. In Canberra Jeff Hart, Mario Fierro, and Stuart Fish sharpened my arguments with their skepticism and made sure that I was wined and dined to an epicurean standard at moments when my absorption in writing made meals seem like a distraction. Jonathan Curtis helped to maintain my spirits with his lively company and installments of *The Lord of the Rings,* the perfect allegory of fortitude in adversity. As the Roman historian Tacitus remarked, "Precipuum munus annalium reor ne virtutes sileantur, utque pravis dictis factisque, et posteritate et infamia metus sit" (The primary function of history is, I believe, that virtues should not be passed over in silence, and that vicious words and deeds should be opposed for fear of future infamy).

No one is more conscious than I of the limitations of this study, dictated by the conditions of its origin and composition. When I began to research the emergence of male circumcision in Britain I was planning to write no more than an introduction (the British background) to a history of the rise and decline of routine circumcision in twentieth-century Australia. But one issue led to another, and soon the introduction not only became longer than the intended book but displaced it entirely. I have published a preliminary account of the rise of circumcision in late nineteenth-century Australia (2001), however crude and inadequate it seems now, and I hope that a full-length study of the Australian experience will be my next project. The second factor is my location in Australia, where I have not had access to the wealth of material that would have been at my command had I been working in London or Washington. Australian libraries have surprisingly good collections of nineteenth-century medical texts and journals, scattered between Melbourne, Sydney, Canberra, and Adelaide, and the library of the Royal Australasian College of Physicians holds an invaluable collection of books and pamphlets. But Australia has nothing like the Wellcome Library, the National Library of Medicine, or even the resources of a major university library in the United States or England, and research here necessarily involves the burning of much petrol, the licking of many stamps, and the sending of countless e-mails. Colleagues overseas provided invaluable help by sending me photocopies of material not available in Australia, and I was able to purchase a number of texts, but I am conscious that had I been writing this book in the United States or Britain, the outcome would have been a richer background and fewer gaps in the narrative. I would have liked to devote more space to the slow development of accurate knowlege of the penis, the advice given in child-care manuals and to the treatment of children, especially at those character-building institutions known euphemistically as boarding schools, and I am well aware that the section in chapter 13 that deals with the personal impact of circumcision could have been expanded into a book in its own right. But research must stop somewhere, and there is a limit to every publisher's patience. I hope that readers will accept this study as a pioneering essay, and that others will go on to write more comprehensive, more detailed, more refined, and perhaps less indignant accounts of the extraordinary process I have attempted to analyze.

Part I

The European Background

The controvertists, answered my father, assign two and twenty different reasons for it:—others indeed, who have drawn their pens on the opposite side of the question, have shewn the world the futility of the greatest part of them.

Tristram Shandy, vol. 5, chap. 28

1 · Introduction

The Willful Organ Meets Fantasy Surgery

[The penis] disputes with the human intellect, and sometimes has an intellect of its own. And though the will of man may wish to stimulate it, it remains obstinate and goes its own way, sometimes moving on its own without the permission or intention of a man. . . . Many times a man wants to use it, and it does not want to; many times it wants to, and man forbids it.

LEONARDO DA VINCI

It has been urged as an argument against the universal adoption of circumcision that the removal of the protective covering of the glans tends to dull the sensibility of that exquisitely sensitive structure and thereby diminishes sexual appetite and the pleasurable effects of coitus. Granted that this may be true, my answer is that . . . sensuality in our time needs neither whip nor spur, but would be all the better for a little more judicious use of curb and bearing-rein.

E. HARDING FREELAND, "Circumcision as a Preventive of Syphilis and Other Disorders," 1900

The condition of our organs and our senses greatly influences our metaphysics and our morals, and . . . our most purely intellectual ideas . . . are largely derived from the shape of our bodies.

DENIS DIDEROT, "Letter on the Blind"

This study is an attempt to explain the sudden vogue for male circumcision in Victorian Britain. Although the causes reach deep into the history of medicine, disease, religion, and morality, the fundamental reason was a change in attitude toward male sexuality and the male body: between the mid-eighteenth and the late nineteenth century, the foreskin was transformed from an adornment that brought pleasure to its owner and his partners ("the best of your property") to "a useless bit of flesh" and an enemy of society. Much of the responsibility for this development lies with the efforts of Victorian physicians as "norm entrepreneurs," as Geoffrey Miller calls them, who set out consciously and resolutely to convince parents that their little boys would be better off without a feature their fathers had enjoyed. The result was that "during the last decades of the nineteenth century . . . a remarkable shift occurred in the English-speaking world. Physicians acting as norm entrepreneurs reconceived the phallus." Where the uncircumcised penis had been regarded as pure, healthy, natural, beautiful, masculine, and good, writes Miller, they succeeded in portraying it as "polluted, unnatural, harmful, alien, effeminized and disfigured," while spinning the circumcised penis, formerly regarded as ugly and chaotic, as "true, orderly and good."[1] The demonization of the foreskin as a source of moral and physical decay was the critical factor in the emergence of circumcision and its acceptance as a valid medical intervention,[2] and it is the central theme of this book. Necessary conditions were the rise of medical objections to masturbation; the conceptualization of "congenital phimosis" and spermatorrhea as pathological conditions; confused and erroneous theories of infectious disease; dread of syphilis; an atmosphere of sexual Puritanism in which non-procreative sex was regarded as immoral and sexual pleasure feared; and the emergence of a new professional elite keen to assert its social authority by proving such pleasures were dangerous as well. In their construction of sex as a risky business for men, doctors characterized the normal male sexual function—the production and emission of sperm—as a life-threatening illness that demanded drastic treatment if there was to be any hope of cure.

These developments were such a surprising departure from traditional attitudes to male sexuality that they demand detailed explanation.

Until Victorian physicians discovered its moral efficacies, circumcision was scarcely known in the Western world. Revering the male body, the Greeks and Romans admired the foreskin and tried to ban the operation among the few of their Eastern subjects who performed it. Although Genesis enjoined the rite on the children of Abraham, the early Christians decided that it was not necessary for converts; the Church Fathers condemned it; and in 1442 the Catholic Church determined that circumcision was incompatible with salvation. Renaissance artists celebrated Christ's unscarred penis in their many paintings of Madonna and naked child, and until the nineteenth century anatomists and advisers on sexual matters held that the foreskin was necessary for normal sexual function and the satisfaction of both partners, and that circumcision was thus contrary to the intent of nature. In the eighteenth century British men valued their foreskin as "the best of your property," and Edward Gibbon described circumcision as "a painful and often dangerous rite" and the result as "a peculiar mark."[3] Well might Sir Richard Burton comment that "Christendom practically holds circumcision in horror."[4]

The sudden transformation of this attitude is reflected in successive editions of the *Encyclopaedia Britannica*. In the third edition (1797) circumcision is described as "the act of cutting off the prepuce; a ceremony in the Jewish and Mahometan religions." The entry makes reference to remarks by Herodotus on the strange customs of Middle Eastern tribes; expresses uncertainty as to whether circumcision was practiced among the ancient Egyptians; and considers female circumcision to be no different from male: "Circumcision is practised on women by cutting off the foreskin of the clitoris, which bears a near resemblance and analogy to the praeputium of the male penis." The ninth edition (1876) maintains this perspective: it makes no mention of circumcision as a medical procedure and rejects sanitary/hygienic explanations of its emergence in favor of religious ones: "Like other bodily mutilations . . . [it is] of the nature of a representative sacrifice. . . . The principle of substitution was familiar to all ancient nations, and not least to the Israelites. . . . On this principle circumcision was an economical recognition of the divine ownership of human life, a part of the body being sacrificed to preserve the remainder." By the eleventh edition (1910) the entry has been turned on its head: "This surgical operation, which is commonly prescribed for purely medical reasons, is also an initiation or religious ceremony among Jews and Mahommedans." Suddenly circumcision is primarily a medical procedure and only after that a religious rite. The entry explains that "in recent years the medical profession has been responsible for its considerable extension among other than Jewish children . . . for reasons of health." By 1929 the entry is much reduced in size and consists merely of a brief description of the operation, which is "done as a preventive measure in the infant" and "performed chiefly for purposes of cleanliness"; readers are then referred to the entries for "Mutilation" and "Deformation" for a discussion of circumcision in its religious context.

What accounts for this dramatic shift in sensibility? It is a remarkable fact that although there is a substantial anthropological literature on tribal circumcision practices, our ignorance about the rise of medically rationalized circumcision in Anglophone countries is still profound; as Ronald Hyam remarked in 1990, we know less about the history of routine infant circumcision in Britain (and its colonies) and the United States than about the rituals of some of the most obscure African tribes.[5] In this study I hope to dispel some of this darkness, at least in relation to

Britain, and explain how an operation formerly regarded as a humiliating disfigurement came to be seen as a mark of manliness, respectability, and health. It was one of the most rapid and surprising developments in Victorian bodily management practices, and in Britain one of the most short-lived: rising to prominence in the 1890s, routine circumcision of young males reached its peak of popularity in the late 1920s, declined in the 1930s and 1940s, and all but vanished in the 1950s. As well as explaining its rise, I hope to shed light on its rapid fall from grace. Although the direct literature on this process is slight, I have been assisted by a number of important studies that have appeared over the past decade: Ronald Hyam's survey of sexuality and empire; Frederick Hodges' research into the history of spermatorrhea and circumcision in the United States; and important studies by David Gollaher.

Although several studies have analyzed the survival of routine circumcision in the United States,[6] the first serious attempt to account for the rise of the practice in Britain was made by Ronald Hyam, who relates the popularity of circumcision at the turn of the century to three main factors. The first was the fear of racial decline and falling physical fitness standards, giving rise to a host of anxieties and countermeasures, including the belief that circumcision would produce healthier and more self-confident males and "contribute to the general improvement of the . . . manliness of the future guardians of empire." The second was the sudden enthusiasm for Jewish child-rearing practices in response to reportedly low rates of syphilis and masturbation among Jewish (and thus circumcised) men and boys, and especially following the discovery by the Committee on Physical Deterioration in 1904 that such children were better nourished and healthier. The third was the necessity for colonial administrators to work in hot or humid climates, where hygiene of the uncircumcised penis was presumed to be difficult. Hyam notes that it was widely believed that normal males were more susceptible to venereal disease in hot climates and that British Army doctors in India were vigorously in favor of the procedure and operated on their soldiers at the first sign of trouble.[7] Hyam's account is constructive but not without serious gaps. He does not explain why hygiene in hot climates came to be seen as a problem only *after* the rise of circumcision in a cool climate, nobody having worried about the issue when the British first entered India in the eighteenth century; nor does he explain why it was believed that removal of the foreskin would produce healthier males; and he discounts the supposed value of circumcision in curbing masturbation as an explanation for its rise. On this point he is seriously mistaken, and his own discussion makes little sense without the conviction that masturbation was in itself a major health hazard and one of the factors contributing to national decline. The main reason for the sudden enthusiasm for Jewish child-rearing practices was the impression that Jewish boys did not masturbate, a contention that would have surprised Alex Portnoy but one that was widely debated in the medical journals of the time and eagerly confirmed by Jewish physicians, who were understandably pleased that the gentile world was at last beginning to see virtue in a rite it had traditionally abhorred. More convincing on this point is Ornella Moscucci, who shows that circumcision was increasingly recommended as a cure for male masturbation from the 1850s onward. She points out that part of this process was the demonization of the foreskin as a source of nervous and physical disease and agrees with Hyam that circumcision was central to the late Victorian redefinition of manliness in terms of self-restraint and cleanliness: "Widely believed to dampen sexual desire, circumcision was seen positively as a means of both promoting chastity and physical health."[8] Moscucci also discusses the contrasting case of female circumcision and clitoridectomy, and explains how, after a brief vogue in the early 1860s for treating masturbation, "hysteria," and epilepsy, the procedures fell rapidly into disfavor. Although the latter operation continued to be performed in the United States until the 1950s, it disappeared from the English surgical repertoire following the disgrace of its chief advocate, Isaac Baker Brown, in 1867. The debate over clitoridectomy was a vital stage in the acceptance of circumcision for naughty boys.

Frederick Hodges locates the origins of circumcision in Europe and Britain specifically in the masturbation phobia of the eighteenth century and in theories of reflex neurosis, which held that disturbances of nervous equilibrium could cause disease and which thus targeted sensitive parts of the body as the guilty parties.[9] In this scenario, particularly according to the work of Claude-François Lallemand on spermatorrhea, erotic sensation was redefined as irritation, prepubertal orgasms misinterpreted as epilepsy, and erections viewed as pathological; as the dynamic and most sensitive part of the penis, the foreskin was particularly suspect. Hodges confirms Hyam's argument that Jewish practice offered inspiration to English doctors: they sought evidence for the effects of circumcision in the only available circumcised population, whose doctors assured them that their boys did not masturbate, or not as much as Christians. Support for preventive circumcision was strengthened by reports that Jewish men also presented with lower rates of syphilis and cancer of the penis, and it was assumed that the absence of the foreskin must account for the difference. These were powerful selling points in Abraham Wolbarst's influential call for universal male circumcision in 1914, but he was equally insistent on its value as a "prophylactic against masturbation."[10] Hodges has also emphasized the importance of erroneous theories about penile development in infancy and childhood ("congenital phimosis"), emerging during the 1840s, in legitimizing the demand for early circumcision.[11]

In his essays on "the world's most controversial surgery," David Gollaher also stresses the importance of reflex neurosis theory, particularly as developed by the orthopedic surgeon Lewis Sayre, in explaining the rise of circumcision in the United States. Sayre claimed that many childhood illnesses were caused by a long or constricted prepuce ("phimosis") and could be cured by circumcision and that the same result in girls could be achieved by separation (sometimes removal) of the clitoral hood. He performed the operation on many boys suffering from various forms of paralysis, all of whom were apparently restored to health, and the future of the treatment was assured. Gollaher recognizes the importance of their determination to prevent masturbation in doctors' efforts to introduce widespread circumcision, but he is imprecise as to the chronology and does not seem to appreciate that it was their prior conviction that masturbation was harmful that inspired them to seek the etiology of common diseases in the condition of boys' genitals. He places the masturbation issue after the work of Sayre (1870s) and the hygiene fad that followed the discovery of germs (1890s onward), but medical concern with masturbation dates back to the eighteenth century: to *Onania* (ca. 1716), and Tissot's *Onanism* (1758), from which much of the nineteenth century's invective against the practice can be sourced. The proposition that circumcision could be used to discourage masturbation was first suggested by Lallemand, and later physicians recommended chastity devices, cauterization of the urethra, blistering of the penis, and even castration. Gollaher recognizes the puritanism and indeed the sadism of many doctors from this period, but he does not relate masturbation to the wider problem of spermatorrhea, an imaginary disease that designated almost any loss of semen other than in intercourse with one's wife as pathological, and of which masturbation or a long foreskin was held to be an important cause.

Gollaher is particularly revealing on the cultural pressures to which doctors were subject. He shows that they were not detached scientific observers but professionals who delivered a service in return for a fee. They complained that their quack rivals, in the days before the profession secured a legislative monopoly over health provision, stirred up people's fears about genital disorders in order to sell them patent medicines, but Gollaher notes that the doctors did much the same thing: projecting lurid scenarios of the disasters that would befall a child in later life unless they were paid to remove his foreskin in infancy. What emerges clearly from Gollaher's book is how much opposition there has always been to the procedure from those whom it is meant to benefit. Despite their enthusiasm for the health benefits of circumcision, doctors were unable to convince more than a few adult men to undergo the procedure, and they thus focused their attention on the younger generation. What emerges from this analysis is that the operation was less about health than power: priests over laymen, parents over children, doctors over parents. "Circumcision became a token of the medicalization of childbirth [and] a symbol of the rising authority of the medical profession over the laity," he writes.[12] Gollaher also shows that doctors knew little about the anatomy and physiology of the penis, were heavily influenced by their religious values, and had an opportunistic attitude to scientific evidence. They embraced circumcision as a miracle-working cure-all with much the same thoughtless enthusiasm with which they would greet Thalidomide in the 1960s, and sometimes with comparably tragic results: until surgical techniques were refined and aseptic conditions achieved, the incidence of complications (bleeding, gangrene, transmission of disease, loss of the glans, ulcers, and scarring) was high, and as late as the 1940s some sixteen boys a year in Britain died as a direct result of the operation.[13] One might think that the surprisingly blasé attitude toward this wastage was the result of the fact that, before effective antibiotics, all operations had a high casualty rate, but to this day remarkably little attention is paid to the risks of such a "safe" operation, even in South Africa, where ritual circumcision claims dozens of teenage lives each year.[14]

This study is intended as a contribution to our understanding of the history of the body, and specifically of the male sexual function as pictured by and expressed in society; to the history of moral attitudes; and to the rise of modern medicine. Of these three fields, as Roy Porter has observed, the first is certainly the most neglected. Referring to Leo Steinberg's remarkable book, *The Sexuality of Christ in Renaissance Art and in Modern Oblivion* (1984, 1996), he points out that the sexuality of Christ's body "had become invisible because scholars work within an interpretive tradition which gives priority to spiritual and ideal meanings, at the expense of material, corporeal and sensual matter."[15] Porter urged historians to pay greater attention to the body but warned against turning its history into a disembodied account of mere representations: "it is important to avoid floating off into the stratosphere of discourse analysis and neglecting the more everyday and tangible materials available."[16] I have sought to follow this advice: if anyone thinks my own account is too earthy, I have an unimpeachable authority to blame. My theme is not the body in general but the male genitals and specifically the penis—an important accessory to most men, but one about which few historians have ventured to write in a frank and objective spirit. By male sexuality, therefore, I do not mean sexual preference or gender identity but something similar to Steinberg's usage—the male genitals in all their anatomical and physiological detail, and the ways in which they have been perceived and managed over several centuries. My focus is the male sexual function in a physical sense, including the processes of secretion, erection, and ejaculation in all their complexity, irrespective of the provoking stimuli or the identity of sexual partners (if any); as Diderot implied, however profoundly sexual behavior is structured by social custom, the same physical organs have to do the dirty work. I hope this perspective will be seen as a corrective to the approach of too many of the books on the body that have appeared over the last decade, most of which seem not to have heeded Porter's advice to eschew the spirit in favor of the flesh. Instead of taking maleness as a whole, many such texts rarely venture below the neck, apparently assuming that masculinity is mostly in the mind and has little to do with the body, let alone the genitals. Some of those authors who do allow their gaze to drift below the navel seem unaware that penises come in many shapes and sizes, including complete and economy versions, and that there are significant objective and subjective differences between the normal and the circumcised manifestation. To ignore these differences would be like overlooking the fact that the English Civil War was fought between Cavaliers and Roundheads (as Australian schoolboys used to designate uncut and cut penises) and to write of it as though it was a struggle among undifferentiated Christians. Recognition of the real differences will tell us more about the history of maleness, medicine, and morality than remaining blind to such phenomena.[17]

If the history of the body is but roughly mapped terrain, the history of masculinity is terra incognita. Lesley Hall has pointed out that although there was "an upsurge in historical writing about sex in history" during the 1980s and 1990s, much of it focused on women and sexual minorities, while the average male received less attention. Unfortunate effects of this neglect have been the easy assumptions that "sexual discourses operated exclusively for his benefit,"[18] and that Victorian sexual anxieties fell far less heavily on men than on women. Apparently unaware of spermatorrhea and the discourses of masturbation, W. F. Bynum writes that "maleness was rarely pathologised; femaleness could be and was," while Thomas Laqueur, after denouncing the craze for ovariotomy, states blandly: "There was no male castration, no removal of healthy testes, except in a few rare and quite specific instances of criminal insanity or to treat cancer of the prostate."[19] Although it was far less common than ovariotomy, castration was occasionally recommended in Britain, and sometimes employed to treat spermatorrhea and masturbation, especially in U.S. mental hospitals and orphanages—although it never achieved anything like the level of acceptance won by circumcision, a topic about which both Laqueur and Peter Gay, in his study of Victorian sexuality, are strangely silent.[20] In his history of psychosomatic illness, Edward Shorter notes in passing that reflex neurosis theory led to the introduction of operations on the male genitals but seriously underestimates their prevalence, and he states quite wrongly that "male surgeons . . . probably shrank back psychically from mutilating patients of their own gender in a way they were perfectly willing to do to women." The truth is closer to the reverse; when it came to operations on the male genitals, Victorian surgeons were anything but shrinking violets.[21] In their study of sexual surgery, Andrew Scull and Diane Favreau make no mention at all of circumcision, infibulation, cauterization, or castration as treatments for male sexual problems, and they entirely suppress the fact that some of the authorities they cite were as keen to take the knife to men as to women—for example, E. H. Pratt, one of the loonies associated with the fringe American group the Orificial Surgery Society. They write that he viewed "orificial surgery" (operations on the rectum and genitals) as "an almost universal panacea for all the ills to which *female* flesh was heir" but seem unaware that he advocated such operations just as vigorously for male problems. They quote Pratt as urging circumcision of women as a remedy for infantile convulsions, hip-joint disease, kidney disease, paralysis, eczema, stammering, dyspepsia, pulmonary tuberculosis, constipation, locomotor ataxia, rheumatism, idiocy, insanity, and lust, without pointing out that he urged circumcision of males for the same conditions,[22] and without seeming to realize that circumcision was approved as a treatment for these conditions in males by the mainstream medical profession as well. Pratt was probably applying to women the list of "indications" for male circumcision, published in the *Medical Record* in 1896.[23] Even the authors of recent works on such relevant topics as masturbation and spermatorrhea seem to have developed a blind eye when it comes to circumcision. Although scholarly articles on these subjects in the 1970s were aware of the intimate connection between control of masturbation and the rise of circumcision,[24] the perception seems to have faded over the following decades. Neither Thomas Laqueur, in his recent history of masturbation, nor Ellen Rosenman, in her valuable survey of spermatorrhea in nineteenth-century Britain, so much as mention the word.[25]

The focus of much work in sexual history on women has led even careful scholars to overlook what many contemporaries actually wrote about men and sex. In an influential essay published in 1977, Barry Smith suggested that nineteenth-century medical opinion was not as repressive as Steven Marcus had represented it, and in particular not as alarmed by seminal loss as William Acton had been. In opposition to Marcus, Smith cites a comment from Charles Knowlton's *Fruits of Philosophy* (a popular birth control manual, famously prosecuted for obscenity in 1877) to the effect that nocturnal emissions were harmless, and claims that both Knowlton and Robert Dale Owen stated that masturbation "did no demonstrable harm."[26] These claims are incorrect. Knowlton did affirm that "occasional nocturnal emissions" were not a disease,[27] but this was Acton's own view, and indeed that of the medical mainstream. Equally orthodox were Knowlton's warnings that early gratification of the sexual instinct (before the age of twenty for males) stunted growth and wrecked health; that excessive indulgence (more than twice a week) sapped male energies and induced consumption; and that onanism not only impaired the bodily powers but often led to insanity. He warned that "the male system is exhausted in a far greater degree than the female" and even cited Tissot on the dire fact that an ounce of semen was the equivalent of forty ounces of blood.[28] It takes a while for specialist knowledge in sexual history to get into the canonical texts, but they eventually catch up. In a recent volume of the *New Oxford History of England* (1998) the author, citing Smith's essay as his authority, states that Acton's view "that masturbation produced physical cripples was by no means universally held" and that popular books such as Richard Carlile's *Every Woman's Book* "spoke as much of the joys of sex as the dangers of over-indulgence."[29] These derivative assertions are highly misleading. Carlile was hardly a respectable figure but a radical republican who had spent several years in jail for distributing banned works by Tom Paine. *Every Woman's Book* was primarily a manual of birth control, the legitimacy of which he advocated against Malthus as a means of helping the poor to limit their families, and thus both to alleviate poverty and reduce the incidence of vice and misery as population checks. It is true that he praised love as "the most delightful of our passions," but he added that it was precisely because it was "so great a part of human happiness" that it ought to be "purified . . . from all alloy."[30] This was little different from the opinion of Malthus himself, who had vigorously defended sexual passion against William Godwin's claim that it would fade away with the advance of civilization.[31] But politically radical as Carlile was, there were limits to his sexual radicalism:[32] the alloys he had in mind were irregular modes of sexual gratification, such as onanism, which he condemned as unnatural. In fact, he sought "to extinguish all these bad and disease producing practices by natural and healthy commerce between the sexes"; onanism was a "base artifice" that "generate[d] disease, and all that is degrading, painful and disgraceful to those who practised it." While moderate intercourse would promote health and happiness, "sexual excess" would produce debility in both men and women."[33] As for Owen, his *Moral Philosophy* warned that in sexual gratification, "the exhaustion to the man is much greater than to the women," ignorance of which fact has "caused more than one husband to forfeit his health, nay his life." He repeated the forty ounces story and assured readers that even of the healthiest man, "nature does not demand connection more than once a month"—a meaner allocation than Acton was willing to permit.[34]

It is safe to say that no Victorian medical authority, whether popular, quackish, or mainstream, challenged any of these dogmas, which were in fact the foundation stones of nineteenth-century sexual medicine. Even at the extreme sexual left, George Drysdale took the assumption that masturbation was deadly as an argument in favor of casual premarital sex and advocated the use of contraception as a way of making it possible to have more intercourse without fear of pregnancy.[35] His view represented such a radical dissent that those who agreed with his endorsement of birth control did not care to associate publicly with him, and even those who denounced his suggestions as incitement to debauchery dared not refer to him by name. This obsession with male sexual energies, and men's greater risk of exhaustion as compared with women, emphasizes the point that the most serious sexual problem of the period was not how to keep women under the patriarchal thumb, nor even prostitution or venereal disease, but the male sex drive and how to control it. When William Acton, in his best-known and most misunderstood remark, wrote that "the majority of women (happily for them) are not very much troubled with sexual feelings of any kind,"[36] he was not primarily making a comment about women at all; he was dramatizing the problem facing men. The key words are *happily* and *troubled.* He did not mean that women lacked sexual feelings or could not enjoy sex, but that, unlike men, they were not *troubled* by sexual urges. Unhappily for them, men *were* troubled by sexual desire: they woke up in the middle of the night with throbbing erections that ached for relief, yet they had to appreciate that yielding to the temptation (no matter how gratified) was dangerous to health and character. Women were fortunate in that they were not under the obligation to exercise such rigid self-control and thus did not have to endure the same torment. By the 1860s men's desire for sex was seen as a want rather than a need; while many considered sex to be necessary for women's health, for men it was increasingly regarded as a threat.[37]

Exceptions to the tendency to assume that sexual history means women and to ignore the things that doctors did to men include Alex Comfort in his largely forgotten but reliable *The Anxiety Makers* (1967) and several more recent female scholars. Showing that there were two sides to the Victorian double standard on sexual morality, Gail Pat Parsons took issue with arguments that, while women were the victims of humiliating surgical procedures at the hands of (male) doctors who left them raw and bleeding, men were treated with more respect. She points out that "men as well as women suffered excruciating treatment at the hands of physicians, whose limited knowledge reduced them to punitive, at times brutal, methods," including chastity devices, circumcision, and castration.[38] Although she underestimates the prevalence of circumcision and other genital surgeries, Janet Oppenheim also acknowledges that Victorian sexual repression "fell heavily on men," reminding us that "more printers' ink was devoted to censuring . . . masturbation than to any other topic."[39] It was not only ink, of course, that was spilled in the battle against masturbation. More recently, in a number of illuminating works, Lesley Hall has argued that the power of male sexuality made it *the* sexual problem of the nineteenth century, responsible not only for prostitution (called into existence by the demands of male lust) and thus venereal disease, but all the additional health problems supposedly caused by masturbation and sexual excess. In an era that applauded "the march of mind," valued self-control, and expected the "higher faculties" to rule the animal passions in much the same way as science was extending its dominion over nature, nothing was more worrying than the lawless libido. Hall writes that "the fear of unbridled male sexuality led to . . . anti-masturbation literature and other propaganda in favour of male purity"; mastery over "baser lusts" was seen as appropriate in all men but particularly necessary in the middle and would-be respectable classes.[40] *Unbridled* is the right word. Leonardo da Vinci had described the penis as having a mind of its own, but by the end of the nineteenth century there were plenty of doctors whose professional program was to bridle it, as the comment by E. Harding Freeland indicates (see the epigraphs to this chapter). The central aim of nineteenth-century sexual medicine was to control and regulate the penis, to make it more predictable and better behaved—leading to the improbable claim that circumcision could fix both priapism and impotence.[41]

Particularly acute understanding has also been shown by Ellen Rosenman in her recent account of the spermatorrhea panic. She points out that middle-class men as much as women lived under "the oppressive abstractions of 'patriarchy' and 'masculinity'" and that "their bodies were equally subject to appropriation in the name of the phallic ideal. Spermatorrhea surgeons objectified, dismembered and invaded middle-class male bodies as quickly as they did those of prostitutes and paupers. The spermatorrhoea panic is a concrete reminder of the virulent antipleasure ideology that literally made itself felt on the bodies of real people." She even remarks that although they endorsed conjugal intercourse "in controlled doses," Victorian surgeons "pathologized other forms of erotic pleasure in hierarchies of deviance, ranging from extramarital sex with a single partner, through promiscuity and prostitution, to the ultimate sin of masturbation."[42] The prostitute might have been a Victorian Other, but the otherest Other was the male masturbator—as they themselves often believed. Hall has shown how anxious men of all classes were about their own sexuality throughout this period, and right up until the 1950s. Many took the warnings of the quacks and mainstream physicians very much to heart, while others were concerned about impotence, lack of libido, the size and structure of their penis, or their ability to satisfy their partner. Many of the men who wrote to Marie Stopes in the 1920s either confessed to self-abuse as a likely explanation for their problems or assured her that they had not engaged in it, or not very much, or not for a long time. Few expressed skepticism as to its harmful effects.

The conviction that circumcision would alter sexual behavior was thus not a side effect of a procedure adopted as a health precaution but its original purpose. The idea of using surgery to promote moral conduct was certainly not new to Western thinking, but stronger precedents were available in the East. Islamic law prescribed punishment of thieves by amputation of the offending hand, of blasphemers by excision of the tongue, and authorized many forms of genital mutilation as well, while Judaic theology offered the gift of circumcision. Philo of Alexandria, whose writings were known in England through John Spencer's *Laws of the Hebrews* and Sterne's *Tristram Shandy*, had been explicit that the purpose of circumcision was "the excision of pleasures which bewitch the mind," thus helping a man to keep on the straight and narrow.[43] Maimonides had confirmed that its objective was "to bring about a decrease in sexual intercourse and a weakening of the organ . . . so that [it] be in as quiet a state as possible." Bodily pain was not a regrettable side effect but the principal objective: "None of the activities necessary for the preservation of the individual is harmed thereby, nor is procreation rendered impossible, but violent concupiscence and lust that goes beyond what is needed are diminished."[44] Such propositions as expressed in circumcision and clitoridectomy were well understood by the author of a satirical pamphlet published in 1873. The author, "Dr John Scoffern, professor of forensic medicine at Aldersgate College of Medicine," particularly mocked Isaac Baker Brown's "psychological surgery" but accurately caught its essence—that it was surgery intended to modify behavior.[45] Citing Jesus' injunction as reported in the book of Matthew, "If thy right hand offend thee, cut it off," Scoffern praised Brown for giving the precept practical effect; he recognized the "connection between sinning and the organic cause of sinning" and appreciated that "if a tongue resolutely bent on evil speaking be excised, that tongue can speak ill no more." Glossodectomie was in order. Brown realized that complete removal of the tongue was too extreme for English public opinion but had devised an alternative that would keep it within decent bounds: "The patient being under the effects of chloroform, a very fine knife is run through the tongue and rapidly withdrawn. The result is that certain muscular fibres are cut; the mobility of the organ is . . . impaired . . . to the extent of making continuous and violent objurgation impossible, but not of interfering with any temperate conversation." Scoffern had to admit that "even in its temperate state" the tongue was still a mobile organ, so that "perfect quietude of this member was impossible to attain, however much the patient may be willing." Although the operation limited the capability of the organ, it did not prevent "the normal and legitimate limits of temperate conversation and agreeable singing."[46] The parallel with circumcision could hardly be more exact.

If the control of immoral behavior had been the only benefit promised by circumcision it would never have won acceptance beyond a narrow circle of ascetics. The promise for most people, especially parents, was better health; in an age when there was no cure for most afflictions, and children died in droves from a host of ailments, this was a more powerful selling point. But it should be remembered that circumcision as a means of discouraging premature sexual arousal came before circumcision as a precaution against infectious and other diseases, important as the latter was in popularizing the procedure. It is therefore necessary to consider the medical history of the period, especially the development of medical knowledge about sex, and the emergence of modern medicine. A schematic summary of the evolution of medical knowledge of sexuality over three centuries reveals a curious pattern. In the libertine eighteenth century, medical authorities were not much concerned with sex, except in relation to venereal disease, but they knew that most men and women desired sexual relations with each other, that such connections were mutually pleasurable and beneficial to the health of mind and body, that normal genitals required no modifications for optimum function and appearance, and that the foreskin specifically was a valuable feature of the male package. In the nineteenth century they knew that many women did not enjoy sex, and some hated it, that men were governed by animal passions, that sexual activity was always risky and "too much" of it positively harmful, that both the male and female genitals were frequently in need of surgical improvement, that the male foreskin was a menace to both health and morals, and that many diseases and social problems were directly related to sexuality. For all their moralism,

Victorian doctors were obsessed with sex. By the second decade of the twentieth century this obsession had vanished, and the average practitioner seems to have known nothing at all about such a nasty subject, and did not want to. As Lesley Hall has vividly demonstrated, doctors in the first half of the century were abysmally ignorant about sexual matters, and most of them were quite unable, and often unwilling, to help male patients with their most common complaints.

Is this modern or premodern medicine? In his account of its rise and fall, James Le Fanu dates modern medicine from the arrival of penicillin,[47] as a result of which it became possible to kill most of the bacteria that had already been identified as the cause of common infectious diseases. In addition to this epiphany, he locates a premonition in 1935, with the discovery of sulphonamides—a more limited antibiotic that was nonetheless effective against some common bacterial infections, including puerperal fever and gonorrhea.[48] Going further back, Le Fanu detects yet another important moment in the 1830s, when some doctors realized that the old Galenic healing routine—bleeding, purging, diets, poisoning patients with heavy metals—was useless. As the nineteenth century passed, British medicine shed most of these old therapeutic techniques, but it had little to replace them with; by the dawn of the twentieth century, despite steady advances in the understanding of disease causation and the physiology of the body, the medical arsenal was not much better stocked than it had been a hundred years before.[49] There had been some important advances, such as the discovery that silver nitrate would prevent blindness in babies, of an antitoxin for diphtheria, the Wasserman test to diagnose and Salvarsan to treat syphilis, and aspirin for headaches and fevers, but most of the improvement in health observed around the turn of the century is now attributed to better sanitation, cleaner personal habits, and the isolation of tuberculosis sufferers in sanatoriums.[50] The exceptions to the general picture of therapeutic stagnation were vaccination for smallpox and surgery, which had made striking progress as a result of anesthesia and antisepsis. Those seeking new and effective medical techniques to sell the middle-class public naturally looked to where innovation was evident, and a swag of new surgeries was the result: not just circumcision but preventive or curative removal of the appendix, tonsils, adenoids, and even the colon became common. In an arresting phrase, Ann Dally calls this development "fantasy surgery."

Fantasy surgery, she writes, was in vogue from the 1880s to the 1930s and was performed "on normal organs for conditions that, on theoretical and ideological grounds, were held to be responsible for the patient's symptoms." It was a response partly to the relative safety of operations as a result of anesthesia and asepsis; partly to uncertainty over the limits of germ theory, with the result that it was thought that all germs anywhere could be malevolent and that the body could thus be poisoned by its own secretions or by rotting food in the intestines, a theory known as autointoxication; and partly by a vulgar misreading of evolutionary discoveries, which produced the idea that certain organs (such as the colon or foreskin) were "vestigial," and thus useless or troublesome. The rationale for fantasy surgery, writes Dally, "lay in the mind of the surgeon and of the public concerning the origins of symptoms and how to treat them." She mentions floating kidney, displaced uterus, the appendix, adenoids, some endocrine glands, and the internal and external genitals, but the focus of her study is Sir William Arbuthnot Lane (1856-1943), a keen exponent of autointoxication as it affected the colon, and of the colon as a vestigial and unnecessary organ. On the basis that food in the large intestine fermented and produced poisons, which provoked disease symptoms elsewhere, Lane performed dozens of operations in which he removed the colon in order to prevent "chronic intestinal stasis" (constipation).[51] In the first act of *The Doctor's Dilemma* (1906), a skeptic like George Bernard Shaw satirized the vogue for such extractions in the surgeon Cutler Walpole, with his monomaniacal determination to treat any bodily affliction you cared to name by excision of the "nuciform sac":

> I tell you, blood-poisoning. Ninety-five per cent of the human race suffer from chronic blood-poisoning, and die of it. . . . Your nuciform sac is full of decaying matter—undigested food and waste products—rank ptomaine. Now you take my advice, Ridgeon. Let me cut it out for you. You'll be another man afterwards. . . . I tell you this: in an intelligently governed country people wouldn't be allowed to go about with nuciform sacs, making themselves centres of infection. The operation ought to be compulsory; it's ten times more important than vaccination.

Shaw was referring to Lane, but the attitude is remarkably similar to what doctors claimed about the foreskin.

In writing about the place of circumcision in the rise of modern medical practice I am not sure that I have resolved the question about whether the intervention was a fruit of scientific advance and modernity, or whether it was a survival from or a throwback to older conceptions of bodily function and disease. I argue that circumcision was generated by elements of both old and new medical theory and practice, but that the influence of the former was more significant. On the one hand, the introduction of widespread circumcision was based on several medical errors and a loss of knowledge about the anatomy and function of the foreskin: the ideas that masturbation and imbalances in "nerve force" caused organic and mental illness, that spermatorrhea was a disease, and that phimosis in infants was a pathological abnormality. On the other hand, the rise of preventive medicine, the achievement of the sanitary movement in cleaning up the cities, and the emergence of germ theory seemed to provide a new and scientific rationale for the preventive removal of parts of the body thought to be similar to the "dirt traps" that caused epidemics in congested urban areas. The success of the sanitary approach in lowering death rates from important killers such as smallpox, cholera, and typhus won great prestige for preventive medicine and predisposed people to take the more speculative extensions of this approach more seriously than they deserved. The image of the cesspool lent itself readily to corporeal extensions, sanitary science was eager to identify dirt traps in the human body, and it was not long before they were duly found in the large intestine, the appendix, the tonsils, and the teeth,[52] thus confirming everything that had been said against the foreskin. It took British medicine a long time to understand how germs caused disease, and during the decisive period in which circumcision was winning acceptance (1860s through the 1880s) many different theories contended. What they all had in common was the idea that disease was dependent on "filth"; it followed that whether you adhered to miasmatic theory, spontaneous generation, or chemical poisoning, if you believed the foreskin was dirty you could be sure it had a vital role to play in the genesis or transmission of disease. It also took doctors a long time to accept the proposition that specific microorganisms caused specific diseases, and the old idea that all disease was multicausal—the product of both predisposing conditions and exciting stimuli—lingered until well into the twentieth century. All these misconceptions helped to keep alive the idea that the foreskin was a disease agent or risk factor and its removal a step toward better health.

Modern medicine is a relative and problematic concept, and I have tried to use it as a rough yardstick, not a fixed star. Medicine could not begin to modernize until the causes of disease were understood, and this did not really get under way until the discovery of microorganisms in the late nineteenth century and the development of antibiotics in the 1930s. Even though medicine could then base itself on scientific knowledge, it remained a professional practice in which the average doctor had more in common with a lawyer or motor mechanic than a scientist. One of the themes that emerges from this study is how long it took scientific knowledge of disease to affect treatment, either because no treatments were available or because the average medical man found the necessary tests too complex, as Michael Worboys has shown in his recent study of gonorrhea.[53] Despite modernization, practical medicine long retained much from its medieval past, particularly its reliance on the authority of former experts. Nowhere was this tendency more apparent than in the ideologically charged area of sexuality and the workings of the genitals, where moral revulsion held back empirical investigation for decades. It was only when the case against masturbation collapsed in the 1930s (largely as a result of the emergence of a more positive attitude toward sexuality and sexual pleasure generally) that it became possible to investigate sexual function in an objective, and thus truly scientific, spirit—one immediate fruit of which was Douglas Gairdner's demonstration that "congenital phimosis" was not a birth defect. Attitudes toward sexually transmitted diseases (STDs), however, remained colored by moral attitudes, and by the implicit belief that the genitals somehow operated differently from other parts of the body. As the debates over AIDS in the 1990s indicate, such an outlook is far from dead today.

The plan of my book is as follows. Chapter 1 introduces my themes and general argument, while chapter 2 sets out the understandings of male sexuality, the male genitals, and sexual behavior that prevailed before the rise of the masturbation phobia and shows that a radical step such as the introduction of circumcision requires a major explanatory effort. In chapter 3 I outline how the masturbation phobia of the eighteenth century, and the subsequent development of spermatorrhea as a disease entity, problematized and eventually pathologized male sexuality, turning it into a disease for which treatments must be found. The remainder of the book deals with the response to this pathologization in England and provides a full explanation of the context that allowed the development of routine circumcision. Chapter 4 describes the necessary changes in sexual morality and attitudes to the body, while chapter 5 surveys the contribution of differing disease theories and the rise of the medical profession to the acceptance of circumcision as a valid intervention. In chapters 6–12 I cover the ways in which the medical profession dealt with the problem of male sexuality as pathologized: the measures to which they resorted and the specific justifications for circumcision they offered in terms of behavioral modification, disease prevention, and health promotion. Chapter 6 offers a new analysis of William Acton, focusing on what he wrote about male sexuality and how he contributed to the demonization of the foreskin, and concluding with a summary of the case for circumcision to the 1860s. In chapter 7 I take a fresh look at the female circumcision controversy of the 1860s and explain how the rejection of clitoridectomy by the medical profession cleared the way for male circumcision, thus erecting a double standard on genital alteration that has endured to this day in Anglophone countries. Chapters 8–12 cover the specific arguments offered for circumcision: as a preventive of or cure for spermatorrhea, masturbation, phimosis, various infectious (and some noninfectious) diseases, and venereal disease, particularly syphilis. A brief conclusion outlines the reasons for the near disappearance of circumcision in the 1950s and summarizes the rather slower decline of the procedure in the major British colonies Australia, New Zealand, and Canada.

In my final chapter I provide a snapshot of circumcision in its heyday in order to outline the reason for its decline and to offer a glimpse into its personal impact. In his *Making of the English Working Class,* E. P. Thompson famously sought to "rescue the poor stockinger, the luddite cropper, the 'obsolete' hand-loom weaver, the 'utopian' artisan . . . from the enormous condescension of posterity."[54] I have a comparable objective in choosing to investigate a neglected area of medical history and to shine a searchlight onto the indignities forced on men and boys by misguided doctors in the name of health or decency. I have tried to understand as well as judge them, but a critical approach and moral accounting there must be: it is not good enough for scholars to accept the erroneous beliefs of Victorian medicine, with postmodern resignation, as just another way of understanding the world. I thus seek to expose something of the resentment caused by unwanted circumcision, to rescue from oblivion and indifference the victims of this medical fad: the infant forced to endure agonizing retractions of his foreskin and the scrubbing of his hypersensitive glans in the name of hygiene; the toddlers who wailed with a contemporary Australian, "I wish I had my old willy back";[55] the boys who were flogged for masturbating; and the men whose penises were disfigured and whose sex lives were blighted in ways that have rarely been recorded and never studied.

2 · The Best of Your Property

What a Boy Once Knew about Sex

Then Britons be wise at this critical pinch
And in such a cause be not cowards and flinch,
But the best of your property guard ev'ry inch.

Popular doggerel, 1753

I lost with the foreskin of my yard all those benefits of a Christian and an Eng-
lishman which were and ever shall be my greatest glory.

English soldier, captured and circumcised by Sultan Tipu, 1780

By many surgeons the idea of circumcision, unless connected with an immediate
demand for interference . . . such as induced phimosis . . . is looked upon as an
unwarrantable operation, a procedure not only barbarous, painful and dangerous,
but one that interferes directly with the intentions of nature. The prepuce by many
is looked upon as a physiological necessity to health and the enjoyment of life.

P. C. REMONDINO, *History of Circumcision*, 1891

If a doctor had suggested to an eighteenth-century Englishman that he
get himself or even his son circumcised, the reply would probably have
been a punch in the nose. In those days the foreskin was regarded as central to male sexual identity and circumcision as a humiliating disfigurement; sexual activity generally was seen as natural and beneficial; ribald
stories were told in respectable society; gentlemen openly kept mistresses; and there was a flourishing market for all kinds of written and
pictorial erotica, most of which was sold quite openly. Although masturbation was already being stigmatized, the message took a long time to
reach the general population, and both sexes indulged freely on an indi-

vidual and group basis. The eighteenth century was not a sexual para-
dise: venereal disease was rampant, pregnancy was a risk, and those who
engaged in homosexual activities were persecuted by law and mob alike.
But the atmosphere evoked by names such as Tom Jones and Fanny Hill
was more than Victorian nostalgia—a far cry from both the Puritanism
of the previous century and the earnest anxieties of the one that followed. Much has been written about sexual life in Georgian England,[1]
and there is no need to rehearse that here, but in order to appreciate what
a dramatic step the introduction of male circumcision was, it is necessary to know something of traditional attitudes toward the male genitals
and sexual activity. In this chapter I outline the features of the British
heritage that nineteenth-century doctors challenged, including professional and popular knowledge of sexual matters, preferred activities, attitudes toward circumcision, and some of the medical theory that facilitated the introduction of that operation a few generations later.

In a society in which half the population was illiterate, most sexual
knowledge was communicated by word of mouth, but for those who
could read the main source for the facts of life in the eighteenth century
were the anonymous *Aristotle's Master-Piece* and Nicolas Venette's *Tableau
de l'amour conjugal,* translated into English under a variety of titles. Both
were first published in the 1680s and went through dozens of editions
over the next hundred years. Each expressed a characteristically Enlightenment attitude toward sex as natural and enjoyable, included frank descriptions of the sex organs and the sexual act, and until the very end of
the century remained free from the swelling chorus against "excess" and
masturbation, a fact that helps explain why the doctors' warnings took so
long to cause widespread anxiety. Venette's was the racier of the two texts,
enlivened by bawdy jokes, insistence on sexual activity as a cure for common ailments, and a general air of sophisticated Gallic hedonism. *Aristotle's Master-Piece* was more stolid and less witty, but it offered more in
the way of practical advice, particularly on pregnancy and childbirth, as
well as remedies for sickness. As Roy Porter has emphasized, it was more
about how to make babies than to have a good time, but it still pictured
procreative sex as pleasurable for both parties and made no attempt to police individual behavior: sex was presented within a reproductive agenda
but "not presented as stained with the stigma of sin, decadence, libertinism, enslavement to passion or psychological disturbance."[2] It included
warnings against contraception and abortion, but these could be read
backward as advice on how to do what was seemingly being forbidden.
Reflecting the rise of prudery, both texts underwent extensive revision in
the late eighteenth century. Editions of Venette after the 1780s were heavily bowdlerized: most of the bawdy material was omitted, and warnings

against "sexual excess" were inserted. In early nineteenth-century editions of *Aristotle's Master-Piece,* the details of sexual anatomy and the act of intercourse, as well as jokes about virginity, were replaced by words of warning to young men, who were suddenly advised that "eager pursuit of sensual gratification disqualifies [them] for the exercise of the loftier powers" and urged to cultivate "self-command" and abstinence.[3] Walter, the protagonist of the Victorian sexual epic *My Secret Life,* read *Aristotle* and tried to understand it with the help of his schoolmates, but his main source of sexual information was other boys.[4] Oral transmission from mates or older relatives has always been the most important means by which boys have learned about sex, and the most significant element in this lore, as I show later, concerned techniques of masturbation.

In their discussion of male sexual anatomy, both Venette and *Aristotle's Master-Piece* take the penis as a whole and, unlike the doctors of a later period, do not try to separate it from its (fore)skin. As Venette recorded:

> Considering this part in gross, 'tis apt to be taken for one piece; but being examined piece-meal, 'tis found to be covered by a little loose skin, and with another somewhat thicker furnished with veins and arteries, as also encompassed by a fleshy membrane, which shuts up, like a case. . . . The glans cover'd with its prepuce, which is at one of its extremities, has such tender and sensible flesh, that nature hath there established the throne of sensitivity and pleasure in women's embraces.[5]

Aristotle viewed the matter similarly:

> the glans, which is at the end of the penis, [is] covered with a very thin membrane, by reason of which it is of a most exquisite feeling. It is covered with a preputium or foreskin, which in some covers the top of the yard quite close, in others not so, and by its moving up and down in the act of copulation brings pleasure both to the man and woman.[6]

It is clear from these passages that the foreskin was regarded as an integral part of the penis and vital to the enjoyment of both male and female: Aristotle's opinion that the movement of the foreskin over the glans brings pleasure to both parties in sexual intercourse should particularly be noted. But although all the elements of the organ were seen as operating together, there was some uncertainty as to whether the greater source of erotic sensation was the foreskin or the glans. Following the lead of the Renaissance anatomists, especially Berengario da Carpi and Gabriele Falloppio, English writers of the seventeenth century such as William Harvey, John Bulwer, and Jane Sharp, author of a well-known midwifery textbook, considered the foreskin to be the locus of the most intense pleasure. Da Carpi had written that the glans was "compact, hard and dull to sensation so that it may not be injured" but that "the functions of the prepuce ... are to furnish some delight in coitus and to guard the glans from external harm."[7] Bulwer condemned circumcision as spoiling both the aesthetics of the body and male and female pleasure, and Jane Sharp described the glans as "not very quick of feeling," emphasized the role of the foreskin in facilitating erection and sexual activity, and criticized circumcision as the action of a madman.[8] The future trend, however, was to forget about the foreskin and concentrate on the supposed sensitivity of the glans. A transitional view was expressed by the English surgeon John Hunter (1728–93), who considered that the foreskin contributed significantly to erotic sensation, but that this was achieved through its role in protecting the glans: "The prepuce is no more than a doubling of the skin of the penis when not erected, for then it becomes too large for the penis, by which provision the glans is covered and preserved when not necessary to be used, whereby its feelings are probably more acute. When the penis becomes erect it ... fills the whole skin, by which the doubling forming the prepuce in the non-erect state is unfolded, and is employed in covering the body of the penis."[9] Like Sharp, and unlike many later experts, Hunter noticed that the foreskin provided the slack necessary for comfortable erections. During the eighteenth century it was well understood that the clitoris was the center of women's sexual pleasure, and the idea that the glans was the G-spot in men arose from the analogy of the clitoris with the penis. As Venette expressed it, in the clitoris "Nature has placed the seat of pleasure and lust, as it has . . . in the glans of man"; it stiffens like a man's member and is covered similarly by a prepuce, and Aristotle thought likewise.[10] Anatomical understanding in the eighteenth century was moving from a "one-sex" model of the human body, whereby the female genitals were conceived as inverted male ones, to a "two-sex" model in which the genitals, like the sexes who wore them, were regarded as radically distinct. In the process there was much confusion about which part matched up with which: the male foreskin was variously compared to the clitoral hood and the labia, and the clitoris both to the glans alone and the penis as a whole.[11] These analogies might seem scholastic, but they became critical in the 1860s, when doctors were debating whether it was legitimate to treat masturbation by excision of the clitoris in women and the foreskin in men.

In striking contrast to the nineteenth century, there was no concern that a man's well-being was somehow threatened by his foreskin, and no sign of the "congenital phimosis" that suddenly became so common in boys after the 1860s. Quite the contrary: in the sixteenth century Falloppio had observed that it was considered shameful and unhealthy for the glans to be uncovered (in classical times this was regarded as a pathological condition known as lipodermos) and prescribed means for lengthening inadequate foreskins. He thought that a penis with an exposed glans looked like a horse's rump.[12] William Harvey wrote that in some men "the glans is never uncovered," without regarding this as a problem in need of surgical correction.[13] The concept of phimosis as a pathological condition requiring medical treatment emerged only in the late seventeenth century, probably as a result of the syphilis epidemic, since the disease often produced scabs that fused foreskin to glans. One of the first to notice phimosis was perhaps the French surgeon Pierre Dionis (d. 1718), who defined it as a condition in which "the extremity of the prepuce is so tight that it will not permit the glans to be uncovered." He observed that it could occur naturally but more commonly arose from a wound or venereal chancre that caused the preputial orifice to shrink. The condition was normal in infants and boys, but if it persisted into adulthood and was troublesome, the patient should treat it himself by pinching the foreskin shut while urinating and allowing the pouch to fill with urine. In cases where the condition arose from an accident or disease, treatment involved nicking the lip just enough to permit retraction.[14] In his *Medicinal Dictionary* (1743-45) the English physician Robert James (1705-76) included an entry for phimosis in which he pointed out that this was usually a natural condition that demanded no medical attention at all: "Some . . . have the foreskin naturally so long and so straitened [i.e., narrow] that the glans can either be not at all or very little uncovered; but as this neither occasions trouble in discharging the urine, nor any impediment in procreation, it requires no aid from the surgeons, unless it be attended with an inflammation, violent pain or any remarkable inconvenience in coition."[15] Phimosis became a medical problem only if the foreskin became "so contracted by a violent inflammation that it cannot be drawn backwards behind the glans," the usual cause of which was "impure coition" (i.e., venereal disease), producing a chancre that caused inflammation and possibly adhesion of the foreskin to the glans. The first line of treatment was to bathe the parts in a decoction of "barley mixed with honey of roses," followed by bleeding and fomentations; only if these measures failed was surgical intervention required—first by slitting the foreskin and, in desperate cases, by an operation similar to "the Jewish circumcision" but noticeably less radical. Cutting was never indicated for paraphimosis, cases of which occurred most commonly in young husbands with tight foreskins who exerted themselves vigorously during intercourse, and in similarly endowed boys who "lasciviously" drew their foreskin back while the penis was flaccid but found they could not return it after the ensuing erection. The only treatment needed was cold water to make the erection subside, lubrication of the penis with olive oil or butter, and manual manipulation if that was not sufficient.[16] Such benign and simple therapies naturally became unthinkable as the masturbation taboo tightened its grip on medical profession and public alike from the late eighteenth century onward. John Hunter gave similar advice and tended to regard all true phimosis as arising from venereal disease, particularly chancres and syphilis.[17] He also observed that the nonretractability of the foreskin in many boys before puberty was perfectly natural and was often overcome by the boys' own manual explorations and fondling: "This natural phymosis is so considerable in some children as not to allow the urine to pass with ease, but in general becomes larger and larger, as boys grow up, by frequent endeavouring to bring it over the glans, which effect often prevents the bad consequences that would otherwise ensue in it when affected by disease."[18] This is an interesting comment, revealing what a down-to-earth observer Hunter was. What he is suggesting is that no treatment was needed for phimosis because boys naturally stretched their foreskin when playing with their penis, gradually loosening it and achieving retractability at their own pace. With the masturbation scare, genuine phimosis at older ages might have become more common, since boys were now instructed not to play with or even to touch their penis, with the result that these manipulations could have become less frequent and this gentle process of loosening disrupted.

What did men do with their equipment? Sexual intercourse is the only activity discussed in the manuals, but there is likely to be a difference between what they advised and what people actually did, and it is reasonable to assume that many indulged in activities against which they were being warned: masturbation, fellatio, and contraception, to name a few.[19] Fellatio was condemned with the sort of invective usually reserved for sodomy: "a Man's putting his erected Penis into another Person's Mouth . . . using Friction etc between the lips" was "so very beastly and so much to be abhorred as to cause . . . the utmost detestation and loathing," wrote John Marten, the same authority who introduced the idea that masturbation caused organic disease.[20] Despite this, Randolph Trumbach found that although it was not common, fellatio was regularly indulged in, particularly by men anxious to avoid venereal infection from prostitutes.[21] Tim Hitchcock argues that premarital sex was normal and ubiquitous but that it rarely went beyond kissing, fondling, and mutual masturbation; intercourse, which could lead to pregnancy and was associated with marriage, was comparatively rare.[22] He cites the case of John Cannon (b. 1684), one of very few eighteenth-century men who left an autobiography that included details of his sexual habits. Cannon reveals that he did not engage in intercourse until after he married, and that even when he was in love with a servant girl for two years they confined their sex play to kissing, caresses, and what in a later age would be called "heavy petting"; it certainly included Mary masturbating him to ejaculation.[23] This picture is confirmed by a few other diary references cited by Lawrence Stone. Samuel Pepys seems to have had a very strong sex drive, keeping several mistresses successively as well as enjoying numerous brief affairs and one-night stands. Because he was afraid of venereal disease he rarely patronized prostitutes, and on the few occasions when he did he was more likely to get the women to masturbate him than to engage in intercourse. In his extramarital affairs he was equally wary of intercourse, but in these cases the concern was pregnancy; prolonged fondling, mutual masturbation, and the repertoire of "foreplay" were the rule.[24] William Byrd, a gentleman from Virginia whose diaries cover the years 1709-12, 1717-21, and 1739-41, masturbated regularly with no sense of shame or guilt, and when he moved to London in 1717 enjoyed "a sexual feast" with many women, but his pattern of sexual activity was similar to that of Pepys. He recorded that in 1718 he achieved orgasm 26 times by intercourse and 27 times by masturbation; the following year, after he had found a discrete brothel that appealed to his taste, the figures were 67 and 22 times, respectively.[25] If James Boswell's experience is any guide, it was not unusual for groups of young men and women to meet by chance and then go somewhere secluded for a single session of sex, and he regularly engaged in threesomes.[26] It is, of course, impossible to categorize sex acts as neatly as these descriptions imply: most encounters must have involved a selection from an extensive range of possibilities, each one merging into another as the fancy took the players. One of Thomas Rowlandson's naughty drawings, "The Finishing Stroke," shows a young couple making love. The man has withdrawn his penis and is bringing himself to orgasm by rubbing it between the woman's breasts, while tickling her vagina with his fingers; some appended verse suggests that she might have had more fun with something thicker, but they both look reasonably happy: does that count as masturbation or coitus?[27] The officially approved sexual repertoire tended to shrink as the century advanced, particularly as masturbation and sex outside marriage became more heavily stigmatized, with the result that marital intercourse eventually came to be seen as the only legitimate way to achieve orgasm. As the nineteenth century drew on, marital intercourse itself was increasingly defined as vaginal penetration, man on top, no foreplay, no touching of each other's parts, and all in the dark.[28]

Venette celebrated the fact that man was "the most lascivious of creatures, because he is disposed for the delights of love at any hour, and in every season."[29] On this issue he is so remote from the medical wisdom of the next century that he might have been living on another planet: while Victorian doctors asserted that "excessive" sexual activity caused impotence and sterility, he considered that it was abstinence that had these effects and actually caused the genitals to atrophy: "Mortification of the flesh and chastity are powerful causes of the diminution of those parts. The example of St Martin convinces us of this truth. He macerated his body by unheard austerities to that degree, and stood up so zealously against the libertines of his age, that after his death . . . his yard was so diminished, that 'twould hardly have been found, if its situation had not been known." Chastity will lead to loss of interest in sex and a general weakening of spirits: "the parts of our body not exercising in the actions nature has made them for, wither and dry up."[30] William Harvey similarly commented that in "those who practise abstinence and chastity the testicles are meagre and the penis retracted into the belly, and they are completely frigid."[31] These ideas were in accord with traditional Western medical teaching and retained their place in popular lore during the nineteenth century, as doctors frequently complained, but among the professional classes it was only a few radicals like George Drysdale who tried to keep them alive.

Although we can never know as much about actual sexual behavior as about what was recommended, masturbation was undoubtedly popular among eighteenth-century men and women. The thriving market for erotica certainly catered to a taste for one-handed reading, and the masturbation scene was a stock episode in eighteenth-century erotica, usually showing a woman doing it rather than a man.[32] Contrary to the impression given by the disparaging names bestowed on the activity, however, it was not always a solitary vice: it was just as often a mutual or collective one, between couples and among both teenage boys and adult men. Hitchcock reports the existence of a homosocial world of private clubs centered around group wanking, a world of male libertines not unlike an American college fraternity, with lots of drinking, a bit of horseplay, and perhaps a female stripper. One of these, the Beggars Benison, held meetings twice a year at which the members dressed in monkish gowns, greeted each other by rubbing their penises together, and collectively masturbated into a ceremonial cup.[33] John Cannon learned to masturbate at the age of twelve from his seventeen-year-old cousin, who showed a group of younger boys who had gone swimming after school: "what he could do if he had a female in place, and withall took his privy member in his hand rubbing it up and down till it was erected and in short followed emission. The same as he said in copulation, and withall advised more of the boys to do the same, telling them that altho' the first act would be attended by pain yet by frequent use they would find a deal of pleasure on wch several attempted and found as he said." Cannon masturbated regularly throughout his adolescence, and although he condemned the practice when he came to write his memoirs toward the end of his life, there is no guilt or anxiety evident at the time, suggesting that the influence of alarmist literature did not become apparent until the second half of the century.[34] If any letters sent in to the author of *Onania* may be regarded as genuine, Cannon's experience was shared by many other boys. One sinner wrote in:

> when I went to school, I and three or four more, on a holiday, went a bird-catching; when we were sat down, one of our companions, who was about 20 years of age, the rest of us not being above fifteen, asked us, whether we ever saw the seed of man? We reply'd, we never did. He told us, if we would reach him a leaf of a cabbage, he would shew us, which he did, by self-pollution; and which, though it fired my inclination, yet I attempted it not until a year after.[35]

Apart from the touch of moralizing, there is enough naïveté and circumstantial detail in the account to suggest that it might be authentic.

Despite the growing chorus of disapproval, if *My Secret Life* can be believed, things were not much different in the first half of the following century. Walter first learned of masturbation from a teenage relative who had come to stay and soon after that encountered a set at school in which the boys masturbated together.[36] Walter tried to join in these activities but was held back by his tight foreskin; the more he worked on the problem, however, the looser it became, and he eventually achieved success in both retracting it and masturbating to orgasm; he reported the good news to two schoolfellows, and "we all went into the garden, each pulled my prepuce back, I theirs, and then we all frigged ourselves in an out-house" (45). Even when he got older Walter did not lose his taste for individual and group activity of this sort. In his late teens he held circle jerks with workmates (111–12), and he enjoyed masturbation with female partners and prostitutes (126, 146, 147, 416, 474–75): indeed, despite his having regular sex partners from the age of about seventeen onward, masturbation seems to have been Walter's most common form of sexual release. Now it may be true, as Ian Gibson has suggested, that *My Secret Life* is a work of pornographic fiction rather than a genuine autobiography,[37] but the chapters on Walter's childhood and adolescence seem so full of misadventure, and so remote from the later world of "pornotopia" analyzed by Steven Marcus, that it seems likely they are at least partly based on experience. If it is mainly a work of fiction, written in the second half of the nineteenth century, when the stigmatization of masturbation was at its peak, it may well be that the author regarded the most transgressive and fantastic elements of his daydreams to be the uninhibited pleasure Walter took in the forbidden vice, so much more wicked and dangerous than raping servant girls or fucking twelve-year-old prostitutes.

His foreskin was certainly central to Walter's experience of sex, and particularly to his enjoyment of masturbation. He refers to it repeatedly when writing about his penis, noting its extreme sensitivity, his delight in pulling it back and forth, and the interesting smell he began to produce when he reached puberty. It was while cleaning this off one time that he had his first experience of masturbating to ejaculation: after he had washed it he "had a cock-stand, and felt again my prick sore, and was washing it with warm water, when it swelled up. I rubbed it through my hand, which gave me unusual pleasure, then a voluptuous sensation came over me quickly so thrilling and all-pervading that I shall never forget it" (44).

Whoever the author was, he either knew something about masturbation or had read the standard medical warnings on how cleaning under the foreskin could give rise to that practice. Having a particularly tight foreskin, Walter had to put up with taunts from other boys because he could not "unskin" his penis in what was obviously an important adolescent rite of passage (15). Despite the difficulties this condition caused him, he had no interest in surgical correction and was horrified when the suggestion was made. After his first intercourse, his foreskin was so sore that he thought he might have a disease; an apothecary advised that "there was nothing the matter with me, that the skin was too tight, that a snip would set me to rights, and advised me soon to have it done, saying, 'It will save you trouble and money if you do, and add to your pleasure.' I declined" (60–61). It is not clear whether the chemist recommended circumcision, or merely an incision to free the preputial sphincter, but the significant point is Walter's recoil from whatever was proposed. He soon realized that he had merely torn the skin in the heat of passion and reports that his penis quickly healed. As his foreskin loosened up as a result of frequent masturbation and intercourse, he found that girls also liked playing with it: "I see her now, making my cock stiff under my direction, her amusement at pulling the prepuce up and down was great" (208). Sex without such a feature was unimaginable.

Walter's adamant rejection of surgical intervention was partly conditioned by knowing that his foreskin was a source of delight and partly by the abhorrence with which Western Christendom had traditionally regarded circumcision. In today's global village, when circumcision of male infants is still common in the United States, and controversy over female circumcision among some African peoples and Islamic cultures is daily news, it is difficult to recapture the shudder of horror that the word would have aroused in eighteenth-century England. Understood as a defining characteristic of such alien people as Turks, Moors, and Jews, circumcision was regarded as a mutilation that left the victims aesthetically disfigured and partially emasculated. The Greeks and Romans had detested circumcision and even tried to ban it among the few of their Middle Eastern subjects who practiced it.[38] Beginning with Saint Augustine and Saint Ambrose, Christian tradition held that baptism had replaced circumcision as the appropriate initiation for members of the church and that it had the same or greater effect in cleansing the infant of original sin, without the need for any shedding of blood.[39] Thomas Aquinas formally restated the Christian ban on circumcision in the *Summa,* but the peak of the Catholic Church's opposition was probably reached in the Bull of Union with the Copts (1442), which prohibited circumcision outright and declared that it "cannot possibly be observed without loss of eternal salvation."[40] This policy was embodied in the attitude of Erasmus, who included circumcision among the Jewish customs on which "we cry shame," in sixteenth-century references to circumcision as a "mutilation," and in Goethe's comment on a painting of Christ's circumcision, seen while traveling in Italy in 1786: "I forgave the intolerable subject and enjoyed the execution."[41]

To most Englishmen, circumcision was a threat from which they had been saved by the defeat of Islamic armies. Their literature offered many reminders of the contest between Christianity and Islam, which had made several determined assaults on the West between the eighth and the seventeenth centuries, beginning with the Saracen invasion of Spain. For Edward Gibbon, the prospect that "the Koran would now be taught in the schools of Oxford, and her pulpits might demonstrate to a circumcised people the sanctity and truth of the revelation of Mahomet" was the greatest of the "calamities" from which the genius of Charlemagne delivered Europe.[42] When, in the 1870s, Richard Burton remarked that Christendom "practically holds circumcision in horror," the observation was ceasing to be true, but it was certainly the case before the nineteenth century. In the seventeenth century a steady stream of British sailors and travelers were captured by North African pirates and sold into slavery in Tunis or Algiers, and some of these were forcibly converted to Islam and probably circumcised. Although most were dismayed, a few were quite glad to abandon Christianity and serve new masters with whom fresh opportunities for winning wealth and prestige might be found. The expression "turn Turk" arose to signify such conversions, and at a time when Islam was the major enemy of and still a significant rival to the Christian West, they had much the same significance as a defection to Moscow during the Cold War. The loss of the defector's foreskin was then seen not merely as a physical deprivation but as a permanent mark of the convert's new allegiance.[43] It was a similar story in Muslim India, where some servants of the East India Company deserted to the Mughals in the hope of a better career path. In 1649 a company official sadly reported the defection of a Josiah Blackwell, who "most wickedly and desperately renounced his Christian faith and professed himself a Moor, was immediately circumcised, and is irrecoverably lost."[44] Forced conversions (meaning forcible circumcision) were more common than the voluntary sort—the fate of several hundred British soldiers captured after the Battle of Pollilur in 1780, who were circumcised and enslaved by Tipu Sultan of Mysore. One of the men, Cromwell Massey, secretly kept a diary in which he recorded the fears of his comrades and their reaction to the various humiliations forced on them. Of himself he wrote: "Terribly alarmed this morning for our foreskins"—as well he might have been, since many of the men were restrained, drugged, shaved, circumcised, fitted with silver earrings, and drafted into the sultan's service. One ensign recorded his shame in bitter terms: "I lost with the foreskin of my yard all those benefits of a Christian and Englishman which were and ever shall be my greatest glory."[45] The teenage James Bristow and his mates were so distressed at what had been done to them that they later caught dogs and circumcised them, knowing that this would incense their captors because Muslims regarded dogs as unclean. The action brought further punishment, but Bristow felt it was justified because "compelling us to undergo an abhorred operation [was] so base and barbarous an act of aggression, that it was impossible to reflect on it with temper."[46] To emphasize the emasculating element of the operation, several adolescent captives were not only circumcised but made to wear female clothes and serve as dancing boys in the sultan's court.[47]

As a Christian country England had no history of circumcision, but there were strong "Judaizing" tendencies in Puritanism, as fundamentalist radicals turned to the Old Testament in their quest to purge Christianity of its popish accretions. Some of these went so far as to adopt Jewish customs such as Sabbath and dietary observance, and a few even tried to circumcise boys—for which offense a certain Anne Curtyn was jailed in 1649.[48] The overwhelming attitude, however, was disgust, and in his critique of artificial efforts to improve upon nature, John Bulwer condemned circumcision at length and anticipated Aristotle's description of the foreskin's role in sexual functioning:

> That part which hangeth over the end of the foreskin, is moved up and down in coition, that in this attrition it might gather more heat, and increase the pleasure of the other sexe; a contentation of which they are defrauded by this injurious invention. For, the shortnesse of the prepuce is reckoned among the organical defects of the yard, . . . yet circumcision detracts somewhat from the delight of women, by lessening their titillation.[49]

Jane Sharp wrote that a few people believed that the "Venerious action" might be performed better without the foreskin but pointed out that circumcision had been forbidden by Saint Paul and hoped that

> no man will be so void of reason and Religion, as to be Circumcised to make trial which of these two opinions is the best; but the world was never without some mad men, who will do anything to be singular: were the foreskin any hindrance to procreation or pleasure, nature had never made it, who made all things for these very ends and purposes.[50]

The hostile English attitude toward the operation also emerges starkly from a description of the Jewish rite witnessed by John Evelyn in Rome in 1645:

> The infant now strip'd from the belly downewards, the Jew tooke the yard of the child and chaf'd it within his fingers till it became a little stiff, then with the silver instrument before describ'd . . . he tooke up as much of the praeputium as he could possibly gather, and so with the razor, did rather saw, then cutt it off; at which the miserable babe cry'd extreamely, whiles the rest continu'd their odd tone, rather like howling then singing: then the Rabby lifting the belly of the child to his face & taking the yard all blody into his mouth he suck'd it a pretty while, having before taken a little vinegar, all which together with the blood he spit out into a glasse of red-wine. . . . This don he stripp'd down the remainder of the foreskin as farr and neere to the belly as he could, so as it appeared to be all raaw, then he strwe'd the read powder on it to stanch the bleeding and coverd it with the paper-hood, & upon this a clowte, and so swath'd up the child as before.[51]

The editor of Evelyn's diary states that aspects of this description are inconsistent with the normal rules for the ceremony, but whether Evelyn's observations or the celebrant's procedure is at fault is hard to say. What comes vividly across is the diarist's revulsion at what is being done to the child, and the same recoil is apparent in the controversy that erupted over the Jewish Naturalisation Act a century later, when popular pamphleteers fortified their propaganda with hoary old myths about knife-wielding Jews, intent on cutting gentile flesh, and drew on deep-seated fears of circumcision. Stories that Jews abducted Christian boys and murdered them after ritual circumcision first appeared in the thirteenth century and played a role in the decision to expel the Jews from England in 1290. They were still circulating in the seventeenth century, and when William Prynne argued against the readmission of the Jews in 1656, he purported to document actual cases of their traditional crime of "circumcising and crucifying Christian children." In his analysis of this literature and its influence on Shakespeare's *Merchant of Venice*, James Shapiro notes that other contributors to the controversy claimed that Jews also captured and circumcised boys without killing them and comments that this obsession with circumcision was peculiarly English: accusations of Jewish crimes in Europe did not stress this offense to anything like the same degree.[52] The figure of the knife-wielding Jew, intent on carving off a gentile's foreskin, was a stock image in written texts and popular illustrations, and it helped provide the model for the moneylender in *The Merchant of Venice*. As Shapiro points out, it is not until the last act that the audience learns that his bond allows Shylock to cut the pound of flesh from near Antonio's heart (6.1.228–30); for most of the play the source of the penalty is unspecified (wherever "pleaseth" Shylock), allowing viewers to speculate as wildly as their imaginations dictated. Given the popular stereotype of Jews as emasculators, it is likely that many would have jumped to the obvious conclusion that Shylock was planning to take his forfeit from Antonio's genitals, particularly as the word *flesh* was a common term for the penis at that time.[53] Some of the bawdier playgoers down in the pit might even have guffawed at the weight of the penalty as a hyperbolic tribute to Antonio's virility. The stock response to these images today is to deplore the anti-Semitism, but what is equally worthy of note is their testimony to the high valuation placed on bodily completeness and the fear of its violation.

The Merchant of Venice was revived in 1741, became one of the main sources of English attitudes toward Jews in the mid-eighteenth century, and contributed to the hysterical atmosphere in which the campaign against the "Jew Bill" was conducted. The Jewish Naturalisation Act of 1753 permitted Jews who had lived in Britain for three years to become naturalized citizens without having to join the Church of England, thus giving them more opportunity to engage in commerce—a progressive reform for the period and one passed by both houses of Parliament without much debate. Despite this, the legislation generated enormous opposition among the public, and its opponents launched such a vigorous campaign against it that it was soon repealed. What is significant about the paper war is that the pamphleteers made circumcision central to their polemic and pictured the widespread introduction of the practice as the most disastrous imaginable consequence of giving Jews citizenship. One broadside emphasized possession of a foreskin as the sign of a "true born Briton":

> Though circumcision now will be
> Within this realm made known
> Yet every true born Briton he
> Will surely keep his own.[54]

Shapiro points out that, although a few pamphlets rehashed the old stories about ritual murder, the main theme of the propaganda was the threat to Englishmen's foreskins.[55] Opponents of the legislation mocked its supporters by showing them having to undergo the procedure and suggested more sinister scenarios, such as forced circumcision of children instead of baptism, and men wanting to do business with Jews having to submit to the operation as the price of a deal. Men were urged to protect "the best of your property" and to guard their threatened foreskins:

> Then Britons be wise at this critical pinch
> And in such a cause be not cowards and flinch,
> But the best of your property guard ev'ry inch.

Wolper describes the pamphlet war as an outburst of "virulent anti-Semitism,"[56] but the severity of this assessment is not borne out by his own evidence. There seems to have been no violence during the campaign, and London theaters actually suspended performances of *The Merchant of Venice* at the height of the controversy in case it proved an incitement.[57] The propaganda overall was good-humored and often funny, expressing hostility to circumcision as cruel to the baby and a mutilation in men, and revealing a high valuation of the foreskin as a vital element in normal male sexuality. The *London Evening Post* visualized the then remote fantasy of "twenty-five children . . . publicly circumcised at the lying-in hospital in Brownlow Street" and projected a grim scenario for the future of England in which "every male" was ordered "to be circumcised: which was accordingly done . . . . And it came to pass on the third day, whilst their private parts were sore, that the Jews took their swords, and slew every male of the Britons."[58] Wolper calls this a "vicious image,"[59] seemingly unaware that it could not have been intended literally but was merely a cheeky retelling of the Hebrews' revenge against the Hivites following the defilement of Dinah (Gen. 34:1-25), a story that would have been well known in an age that knew the Bible and flocked to Handel's oratorios. Incredible as it may seem, the striking thing is that the first part of the *Post's* baleful fantasy was pretty much the scenario that did come to pass in the late nineteenth century—not as the result of a Jewish plot, however, but on the authority of the British medical profession.

In contrast to the substantial advances made by the biological sciences and the humanities, medicine made little progress in the eighteenth century. In his *Domestic Medicine* (1772), William Buchan commented that "improvements in medicine, since the revival of learning, have by no means kept pace with those of the other arts," and he felt that medical discoveries had "either been the effect of chance or of necessity, and have been usually opposed by the faculty till everybody else was convinced of their importance. . . . An implicit faith in the opinions of teachers, an attachment to systems and established forms, and the dread of reflections, will always operate upon those who follow medicine as a trade." Buchan offered several reasons for this backwardness: that medicine was studied only by those who intended "to live by it as a trade"; that practitioners had tried to keep the art wrapped in mystery; and that ordinary people had not been stimulated to think about medical matters by public controversies, unlike religion. He felt it would be a good thing if gentlemen learned some medicine as part of a general education, if only so as "to guard themselves against the destructive influences of Ignorance, Superstition and Quackery."[60] Roy Porter similarly describes eighteenth-century medicine as characterized by formalist theorizing, failed hypotheses, and therapeutic stagnation, and observes that advances in anatomy were not matched by improvements in therapy, though they did contribute to improvements in the treatment of injury.[61] Despite the scientific revolution of the seventeenth century, medical treatment remained largely based on the theories of Galen (129–ca. 216), which held that the "four humors" governed bodily development; the flow of blood, phlegm, yellow bile, and black bile, corresponding to hot, dry, wet, and cold characteristics, respectively, regulated organic functions and appearance: balance meant health, imbalance meant illness.[62] Therapies thus aimed to restore health by purging the body of whatever humor was overweight (bleeding, vomiting, enemas) or adding what was lacking (particular foods thought to strengthen the humor in short supply). As Porter comments, "the enduring popularity . . . of purging and phlebotomy [bleeding] hinged on the old conviction that sickness followed plethora (excess) or the build-up of peccant humours in the system, requiring periodic discharge." Bleeding was by far the most widely used treatment, prescribed for anything from drowning to head wounds; the practice was still common in the 1830s, when country patients were often bled till they fainted. On the restorative side, physicians offered a bewildering array of chemical and herbal concoctions, some of whose ingredients would have challenged the ingenuity of even the most resourceful apothecary: the revised edition of the London Pharmacopoeia (1746) dropped spider webs, moss from human skulls, unicorn's horn, and virgin's milk but retained mithridate, wood lice, bezoars, vipers, and coral.[63] As late as the 1860s William Acton gave recipes intended to promote continence in men, and all those who sought to discourage sexual excess urged abstention from red meat, wine, and other stimulants.

The influence of humoral concepts is apparent even in the scientific advances that emerged to challenge Galenism, the most important of which were the theories of nervous force developed by Albrecht von Haller (1708–77) and William Cullen (1710–90). Haller, professor of medicine at Gottingen, made important discoveries about how the nerves controlled the action of muscles, showing that muscles possessed an intrinsic power to contract and that they did so under the stimulus of a nerve impulse.[64] Unfortunately, his word for this capacity (contractility) was often translated as "irritability," a term that was later improperly extended to explain any bodily phenomenon not understood, from muscular paralysis to seminal loss. The foundation for Haller's teaching and nerve force theory generally was laid by Friedrich Hoffmann, a professor of medicine at the University of Halle, who revived ancient ideas about the influence of the nerves on health and created a system in which a "nervous ether" radiating from the brain set the rest of the body in motion. Illness occurred when contractions blocked the pathways of this fluid, especially along the spine.[65] Haller distinguished between nerve impulse (sensibility) and muscular contraction (irritability), but later authorities on male sexuality misapplied these terms and came up with concepts like *genital irritability* to mean the responsiveness of the penis to tactile pressure and its capacity to convey erotic sensation, and by the mid-nineteenth century *irritability* had become a key term in the vocabulary of the crusaders against the most sensitive part of the penis. Haller's discoveries were also extended to authorize the view that there was something that could be called nerve force, which circulated in the body in a manner comparable to the motion of the four humors, imbalances of which could likewise cause illness. Cullen, professor of medicine at Edinburgh and an influential teacher, saw life itself as a function of nervous power and came to argue that all diseases were ultimately nervous in origin. His pupil John Brown (1735–88) went further to argue that "in certain view almost the whole of diseases of the human body might be called nervous." A balance of nerve force meant health, whereas disease was caused by an excess (sthenic) or a deficiency (asthenic) of nervous excitability; all diseases tended to become asthenic as exhaustion set in.

It was really a nerve-based version of humoral theory: sthenic diseases were treated by tranquillizers (bleeding, emetics) and asthenic by stimulants, of which alcohol was the most prominent.[66] Brown asserted that at birth every person was "endowed with a fixed quantity of excitability," which provided the "necessary energy to live," a concept that was much developed by the fixed-sum theories of nervous energy dominant in the mid-nineteenth century.[67] Shorter suggests that Brown's theorizing represents a "mere caricature of research and medical advance," leading physicians to ask whether disease was the result of irritation, and that this concept acquired a "spurious legitimacy" because it was conflated with inflammation, a genuinely pathological process usually caused by infection.[68] The misapplication of these propositions played an important part in the claim of late eighteenth-century doctors that masturbation caused many physical and mental diseases, and of their nineteenth-century successors that circumcision could prevent or cure them.

The eighteenth century was not a good time to get sick. Hospitals were few and more often centers of contagion than healing; diseases such as smallpox, typhus, tuberculosis, and unnamed "fevers" were common and frequently fatal; infant and child mortality was high; cuts and injuries could easily become infected, leading to gangrene and the choice between amputation and death; venereal diseases were rampant, giving rise to a thriving market for pox doctors and other quacks, each with his own patent remedy, often dispatched by mail order.[69] As Robert James observed in his *Medicinal Dictionary*, "mankind is every way surrounded with so many and so great miseries, that inexpressible care, solicitude and diligence are necessary in order to avert the violence of so many diseases to which we are subjected."[70] No quantity of solicitude, however, could make up for the fact that there was very little that doctors could do about most diseases, the causes of which were not understood and remedies for which did not exist: given such ignorance, it is not surprising that personal characteristics or behavior, such as constitutional susceptibility or overindulgence, were often blamed. As Roy Porter comments, "even with rampant infections like smallpox, some individuals were afflicted, some were not"; with no concept of immunity, doctors drew the conclusion that personal conduct was the key to the avoidance of illness and proposed "strategies of containment through self-discipline."[71] Where treatment was attempted, it often involved the administration of purgatives intended to rid the body of whatever alien substance was thought to be causing the problem, but since these were usually based on mercury, antimony, and lead, they often added the agonies of heavy metal poisoning to the effects of whatever disease they were meant to alleviate. The standard treatment for syphilis (and sometimes gonorrhea) was mercury, with the result that the symptoms of those diseases were often confounded with the manifestations of mercury poisoning.[72] The difficulty of making sense of the cases described by eighteenth-century doctors is aggravated by the fact that neither they nor their patients described symptoms or syndromes that correspond to the diagnostic categories of today. Doctors rarely performed physical examinations, relying instead on patients' own descriptions of their problem, but all they could do was report their experience of mysterious, uncontrollable, frightening, and often painful changes in their bodies.[73] They sought explanation as much as cure.

Although there were few significant advances in medical understanding or treatment during the eighteenth century, the spread of a materialist approach to life and the development of a prosperous middle class laid the foundations on which doctors were able to establish a profession that achieved unprecedented prestige and social authority by the middle of the Victorian age. Surgery made great progress thanks to advances in anatomical knowledge, and by the early nineteenth century the art was considered to be ordered according to "fixed and rational principles"; it was still confined to the amputation of limbs, however, and a very few invasive procedures such as lithotomy; the internal organs remained beyond reach.[74] More people were dying with a physician rather than a priest in attendance, and by the end of the century, as Hitchcock writes, "a tradition of personal control by the patient over the course of an illness and its treatment was being replaced by a system in which the professional, and now male, doctor was in control."[75] These developments represented the beginnings of the "medicalization of life," which would reach its peak in the mid-twentieth century; medicine was replacing religion as the chief source for the rules of living and the meaning of existence itself.[76]

Eighteenth-century medicine remained particularly backward, and actually regressed, in its understanding of reproduction and sexuality. William Harvey had famously solved the mystery of the circulation of the blood, but his attempt to explain generation remained within the old paradigms.[77] The period's most significant discovery, that a major cause of organic diseases was masturbation, was an error with monumental consequences, and there were three specific ways in which understandings of male genital anatomy and function prepared the ground for the acceptance of circumcision as a valid medical procedure. First, in accordance with ancient medical teachings, sex was seen as tiring and potentially debilitating for men, since emission of semen meant loss of the hot, dry humor, leading to pale complexions, lassitude, and debility.[78] As a later version (1776) of *Aristotle's Master-Piece* put it, "why is immoderate carnal copulation hurtful? Because it destroys the sight, dries the body, and impairs the brain; often causes fevers, as Avicenna and experience shew; it shortens life, too, as is evident in the sparrow, which, by reason of its often-coupling, lives but three years."[79] This concern about male exhaustion arose from belief in the greater sexual appetite of women and the consequent fear that men would wear themselves out in attempting to satisfy their limitless desire.[80] Paradoxically, this belief faded toward the end of the century, to be replaced by the completely opposite view by the 1850s: that women were not much interested in sex and submitted to their husbands only as a conjugal duty or out of the wish for children. Second, there was a loss of knowledge about the functions of the foreskin. Renaissance anatomists had appreciated that the glans of the penis was relatively insensitive and that the main source of male sexual pleasure was the mobile tissue of the shaft, particularly the portion that normally covered the glans and slipped back and forth over it, thus generating the sensations that led to ejaculation. By the mid-eighteenth century it was increasingly assumed that the glans was the most erotically significant part of the penis and that the role of the foreskin was merely to maintain its sensitivity by guarding it from friction when not in use; as Robert James expressed it, "the use of the praeputium is to keep the glans soft and moist, that it may have an exquisite sense."[81] This was a fateful devaluation of the foreskin: once it became accepted that the foreskin had no significant function in its own right, it became much harder to mount an effective defense against those who wanted to cut it off. Third, some doctors began to propose a connection between the foreskin and venereal disease: "Those who have their foreskins naturally very long are much more easily infected by impure embraces than others, as we learn from both reason and experience," asserted Robert James,[82] though he did not elaborate. It is possible that James was the first English physician after John Marten (see the next chapter) to make reference to circumcision as a therapeutic procedure, describing it as indicated in cases of gangrene and cancer of the penis. More ominously, he went on to praise the operation generally as a "hygiene" measure in terms that seem more typical of the nineteenth than the eighteenth century: "Circumcision seems to be a very convenient operation in warm countries, for the sake of cleanliness. For the Glandular Odoriferae, lying under the prepuce, discharge their contents, which . . . corrupt and become acrimonious, corroding the glans, and inflaming both that and the prepuce; and this, even in our cold countries, where the humours have not so great a tendency to putrefaction as in warmer climates. The case is often mistaken for a clap."[83] Although there are no glands under the foreskin, and no quantity of accumulating "secretions" can cause the glans to "corrode" or putrefy, the notion that subpreputial moisture was harmful and could generate infection and disease became, and remains, an article of faith among crusaders for routine circumcision.[84] James was clearly a man ahead of his time.[85]

A final factor that might have made circumcision more acceptable was a shift of taste in genital aesthetics. In the ancient world, as Greek and Roman statues attest, the ideal penis was covered with a long, tapering prepuce, and erotic paintings usually showed even fully erect penises so sheathed; the glans was considered so ugly that it was rarely depicted, and exposing it in public was considered obscene.[86] This sensibility was revived along with classical learning during the Renaissance, when artists resolutely refused to depict any penises as circumcised, whether they were painting Madonnas with naked child or sculpting Davids. As Leo Steinberg argues, this policy was partly the result of an obligation to demonstrate the theological doctrine of the incarnation (the word made flesh in all its human detail) and partly because they could not bear to depict an imperfect body. The pain of circumcision was seen as further proof of Christ's love and a prefigurement of the greater pain and bloodletting of the crucifixion. His circumcision was perceived "as both deliverance [from original sin] and deprivation, riddance and loss. A God-framed sacrament . . . to cleanse man . . . of original sin was yet a 'despoiling of the body' (Col. 2:11), an embarrassing defect. The honorific seal of a compact between man and God as manifestly a shameful scar." The artists knew which side of the divide they were on: "Depicting the nude infant Christ at whatever age, they willingly paid the price of inaccuracy to spare the revered body the blemish of imperfection."[87] By the mid-eighteenth century, however, if written and pictorial erotica are any guide, a willingness to see the penis with glans exposed seems to have evolved. Fanny Hill got excited over the vermilion termination of the "uncapped" cock and never makes explicit reference to the foreskin at all, though she delighted in the contrast between the glistening crimson head and the snowy white folds of the sheath from which it emerged: "that capital part of man: the flaming red head as it stood uncapped, the whiteness of the shaft."[88] Of course it is pornography, a world of physical perfection, but Fanny's perspective was hardly likely to be different from that of the readers to whom Cleland was trying to appeal. In the world of pornographic fantasy, the exposed glans seems to have indicated a powerful erection and readiness for action, but the sheathed penis flaccidity and the implication of impotence. The naked glans is equally evident in many of Rowlandson's erotic drawings. Although such a shift in taste would probably not have encouraged circumcision, it might well have helped to reduce objections to the practice on aesthetic grounds.

Behind these developments lay long-term changes in the organization of sexuality and family life. The period from 1680 to 1800 witnessed a slow sexual revolution that transformed public understandings, creating what Hitchcock calls "a phallocentric and increasingly heterosexual culture" in which behaviors beyond the bounds of penetrative sex were seen as unnatural, and giving birth to recognizably modern sexual identities. Hitchcock proposes that as the century advanced, there was a rise in the birth rate as the frequency of intercourse increased; that there was a corresponding decline in other forms of sexual activity, such as petting and masturbation; and that more rigid definitions of male and female natures emerged.[89] Robert Shoemaker has also argued that over this period, gender roles became more sharply defined and women came to be seen as less sexually passionate and more naturally virtuous than men. The concern of moralists shifted from women's lustfulness to male desire, and "sexual practices became restricted to . . . vaginal intercourse, as mutual masturbation and fondling became less common," leading eventually to more restricted sexual opportunities and more rigidly defined roles for both sexes.[90] What is most notable about writings on sex over this time is the decline of explicitly religious works and the rise of medical texts, paradoxically resulting not in richer knowledge of sexuality and greater freedom of activity but in medical delusions that now seem bizarre and new systems of controlling personal behavior.[91] As Hitchcock has further argued, the rise of medical discourse turned an activity previously regulated by the church (through sermons, the confessional, church courts, and community pressure such as the "rough music"—or charivari)[92] into one monitored by the expanding medical profession. Such a transfer of authority had far-reaching consequences: the Christian church had always regarded sex outside marriage, and even nonprocreative sex within marriage, as a sin, but the medical profession turned it into a physical and mental illness, requiring more drastic measures than mere admonishment and penance by way of cure.

3 · Pathologizing Male Sexuality

The Masturbation Phobia and the Invention of Spermatorrhea

Young men afflicted with this disorder [a continual efflux of a "thin, cold, colourless substance"] . . . become old in habit of body, slow, languid, spiritless, dull, silent, feeble, wrinkled, unactive, pale, white, effeminate, of a weak appetite, cold, with a heaviness of the limbs and a numbness of the legs, weak, lazy and indisposed to all manner of action. In many it is the forerunner of the palsy; for how is it possible for the nerves not to suffer under the decay of their forces, when nature . . . is infrigidated? Since it is the vital seed which makes us men, hot, robust, hairy, of a strong and deep voice, bold and courageous, and fit to contrive any enterprise.

ARETAEUS THE CAPPADOCIAN, second century

Did you make fornication with yourself alone . . . I mean that you yourself took your manly member in your hand, and so slide your foreskin (praeputium), and move [it] with your own hand so as by delight to eject seed from yourself?

Confessor's question to penitents, eleventh century

I refer to masturbation as one of the effects of a long prepuce; not that this vice is entirely absent in those who have undergone circumcision, though I never saw an instance in a Jewish child of very tender years, except as the result of association with children whose covered glans have naturally impelled them to the habit.

DR. M. J. MOSES, "The Value of Circumcision as a Hygienic and Therapeutic Measure," 1871

Although routine circumcision was not established until the late nineteenth century, a necessary condition for this development was acceptance of the theory that masturbation was the cause of many organic (and later mental) diseases. While eighteenth-century doctors elaborated this hypothesis with an increasing wealth of detail, it was left to their Victorian successors to answer the question they had posed but failed to answer convincingly: How do we stop boys and girls from doing it? But in order to make sense of the urgency of this demand, we must explore the origins and growth of a phenomenon that is more than a mistaken medical theory and that has been rightly described as "a great fear." It is the depth of the fear that explains the severity of the means eventually adopted to deal with it.

Christian theologians had always condemned masturbation, along with all other nonprocreative sex, but it was not until the seventeenth century that anyone suggested the practice might be physically harmful. Although it makes no specific mention of masturbation, the Old Testament generally regards sex as a disagreeable necessity: intercourse, ejaculation, menstruation, and childbirth all brought about a state of uncleanness that had to be purged by ritual purification (and in ancient times, animal sacrifice). Intercourse was banned during menstruation because there was no possibility of conception.[1] Despite the absence of biblical direction, early Judaic theologians classed masturbation as an abomination characteristic of idolaters and the uncircumcised, and universally regarded it as a sin, or even a crime warranting the death penalty.[2] It is difficult not to connect the Jewish abhorrence of nonprocreative sex with their practice of early circumcision: commentators held that the effect of circumcision was to curb excessive sexual indulgence, and Philo emphasized that its purpose—the "excision of pleasure"—was to remind men that sex was strictly for reproductive purposes.[3] In the second century Rabbi Eliezer prohibited men from touching their penis even when they urinated,[4] and to this day orthodox Jews teach their sons that they must urinate hands free: "Better a bad aim than bad habit!" As Thomas Szasz comments, "for a male to urinate in this manner is a difficult enough feat if he is circumcised. If he is not, it is impossible."[5] The Jewish tradition was inherited by Christianity, which began as an ascetic religion eager to dissociate itself from Pagan sensuality and worldly pleasures. Saint Augustine considered that all forms of sexual passion revealed the inability of the spirit to control the flesh, hence that sex must be original sin, and early penitentials prescribed a penance of psalm singing and a day's fasting for masturbation, a light penalty compared with the seven years' mortification imposed for sodomy.[6] The medieval church took a more serious view of the matter, following Thomas Aquinas's categorization of masturbation as a sin against nature, and thus a mortal sin: penances for the activity in adults became more severe, and some Flemish jurists in the sixteenth century actually considered it a crime that should be punished in the civil courts.[7] The matter was not yet viewed so seriously in newly Protestant countries, and bawdy allusions to "frigging" were common in Elizabethan and early Stuart drama,[8] but with the rise of Puritanism, such indulgences were increasingly frowned upon, and one writer in 1600 warned that willfully shedding sperm would harm a man "more than if he should bleed fortie times as much." As the Rev. William Gouge remarked in his *Domesticall Duties* (1627), "the body must be beaten downe and earnest prayer made for the gift of continency."[9]

At this stage the doctors were inclined to disagree. In accordance with Galenic theory, they believed that a buildup of semen could be harmful to health because of the resulting imbalance in the humors, and they recommended masturbation as a means of restoring equilibrium. Venette was particularly eloquent on the health benefits of seminal discharge: "Woman does not have the ability to pollute herself, as does man, or to discharge her superfluous seed. . . . Unlike man who, by polluting himself frequently, even during his sleep, benefits from a seed that is always renewed and never remains in his canals long enough to become corrupt."[10] He also recommended masturbation as a cure for impotence: "if the hand of a pretty woman, which is the most excellent medicine, has not power enough to cure the lankness of a man's member, other remedies will signify nothing."[11] In an English case of 1723 a patient with "congested testicles" was allowed "mastupration" after bleeding and purges had failed, and was apparently cured. Theologians attacked doctors for advising that masturbation could be beneficial to health, asserting that it was more important to avoid sin and preserve chastity, even at the cost of illness or death; precisely because it was pleasurable, masturbation was never permissible.[12] Religious condemnation had focused on masturbation in adults and been little concerned with the practice in adolescents, let alone in boys before puberty, and no one apart from priests seems to have shown any alarm before the eighteenth century. The Rev. George Trosse (1631–93) recorded in his autobiography that "a lewd fellow-servant led me to practice a sin, which too many young men are guilty of, and look upon as harmless, tho' God struck Onan dead in the place for it."[13] But when Thomas Hobbes was tutor to the young Duke of Buckingham in the 1640s and found one day that the inattention of his young pupil was because "his Grace was at mastupration (his hand in his codpiece)," he reported the fact with evident amusement and no sign of disapproval.[14] It was the calm before the storm: although masturbation is not mentioned in books on child rearing before the eighteenth century, condemnation of the practice begins suddenly around 1750, rising steadily to a peak at the end of the nineteenth.[15] By 1800, as Hitchcock comments, "masturbation had been transformed for both elite and popular audiences into a serious social and medical concern on which many of the social problems of the day could be heaped."[16]

The virulence of the phobia is hard to explain, but it was partly the outcome of a powerful alliance between religion and medicine: doctors took the moral arguments of priests and priests the medical arguments of doctors to fortify their respective positions, and the result was a formidable body of dogma, endorsed by both the theological and the scientific establishments. In 1633 the Puritan Richard Capel condemned "self-defilement" as "a foule sinne much against nature" and worse than murder, but he also flew the kite that it caused the body to "rot and weaken . . . by the curse of God . . . [and] make people unfit for marriage."[17] This helpful suggestion was taken up by late seventeenth-century physicians, who claimed to identify a form of gonorrhea induced by masturbation and manifest in continual emissions from the penis. Richard Wiseman (ca. 1622–76) diagnosed friction and masturbation among boys at puberty as a cause of the "relaxation" of the seminal vessels, leading to their inability to retain semen.[18] This proposition was in turn seized by "two reverend divines," who warned "young gentlemen," in their *Letters of Advice . . . about a Weighty Case of Conscience* (1676), that masturbation was not only sinful but provoked a slackening of the "muscles which extend the penis," leading to a "constant flowing of semen" and eventually impotence. One can imagine the young rakes of the Restoration being far more alarmed at the prospect of impotence than of hellfire, and few would have known that erections are not produced by muscular action. In the early eighteenth century the Society for Promoting Christian Knowledge was energetically distributing short tracts on moral behavior, including *Rebuke to the Sin of Uncleanness* (1704), which denounced fornication, adultery and "mollities"—that is, masturbation.[19] It was in the context of this moral backlash against the license of the Restoration than an enterprising quack published a pamphlet that became one of the most influential texts in medical history.

Onania: Or the Heinous Sin of Self Pollution (1716) said little that was new,[20] but it united the medical and the theological case against masturbation in a plausible synthesis, made all the more convincing by the offer of patent medicines guaranteed to alleviate common ailments. The bulk of *Onania* is a condemnation of masturbation on religious grounds: the corporeal consequences took up only five pages out of an original seventy-six, although the text was later expanded by the addition of lengthy letters, supposedly from readers. Remedies for the diseases could be purchased from the bookseller who distributed the work: a "strengthening tincture" cost ten shillings a bottle and a "prolifick powder" twelve shillings a jar.[21] The author states that his aim was "to promote virtue and Christian purity, and to discourage vice and uncleanness" (*Onania*, 1); to this end he marshals both religious and medical arguments within a common causal framework: just as indulgence in a harmful practice would give rise to bodily afflictions in this world, so the commission of such a grave sin would be punished in the next (28–29, 124). The author explains that he wrote the book because of the frequency of the activity among male youth, and because he was sure that many would not have been guilty of it "had they been thoroughly acquainted with the heinousness of the crime, and the sad consequences to the body as well as the soul" (iii–iv). The author was remarkably candid in acknowledging that nothing would restrain youth from masturbation "if they imagined it could do them no bodily injury, and had no notion that it was an offence to God" and admitted that his aim was to "frighten them from it" (119). Scary indeed was his claim that the physical effects of masturbation were to stunt growth and cause paraphimosis, ulcers, fainting fits, epilepsy, and consumption, as well as "stranguaries, priapisms and other disorders of the penis and testes, but especially gonorrhoeas more difficult to be cured than those contracted from women." Impotence and sterility could arise because "when the seminal vessels are first strained and afterwards relaxed, the ferment in the testes is destroyed, and the seed grown thin and waterish, comes away unelaborated," a distemper that often proved fatal (17–18).

It was an impressive charge sheet, but hardly original even then. Michael Stolberg has shown that it was cribbed almost verbatim from John Marten's *Treatise of Venereal Diseases*.[22] Marten (ca. 1670–1737) was a typical pox doctor—a medical entrepreneur specializing in venereal disease—who consolidated the scattered remarks of late seventeenth-century writers against seminal loss, and coaxed the result into a plausible syndrome that seemed to be based on the observations of reliable authorities and to meet the requirements of the prevailing paradigm for understanding bodily function and disorders. Marten's colorful description of the effects of masturbation was repeated by nearly every writer on the subject for the next two hundred years: "With meagre jaws and pale looks, seldom without scabs and blotches, these loathsome relics of their odious vices, with limber hams, and legs without calves, feeble at mature years as ricketty children, weak and consumptive, when they should by nature be most hail and vigorous; rotten before they are full ripe, and fit for nothing in the prime of their years but to be lodged in an hospital."[23] Acton at his most eloquent hardly put it with such fervor.

It may be that Marten deserves more of the credit for the masturbation anxiety and its sequelae than the better-known *Onania*, and his role as both a surgeon specializing in venereal disease and a moralist eager to condemn sexual sin emphasizes the close connection between fear of syphilis and negative attitudes toward sexuality. Not content with giving

scientific backing to the claim that masturbation was physically harmful, Marten warned that sexual variations such as sodomy and fellatio
were particularly likely to spread syphilis; he also described the symptoms of what was later called spermatorrhea and was the first English
medical writer to suggest that the foreskin might be a curse. His condemnation of fellatio was not merely that it was risky and disgusting but
that it was a heinous sin: "O monstrous! thought I that Men, otherwise
sensible Men, should so vilely debase themselves, and become so degenerate; should provoke God so highly, contemn the Laws of Man so openly,
wrong their own Bodies so fearfully; and which is worse (without sincere repentance) ruin their own Souls eternally."[24] There is not much to
distinguish Marten from the author of *Onania* here. He identified three
types of gonorrhea—one expressed as nocturnal emissions, one arising
from "putrefaction of seed," and one from venereal disease—thus making the conflation between discharges of sperm and of matter produced
by infection that persisted until the late nineteenth century. He then
moved directly into a discussion of what was later called seminal weakness or spermatorrhea, the most common cause of which he attributed to
"too liberal using Friction with the Hand when they were School Boys,"
and the results of which were "weakness . . . debilitation . . . [and] total
incapacity to perform the Conjugal Rite." Marten (quite falsely) claimed
that Diogenes (who famously advocated masturbation as a convenient
form of release) reckoned masturbation "with fornication, Adultery, Incest, to be an abomination in the sight of God," piously adding that he
"can't agree with him in ranking it equally with those sins."[25] Most interesting for my purposes is Marten's equivocal attitude toward the foreskin. Although he reported the medical orthodoxy that its mobility generated pleasure and that circumcision was unnatural,[26] he also asserted
that the foreskin was often troublesome and in need of removal (as it
might have been in many of the syphilitic men he saw in his practice):

> Nature seems not so wanton in any part of her Works as in the make of
> the Yard, especially the Prepuce, because there seems to be no necessity
> for it: In some it is very troublesome, from hence perhaps arose the ne-
> cessity of Circumcision so generally practis'd in all the Eastern Parts of
> the World, as it is among the Jews to this Day. The first of which, use it
> out of cleanliness, and to prevent Diseases, which the detention of the
> Mucus of the Subpreputial Glands which ouze thro' might breed in
> those hot Countries.[27]

Citing the example of the Arabs, he rejected the common view that circumcision made men less lustful, and he went so far as to claim that the
operation was often desirable:

The largeness of length of the Prepuce . . . is an infirmity very trouble-some to some Men, and doubtless very much hinders Procreation, for the Prepuce hanging so much over the Glans or Nut, and receiving the Seed when ejaculated, like a purse, and it staying there, hinders impregna-tion. . . . Those that are troubled with this Infirmity, do frequently pol-lute themselves in making Water. . . . The Cure of this can no way be so well effected as by cutting.[28]

It seems likely that the more respectable Robert James relied on these pas-sages for his own minatory comments on the association between long foreskins and venereal disease (see chap. 2). There is a certain prophetic symbolism in the fact that the first known English medical writer to re-fer favorably to circumcision was also one of the first to identify mastur-bation as a major cause of organic disease, and a sin not quite so bad as fornication, adultery, and incest; to denounce fellatio as an abomination that would send the practitioner to hell; to identify spermatorrhea as a disease and attribute most cases to masturbation; to disparage the fore-skin as an inconvenience to many men and long ones a hindrance to both impregnation and hygiene; and to suggest that circumcision among "eastern nations" had a sanitary rather than a religious rationale. Little did he realize how well worn and how marvelously amplified his draft script would become.

It has been suggested by Thomas Laqueur and others that Marten was the author of *Onania*, but this is denied by Patrick Singy, who argues that Marten was primarily an entrepreneur selling quack cures for venereal disease, whereas *Onania*'s author seems to have been a moralist interested in discouraging sexual adventure of all kinds.[29] The author's fundamen-tally religious motivation is clear from his own declaration, his animad-versions on sex in general, and his response to the other side of the Galenic coin—that good health might necessitate the evacuation of se-men. He shows awareness of this view but claims that other medical writ-ers had exaggerated the harm that arose from retention of semen, and continues: "let us suppose a man really labouring under such a retention, and actually suffering the ill-consequences of it; as dimness of sight, ver-tigo, dullness and melancholy, and whose circumstances hinder him from conversing lawfully with a woman, I cannot see why he should not look upon this in the same manner as he would upon any other affliction sent him by the hand of God, either for trial or chastisement" (*Onania*, 113). This is a position more reminiscent of the book of Job than of a manual on health. Equally fatalistic is his insistence that any kind of sex is wrong unless intended for procreation. Following Saint Paul and Saint Augustine, he asserts that "lustful desires" will arise because "we are conceived in sin," with the consequences that "our chastity is always in danger" and "all carnal temptations ought to be shunned" (21). The object of matrimony is to "prevent the sin of uncleanness, that is, to hinder all people in whom carnal desires are stirred up, from fornication, self-pollution and other sorts of defilements" (91). The author's piety and his alienation from the skeptical mood of his age emerge most starkly in his sharp reply to a woman who had commented that marriage was good and fornication bad because of their social effects: "You imagine that it [fornication] is forbid, not because it is in itself evil, but as it is destructive to the good of society: This is a dangerous assertion, and gives too great a handle for deists and other libertines, who would persuade the world that religion is only a political invention, and no further to be minded, than as it is beneficial to the order and government of society." No, he insists, the duty of a Christian is obedience to the will of God, however inscrutable it might be: "The only rule a Christian is to walk by is the word of God . . . that fornication is forbid, is plain from holy writ; but why it is forbid is arrogance to determine" (88). That was as much an injunction against scientific investigation of the natural world as against recreational sex; indeed, this mood of Job-like submission is so far from the scientific and libertarian spirit of the Enlightenment that it is hard not to agree with Singy that *Onania* represents not "the secularisation of morality," as is often stated, but "the clumsy swansong of the weakened Christian discourse of the flesh"[30]—except for the reference to "swansong." Although the Christian discourse remained muted during the eighteenth century, it never died, and enjoyed a vigorous resurgence in the late nineteenth, especially in the work of William Acton and the later social purity movements.

Influential though *Onania* was, its success was minor compared with that enjoyed by a work written fifty years later, *Onanism: Or a Treatise on the Diseases Produced by Masturbation,* by the Swiss physician Samuel-August Tissot. Unlike the obscure Marten, half quack, half preacher, Tissot was a European celebrity and an important figure in the Enlightenment, with progressive views in some areas of medicine, such as inoculation against smallpox. His book was first published in Latin in 1758, French in 1760, English in 1766, and most other European languages thereafter, and it remained in print until 1905. In 1829 it was consulted by no less a figure than William Gladstone, and in the early twentieth century G. Stanley Hall, in his influential text on adolescence, praised it as an "epoch-making classic."[31] Yet Tissot made no physiological discoveries or medical breakthroughs, developed no antidotes or helpful therapies, cured no one of any disease, and today he represents no more than a medical dead end, studied by historians of popular delusion. What accounts for the influence he exerted for so long? Stengers and van Neck list six factors: his reputation; a dramatic style; spine-chilling case histories; a peremptory and authoritative manner; his display of learning; and his claim of scientific objectivity, which suited the rationalist mood of the times.[32] All these are important, but the crucial factor was probably the last. Although Tissot wrote from a highly moralistic standpoint, establishing that "the crime of Onan" was a sin in the eyes of God before discussing its effects on health,[33] he claimed to be writing a purely objective account and actually disparaged *Onania* as excessively ideological: "truly a chaos, the most unfinished work written for a long time. Only the cases can be read, for the reflections of the author are but theological and moral frivolities" (17). Despite such hauteur, Tissot relied heavily on *Onania* for his own description of the symptoms of masturbatory disease, summed up under six headings: the intellect weakens; the body loses strength; aches and pains; pimples; many harmful effects on the genitals; and intestinal disorders. In explaining why masturbation induced such troubles Tissot relied principally on Galenic/humoral theory, and his evidence consists entirely of statements by medical authorities that loss of semen is harmful: "physicians of every age have unanimously admitted that the loss of one ounce of it enfeebles more than forty ounces of blood" (v). The idea that excessive loss of semen was tiring and could cause illness was ancient, but the statistical precision seems to be a distorted reference to Avicenna's dictum that a single ejaculation was more tiring than forty bloodlettings.[34] Typical of his citations is one from the contemporary Dutch medical authority, Hermann Boerhaave: "The too great loss of semen produces weakness, debility, immobility, convulsions, emaciation, dryness, pains in the membranes of the brain, impairs the senses, particularly that of sight, gives rise to dorsal consumption, indolence and to the several diseases connected with them" (12). For the rest of his treatise he relies on terrifying case histories, all supposedly witnessed in person.

Although the bulk of Tissot's treatise was unoriginal, there were two areas in which he made innovations: the revival of the ancient idea that semen was necessary to maintain masculine characteristics and the proposition that the shock of orgasm could damage the nerves and brain. The traditional Galenic/humoral view was that both excessive loss and excessive retention of semen could be harmful, but early in the eighteenth century medical writers argued that circulation of semen within the body was vital to the maintenance of masculinity and that its loss would therefore lead to eunuchism.[35] Tissot added this point to the reasons why masturbation should be avoided and quoted the opinion of an unnamed expert that "the semen is retained in the vesiculae seminales until it is used or expended by nocturnal emissions. During all this time, the quantity existing there excites the sexual desires of the animal; but the greatest part . . . is resumed by the blood, and produces . . . remarkable changes, the hairs and the beard; it alters the voice and the manners" (vi). Although Tissot was probably just paraphrasing Aretaeus (see the first epigraph in this chapter), the idea is plausible in the absence of knowledge about hormones, which were not discovered until the 1920s.[36] Tissot displayed some ingenuity in explaining why eunuchs, who could produce no semen, did not suffer the same ill effects as "those who are exhausted by venereal debauchery," suggesting that they "do not suffer the spasms of orgasm which derange the nervous system" (44). This idea takes us into the only point in his case against masturbation that was really new: the proposition that ejaculation occasioned a spasm that convulsed the nervous system, leading to an excess of blood in the brain (producing mania) and disorders of digestion, the nerves, and perspiration (32, 37–45). This was also the main reason why masturbation was harmful to women, even though they had no semen to lose (45). It is apparent that Tissot has derived this idea from the nerve force theories then being developed, and he quotes von Haller as stating that intercourse is "very violent, similar to a convulsion which . . . weakens and affects the whole nervous system" (37). Tissot's deployment of such scientific advances to shore up his case is similar to the way in which *Onania* made use of the then revolutionary understanding of the circulation of the blood to help describe the distillation of semen and, in particular, to explain (contra the orthodox Galenists) why no problems could arise from not evacuating accumulations of semen: the surplus simply returned to the bloodstream when the testicles were full.[37]

After his lurid description of such a hydra-headed vice and the hair-raising case histories, Tissot's treatments come as an anticlimax. All he can offer is diet, exercise, sleep, and avoidance of feather beds or lying awake in the morning, supplemented by various cocktails from the pharmacopoeia of the day, but he is forced to conclude that even the most judicious regimen of these, plus the goodwill of the patient, was not always sufficient to effect a cure (53–87). But as Jordanova observes, it may be that Tissot's object was not so much to achieve cures as to institute a system of panoptic surveillance over a person's, and particularly a child's, daily behavior. She points out that he introduced two ideas that remained central to nineteenth- and twentieth-century discourses on masturbation: the sexuality of children, yet the need to repress it; and the proposition that children were often instructed in masturbation by servants.[38] Why masturbation was a problem before puberty, when ejaculation never and orgasm rarely occurred, was a paradox Tissot did not seek to elucidate, and one that later exercised the inventive mind of William Acton.

Whatever its contradictions and inadequacies as a scientific text, Tissot's *Onanism* had immense influence, and in its wake it became "almost impossible to write a popular medical text without roundly condemning the likely consequences of masturbation."[39] Popular English medical works by James Graham, Ebenezer Sibly, and A. M. F. Willich swelled the chorus of disapproval, generating an atmosphere of guilt and anxiety that suited the deepening antisensualism of the early nineteenth century.[40] Graham was a plausible quack who hired out (at £50 a night) a magnetic bed to infertile couples. In his *Lecture on the Generation, Increase and Improvement of the Human Species* (1780) he fulminated against early sexual experience (before the age of twenty), venereal excess in general, and masturbation particularly, indulgence in which would produce "debility of body and of mind—infecundity—epilepsy—idiotism—extreme wretchedness and even death itself." Anticipating Acton's insistence that young men must remain continent until marriage, Graham regarded as "supremely blessed" young men and women who reach twenty "without even once having had even one seminal emission . . . voluntarily or involuntarily."[41] In his *Lectures on Diet and Regimen* (1799), Willich moderated Tissot by warning that "the emission of semen enfeebles the body more than the loss of twenty times the same quantity of blood," but that this was still enough to "weaken the nerves, the stomach, the intestines, the eyes, the heart, the brain . . . [and] the mental faculties."[42] In his *Medical Mirror* (1770) Sibly took on the persona of a grand inquisitor as he forced reluctant youths to confess their secret sins and lectured them on the need to reform their ways.[43] The confessional aura was also prominent in Samuel Solomon's best-selling *Guide to Health, or Advice to Both Sexes in Nervous and Consumptive Complaints* (ca. 1800): if you revealed all, he could relieve even the effects of seminal loss by "the famous and highly exalted medicine, the Cordial Balm of Gilead."[44] Unlike the treatments devised next century, this concoction was probably harmless. Controlling immature desire became an obsession of subsequent medico-moral discourse, the aim being, in Christabel Pankhurst's later words, to make male sexuality "lie dormant until legitimate occasion arises for its use."[45] Possibly the only physician to dissent from the new medical orthodoxy was John Hunter, who questioned the link drawn between onanism and impotence with the logical and (to us) commonsense observation that impotence "appears to me to be by far too rare to originate from a practice so general."[46] He went on to doubt whether blaming impotence and related genital problems on masturbation was useful and asserted his own conviction that "many of those who are affected by the complaints in question are miserable from the idea; and it is some consolation for them to know that it is possible it may arise from other causes. I am clear in my own mind that the books on this subject have done more harm than good. I think I may affirm that this act in itself does less harm to the constitution in general than the natural [i.e., intercourse]." Although many of his patients believed that masturbation was the root of their problems, Hunter observed that they "did not appear to have given more into the practice than common."[47] Hunter's isolation on this issue may be judged from the fact that in the 1810 edition of his book, after his death, the last sentence from the passage just quoted was censored.[48]

An important way in which belief in the harm of masturbation gained popular currency was through new forms of knowledge diffusion. By 1728 *Chambers Cyclopaedia* had an entry for *onanism,* defined as a term "some late empirics [quacks] have framed to denote the crime of self-pollution, mentioned in Scripture to have been practised by Onan, and punished in him with death."[49] The passage was repeated in the second edition of the *Encyclopaedia Britannica* (1781), supplemented by the discoveries of Tissot, and the result was a story that must have terrified many young men, including George Drysdale, who had a nervous breakdown and dropped out of his university course after reading it: "His excited imagination and ignorance of bodily disease at once filled him with terror at these symptoms [constipation and nocturnal emissions]. He read an article on onanism in the Encyclopaedia, written by some antiquated horror-monger, and of course applied all the extreme effects of this disease to his own case."[50] What is particularly interesting about the entry is its discussion of treatment. Tissot had been pessimistic about cure, but *Britannica* suggested that masturbation could be stopped if it were possible to "prevent irritability of the parts of generation," and it offered five means to this end: plain but nutritious food; vigorous and fatiguing exercise so as to reduce the secretion of semen; the bare minimum of sleep; no alcohol; and doses of Peruvian bark (quinine).[51] It seems a fairly pathetic list of expedients, exposing the inadequacy of available remedies when faced with such a new and powerful enemy, but the stage was set for the introduction of more effective treatments. There was no mention of surgery, but if the objective was to "prevent irritability" of the penis, there was a lead for inventive surgeons to come up with new tactics toward that goal.

This panic over masturbation, as Peter Gay has observed, is easier to document than to explain.[52] Stone has commented that the rise of anxiety over adolescent masturbation in the eighteenth century is particularly puzzling, given that it occurred in a context of increasing sexual permissiveness for adults; the nineteenth-century hysteria over the practice makes more sense, "since it coincided with the rise of Evangelical doctrine and the growing sense of horror and shame" about all forms of sexual expression.[53] Porter noted that alarm was whipped up by both quacks and regular doctors and that it was in some way related to the prolongation of childhood in the eighteenth century and the greater care, and thus surveillance, that middle-class parents were bestowing on their children, but that no definite answers to the problem have emerged.[54] Thomas Szasz compared the cruel treatment of masturbators in the nineteenth century with the persecution of witches at an earlier period and related the obsession with masturbation as a illness-generating vice to the decline in the belief that disease was caused by witchcraft; in an age trying to be scientific, but when the causes of most diseases were not understood, blaming them on personal habits was both morally satisfying and consistent with the nerve force theories then emerging.[55] Gilbert suggested that the centrality of masturbation in accounts of organic disease was related to doctors' rising prestige and their tendency to take over the role of the priest; the cycle of sin, confession, penance, and redemption was transferred from confessional to consulting room. At the same time, there was little that they could actually do about most diseases, and blaming them on masturbation was often found more satisfactory than admitting their own impotence.[56] R. P. Neuman related the concern with masturbation to demographic factors, arguing that with the Industrial Revolution the average age of puberty declined while the normal age of marriage rose, creating a longer interval between childhood and adulthood. This was associated with a new concern with child rearing and a closer supervision of sexually mature children, who now spent a longer interval between puberty and marriage. Associated with these developments was the denial that young children had any sexual feelings, with the result that manifestations such as fondling and masturbation were categorized as pathological and attributed to local irritation (such as a tight foreskin), to bad influences (particularly at school), or to servants' tickling of a child's genitals. As Neuman puts it, "in order to preserve the respectable sexual fantasy that sex was for adults, not children, and for the purpose of procreation rather than pleasure, doctors had to explain masturbation in the very young as the product of certain organic problems or as the result of bad habits taught by others. So it was suggested that infants scratched their genitals because of local irritations caused by uncleanness or worms."[57] If any expression of sexuality before puberty was pathological rather than normal, it had to be eliminated, and corrective surgery, including circumcision, was one of the means. It is significant that in the nineteenth century, when antisensualism was in the ascendant, restraint was imposed on everyone, while in the eighteenth century, when the puritans were only a minority pressure group, demands for restraint were directed mainly at "deviants" (like homosexuals) and children. It may thus be seen that they concentrated their efforts toward attempting to restrict the sexual freedom of those most subject to legal or adult authority and least able to fight back; as Spitz observes, "helpless children are suitable objects for retaliation."[58]

Stengers and van Neck are inclined to explain the great fear by reference to salesmanship—the author of *Onania* exploited a market niche, Tissot traded on his reputation, and both aimed to curdle their readers' blood with minatory case studies. They are particularly skeptical toward the class-based hypotheses that seek to relate conservation of sperm to bourgeois thrift and their hatred of nonproductive expenditure, as proposed by Bouce (1982) and, most famously, by Steven Marcus in *The Other Victorians*. Marcus made much of the fact that the nineteenth-century word for *orgasm* was *spend* but seems to have been unaware that the same word was in common usage in the sixteenth and seventeenth centuries,[59] long before those thrifty Victorians began poking their pennies into money boxes. Just as significantly, ancient Judaic and traditional Christian theology was equally set against nonproductive (i.e., nonprocreative) emissions long before the bourgeoisie had begun its seemingly limitless rise, and misers have been found in all ages. The idea that seminal loss could cause illness is an ancient medical principle, not the invention of William Acton, eager though he was to ensure that male energies were cautiously husbanded; spermatic niggardliness is an ancient and religious demand, not a modern or secular ideal. The great weakness in the analogy between sexual continence and economic thrift is that the Victorian economic miracle depended on invention, investment, credit, and spending on a rapidly expanding array of consumer goods, not just saving, and all these requirements are inconsistent with the model. The attempt to relate the masturbation phobia to socioeconomic developments is thus not convincing, at least not if the focus remains on the nineteenth century. As we have seen, however, the syndrome actually developed a hundred years before, and the connection makes more sense in the context of the mercantilist economy of the early eighteenth century than in the industrial and increasingly consumerist economy of the mid-nineteenth. In the mercantilist system a nation's wealth was thought to arise from a favorable balance of trade (hence the need for a growing population, big navies, colonies, and so forth). International trade was seen as a zero-sum game: since one nation's gain was another's loss, it was vital to ensure that you exported more than you imported, or spent less than you earned.[60] The supreme object of this game was the accumulation of trade surpluses in the form of gold specie, the hoarding of which seems to take us closer to the rules of the spermatic economy than those in force after the Industrial Revolution. From this perspective, (solitary) masturbation appears to be a typically capitalist (individualist) activity, and its reprobation a rearguard action by old-fashioned collectivists who wanted to maintain the traditional policing of personal behavior and discourage solitary pursuits as antisocial and dangerously free from the restraints of church and community. The masturbation phobia thus becomes not an aspect of modernity but a reaction against modernization and an attempt to preserve an older ethic of collectivism, group responsibility, and priestly supervision of personal behavior—just the sort of close-knit, rule-bound world still common in many Islamic societies and both Jewish and Christian fundamentalist communities today.[61] The contours of the evolution of the great fear fit Stone's suggestion that the moral or religious mood is the vital determinant, not socioeconomic conditions or class interests.[62]

The most persuasive explanations for the masturbation phobia are thus those that stress its moral or religious dimension, as argued by Peter Wagner and Patrick Singy, and its importance in providing a believable theory of disease, as proposed by Thomas Szasz and Michael Stolberg. Wagner suggests that its origins lay neither in medical discoveries nor economic change per se, but in the reassertion of Christian prohibitions by moralists and purity campaigners alarmed at the spread of nontraditional values and behavior.[63] It was, in short, a typical conservative response to modernity: "The powerful and enduring misconception that masturbation is a specific cause of mental and physical diseases was the brainchild of moral writers in the religious field who ... demanded more strictness in an age which they perceived to be dominated by apostasy and uncleanness."[64] This is particularly clear in the case of *Onania*, in style and content a jeremiad against the libertinism of the Restoration and early Georgian age. What is less obvious is its attempt to deploy some of the claims of the Scientific Revolution against scientific progress and especially against the less restricted forms of personal behavior that logically followed from discoveries about the natural world and the functions of the body. In addition to its argument that masturbation was a sin sure to earn punishment in the afterlife, *Onania* drew on recent knowledge about the circulatory system and the latest information about venereal disease to add the novel idea that it would also harm the body here on earth. Tissot took this process of secularization further, using the arguments of the Enlightenment against the sort of personal liberation promised by the catchwords *sapere aude* and *ecrasez l'infame*. His eschewal of openly theological argument was a response to the rise of skepticism and the decline of belief in eternal punishment even on the part of those who clung to other Christian verities. People of the Age of Reason would not be deterred from masturbation by sermons on how they were risking hellfire, but they might pay attention if a respected physician informed them it would induce impotence or tuberculosis. Members of the clergy thanked Tissot for providing them with "powerful weapons" to intimidate "impetuous youth," who were more deeply impressed by accounts of the physical consequences of masturbation in this world than by "the liveliest descriptions of eternal suffering."[65] This strategy was also made plain by the English gynecologist Lawson Tait in the late nineteenth century: "The best remedy was not to tell the poor children that they were damning their souls, but to tell them that they might hurt their bodies."[66]

Stolberg attributes the success of the campaign to demonize masturbation to several political, ideological, and economic motives, including religious concern with "uncleanness," bourgeois fears about self-control, and the "financial interests of the London venereal trade." He also shows how the symptoms blamed on masturbation addressed contemporary anxieties about virility, gender identity, and selfhood and were consistent with prevailing understandings of bodily function and disease causation. Stolberg particularly mentions the role of medical entrepreneurs eager to increase the sale of their goods and services, and notes that masturbation gave the medical profession "a welcome opportunity to demonstrate the importance of medical expertise for promoting individual as well as social welfare." Observing that the campaign originated in and remained strongest in Protestant countries, he also points out that while it drew on the traditional Christian principle that the spirit should subdue the wayward flesh, it exercised a particularly strong appeal to "puritan and pietistic ideals of introspection and constant control over the workings of the mind." The doctors exploited these concerns by asserting that the masturbator's obvious moral weakness would be followed by a loss of physical control.[67] Stolberg concludes that *Onania*'s condemnation of masturbation on religious grounds drew on a long tradition of moralistic writing and was part of a larger campaign against the increasing sexual permissiveness of the period waged by puritanically minded groups like the Society for the Reformation of Manners, whose target was not just masturbation but any form of nonmarital sex and uncleanness in general. He adds that *Onania* popularized the idea of masturbation as the real cause of common diseases, and that linkage of an alarmist text with the sale of medicines and advice were typical quack tactics, although he points out that there were no firm boundaries between quackery and regular medicine at that time. The only point on which Stolberg's analysis might be questioned is its acceptance of *Onania*'s own reason for particular concern about masturbation—that it was common among the young, easy to do, and the first step toward more serious misdemeanors such as fornication. It seems more likely that masturbation was targeted because children were easier to boss around than their parents: although it might not be possible to pressure adults to curb their own sexual enjoyments, there was a chance of persuading them to restrict the sex lives of their children, particularly if restraint was sold as a means of preserving health. That was in fact the pattern with circumcision in the late nineteenth century, when fathers had their sons cut but left their own penises intact. If the masturbation phobia was the result of a medico-religious alliance, a similar convergence of medical and religious discourse made a powerful case for circumcision in the nineteenth century.

It is important to understand not only the moralism behind the medical argument but the primitiveness of the sexual science that underlay these claims: knowledge of sexual physiology and even anatomy was rudimentary until very recent times. As Stolberg points out, the concept of masturbatory disease was "plausible within the framework of contemporary . . . understanding of the body," and it is unhelpful to dismiss it as a collective neurosis.[68] The theory was supported by nearly all the most eminent physicians of the day, and it continued as an article of faith until the 1930s. But to acknowledge this is to appreciate the scientific limitations of medicine until the discovery of microorganisms provided a correct understanding of infectious diseases and the development of antibiotics an effective means to combat them. Both the theory that masturbation was a cause of disease and the proposition that circumcision was a valid intervention belong to medicine's prescientific phase. Even in terms of eighteenth-century science, masturbatory disease was only a plausible hypothesis, not a connection supported by evidence or verified by experiment; those who observed the symptoms of masturbation-induced illness were interpreting what they saw in the light of their initial assumption in a manner that was markedly nonscientific even by the standards of their time. Consider Tissot's claim that loss of semen would lead to eunuchism. At a superficial level it was not unreasonable to think that semen was the factor responsible for a male's secondary sex characteristics, since the two came together and a eunuch had neither, but careful observation (quite within the scientific paradigm of this period) would have revealed that the appearance of those features (enlargement of the genital organs, growth of body hair, deepening of the voice, and so forth) sometimes preceded the capacity to produce sperm. A controlled experiment along the lines of the disproof of mesmerism by a French scientific commission in 1784 would have shown that visible masculinity did not diminish in response to frequent ejacu-lations.[69] The persistence of the error betrays the predominance of ide-ological concerns and a consequent unwillingness to subject a question hedged with religious taboos to scientific inquiry.

The masturbatory hypothesis had too much explanatory power. As Stolberg comments, it offered "a convenient frame of reference for the interpretation of a wide range of disease cases" and made empirical fal-sification almost impossible: "if some masturbators remained seemingly healthy . . . this could be explained by the fact that they had a particu-larly robust constitution."[70] Doctors did not claim there were any new diseases provoked specifically by masturbation;[71] instead, masturbation was a new explanation for many old diseases, some known, many not yet identified. The masturbatory hypothesis allowed people to put a name to whatever afflicted them and the power to ascribe a cause to those dis-tressing but mysterious conditions. From this perspective the great fear can be seen as a myth: an explanation for bodily phenomena that were not understood and tribulations for which there was no cure. It appealed because it seemed to explain why. The hypothesis offered even greater benefits to the medical profession itself: despite their impotence when it came to cure, it allowed doctors to appear omniscient as to the cause of the problem and blameless if their treatments failed, since the patient had brought his problems on himself by failing to heed medical warn-ings; his fate was literally in his own hands. Paradoxically, the doctors' claim to diagnostic infallibility was enhanced every time a patient died: it was yet further proof of the perils attending the practice they had warned against. As befitted a self-inflicted disease that was also a moral crime, treatments devised to treat masturbation in the nineteenth cen-tury were intended to be punishments as much as cures.

The masturbatory hypothesis was thus a crucial step in the rise of the medical profession and an important stage in the history of theories of disease causation. In primitive societies and the Middle Ages, disease was thought to be the result of the action of witchcraft, evil spirits, or the devil, but with the rise of scientific understanding in the seventeenth century such superstitious beliefs were discredited, and a materialist ex-planation was needed.[72] Traditional Galenic medicine, with its humoral model, was revived in the Renaissance, and this was supplemented by the nerve force theory, based on Haller's research. But for a full expla-nation, those theories required an agent to disrupt the humoral or ner-vous balance, and that agent was provided by masturbation, a suitably concrete activity for an age that demanded mechanical causes. The pho-bia became worse in the mid-Victorian period as Christianity faced the new challenge of Darwinism, sexual Puritanism intensified, other out-

lets (such as prostitutes and mutual masturbation) became less acceptable, and the prestige of the medical profession rose. The fear declined in
the twentieth century as secularism advanced, antisensualism retreated,
and the discovery of germs provided a better explanation of the disease
phenomena previously attributed to masturbation. Although it was a
powerful disease theory for a long period, the masturbatory hypothesis
was a backward step in the understanding of male sexuality. The hypothesis led to further loss of knowledge about the anatomy and physiology of the penis, especially the functions of the foreskin, with the result
that there was little opposition to the introduction of mass circumcision
at the end of the nineteenth century—an ironic outcome in view of the
fact that it was precisely their understanding of the sexual significance
of the foreskin that gave early Victorian doctors the idea that circumcision might be just what a continent society needed.

The most significant figure to make this connection, and thus provide
a link between the eighteenth century's concern with the harm of masturbation and the nineteenth's determination to stamp it out, was the
French surgeon Claude-François Lallemand.

To proclaim that masturbation was the real cause of many common diseases might seem ambitious enough, but in the early nineteenth century
a significant stream of medical opinion went a step further to conclude
that not just masturbation but any seminal emission (except occasionally
within marriage) was damaging, or indeed that sexual excitement and
even erections were suspect. Since the only biological function of the
male animal is to produce and emit sperm, this perspective amounted to
the pathologizing of normal male sexuality itself. To this new and imaginary disease doctors gave the name *spermatorrhea*, a chronic but life-
threatening condition, protean in its manifestations, which required many
visits to the surgery and increasingly drastic treatments if there was to be
any hope of cure. Spermatorrhea had many parents, but it was the particular brainchild of Claude-François Lallemand (1790–1853), professor
of medicine at Montpellier, whose massive study *Les pertes seminales in-
volontaires* (Involuntary seminal losses) was published in three volumes
between 1836 and 1842. Of particular significance in explaining the
emergence of widespread circumcision in the 1860s was Lallemand's
identification of the foreskin as the ringleader of the male genitals' conspiracy against masculine well-being: a danger to health and "source of
serious mischief," as William Acton termed it, which ought, as a matter
of prudence, to be amputated before it could do significant damage.

Havelock Ellis blamed *Onania*, Tissot, Voltaire, and Lallemand for
the masturbation phobia, but Lallemand has not featured in modern ac-

counts of it.[73] In his day, however, he was one of the most widely read and influential authorities on the new scourge that suddenly seemed to be afflicting ever-growing numbers of French and English men: spermatorrhea. His three volumes of case studies bespeak a lifetime devoted to observing and treating the disease, but to the modern eye it is a strange work, more like an anthology of bizarre sex stories than a scientific treatise. The intimate detail in which Lallemand recounts the private lives of his patients as well as the certainty with which all bodily and mental problems are ascribed to a single source are reminiscent of Freud's case histories, and his work shows the same insistence on subordinating the facts observed to the hypothesis with which he started.[74] Consistent with this approach is his rather vague definition of the disease under study: spermatorrhea is "every excessive spermatic evacuation from whatever cause it may arise."[75] Although nocturnal emissions may be beneficial, involuntary discharges become a problem if they are "excessive" or "outlive the state that excited [them]," leading to increased secretion and hurried discharge with neither erection nor sensation. What "excessive" means or how it is to be recognized is never clarified: presumably a man's presenting himself at the surgery or an urgent call from an anxious parent was proof enough. But if Lallemand is weak on definitions he is an adept at classification: although the major general cause of spermatorrhea is "too great excitement of the genital apparatus, following venereal excesses or masturbation" (33), he lists no fewer than eight specific causes of the condition: "blennorrhagia" (another name for the benign gonorrhea identified by Robert James and other eighteenth-century authorities);[76] "cutaneous affections" (eczema, herpes etc); "influence of the rectum" (constipation, fissures, worms); abuse (masturbation); "venereal excesses"; action of medicines; influence of the "cerebro-spinal system"; and "congenital predisposition" (a tight or long foreskin, phimosis, excessive secretion of "sebaceous matter," or an "exuberant prepuce"). For our purposes the most significant of these factors are masturbation and congenital predisposition, although a perusal of the case histories in which spermatorrhea had been caused by venereal excess or the bad influence of the rectum would also provide abundant evidence of the obsessive nature of Lallemand's project.

The most frequent cause of spermatorrhea was masturbation, for even in cases where it is not specified as *the* cause it is frequently mentioned as a contributing factor: nearly all Lallemand's patients seem to be guilty of it. By abuse he meant "any irregular or premature exercise of [the genitals]; any application of them which cannot have, as its results, the propagation of the species" (126). Such a broad definition would seem to cover the vast majority of sex acts, including intercourse with the use of contraceptives or during a woman's nonfertile period, but masturbation was "the most dangerous of all vices" because it was "the most difficult to discover and prevent and . . . does not require any assistance for its consummation" (161). Lallemand laid particular stress on the danger of the vice before puberty because he felt the problem had not attracted sufficient attention: "The most anxious parents" believed there was no need to watch over "the actions of their children with regard to the genital organs," but this was a fatal error, since "numerous causes may give rise to abuses" at an early age (143), and masturbation in childhood "produces exactly the same effects as spermatorrhoea" (290). Putting a stop to abuse among boys was thus a vital first step toward their return to health from whatever disorders their bad habit had provoked, and Lallemand was not afraid to act decisively in such cases. In 1824 he treated an eight-year-old with paralyzed legs and a "disturbed intellect," both brought on by masturbation:

> After two or three trials I found it was no use trusting to the strait-waistcoats and other means usually employed, but I accordingly determined to pass a gum-elastic catheter into the bladder, and to fix it so that the patient should be unable to withdraw it. The presence of the foreign body excited inflammation of the urethra, as I expected. . . . I kept up . . . a constant state of inflammation for a fortnight, which rendered the parts so painful that the child was unable to touch them.

Within a fortnight the boy could run about, and Lallemand sent him away, though not before threatening him with a repeat of the treatment if he relapsed (153–54). The idea of breaking the habit of masturbation by making the penis too sore to touch was eagerly taken up and extended by Lallemand's English followers, and it set a precedent for treating mysterious bodily disorders by means of surgical procedures on the genitals.

In his medical theory Lallemand displays a wavering between Galenism and the new nerve force theory similar to that observable in Tissot. He retains sufficient Galenic terminology to describe patients as exhibiting lymphatic, sanguine, or nervous temperaments and to admit that "excessive spermatic plethora" could be as detrimental to health as excessive loss, and even that is difficult to distinguish between the two conditions (185). He accordingly regards wet dreams (although only in "a healthy and continent individual") as beneficial because they free the bodily economy "from a source of excitement, the prolonged accumulation of which might derange the animal functions" (33). But when he comes to explain why masturbation was harmful in boys before puberty, when there was no emission of semen, Lallemand is forced to jump aboard the nerve force bandwagon and propose that the shock irritated the system and could even cause death: "In childhood seminal emissions are never experienced, but nevertheless the patients fall into a state of marasm,[77] to which some even succumb" (154). Even in young children "masturbation produces the same effects as diurnal pollutions . . . [because of the] power of the nervous system at this early age" (296). Lallemand reports that some authorities had therefore concluded it was not the loss of semen that caused debility but "the nervous excitement and convulsive motion which usually accompany the discharge." He could not allow that the damage arose only from the shock of orgasm, since his whole practice was built on the premise that involuntary discharges (that is, without sensation) were dangerous, but by adding the new nerve force theory to the old Galenic paradigm he was able to have it both ways. Before puberty the harm is due only "to the effects on the nervous system," but afterward the damage of seminal loss is added: "Every excessive loss of semen, even when unaccompanied by sensation, is followed by debility." He concludes that the two distinct sources of injury were "nervous disturbance and debilitating discharges," each of which produced the same symptoms by weakening the economy (154–55). Despite Lallemand's acknowledgment that excessive accumulation of sperm could be as harmful as its loss, none of his patients seems to have sought his aid with the former problem, and none was offered treatments designed to relieve the plethora. Nor do we have reports of cases in which wet dreams helped to preserve health: in all the histories cited, Lallemand seems to regard them as pathological and in need of treatment. There were moral limits to his residual Galenism.

Lallemand's favored therapies were not Galenic at all: acupuncture, catheters, cauterization, and circumcision. He continued to follow some of the traditional prescriptions aimed at restoring humoral balance: special diets, bathing in mineralized waters, enemas, exercise, and bleeding; in one case he treated indigestion by the application of leeches to the epigastrium and anus (162). Occasionally he reports success with such new therapies as galvanism (the application of electricity), but his preferred approaches were resolutely surgical. By acupuncture Lallemand did not mean the gentle Chinese technique of pricking the skin but driving long needles through the perineum and into the prostate:

> After having caused the patient to make water, the first of these needles is to pass through the raphe of the perineum, midway between the root of the scrotum and the margin of the anus . . . so as to traverse the inferior lobe of the prostate, nearly as far as the neck of the bladder. The second is next to be introduced between the first and the . . . anus . . . and

the third may be inserted in front of the first, the point being directed obliquely towards the . . . neck of the bladder. . . . I allow the needles to remain at least one hour, and at most three. . . . The extraction is generally painful. (315)

This was a big step forward from the sissy treatments proposed by Tissot. Catheterism involved the introduction of a catheter through the urethra and into the bladder, a procedure intended to arrest "the nervous phenomena of which the genital organs are the seat, and also of lessening the increased sensibility of the urethral mucous membrane." As to the procedure:

A moderate-sized gum elastic catheter should be . . . employed; the introduction should be performed slowly . . . to allow the pain to pass off and to get rid of the spasm of the passage. . . . Some patients suffer such pain during the passage of the instrument, that the whole body becomes agitated . . . and it is precisely in these cases that the catheter produces the most marked and lasting effects. . . . It is remarkable that notwithstanding the severe pain caused by its introduction, the patients invariably experience a sense of comfort immediately after its removal. (314)

Astonishing indeed! But as we have seen in the case of the eight-year-old, Lallemand could resort to the catheter as much to cause irritation and distress as to alleviate them. His favorite treatment, and the one with which he is particularly associated, was cauterization of the prostatic section of the urethra with a solution of silver nitrate. He gives detailed instructions on the method of effecting this by means of a *porte-caustique,* or hollow metal sound, which should be inserted as far as the neck of the bladder and then slowly withdrawn, spraying a film of the caustic as it retreated. The object of the exercise was to reduce the irritability of the prostate and seminal ducts, and Lallemand reports many "complete cures" as a result of this technique. It was usually a painful ordeal. In the case of one patient whose problems (indigestion, itching of the genitals, and seminal discharges when defecating) had been caused by adolescent masturbation and subsequent excessive coitus after marriage,

I proposed cauterisation as the best means of altering the condition of the affected tissues; and the patient consented. On introducing the catheter I found the canal extremely sensitive; the spasms were so severe . . . that the whole of M. C—'s body was covered by a profuse sweat, and I found it necessary to delay the cauterisation. Three days afterwards . . . I cauterised the bladder near its neck, and the prostatic and membranous portions of the urethra. The operation was performed rapidly . . . but it caused . . . acute pinching pain at the margin of the anus and in the rectum. (171)

Since the man did not return for more, Lallemand pronounced him cured. This ordeal became the standard treatment for spermatorrhea, widely practiced by his followers in England and particularly recommended by Acton. It is hard to think of any other instance in medical history where such an imaginary complaint was treated with such savage doses of reality.

Forcible catheterization of boys as a treatment for masturbation might seem heroic enough, but Lallemand went further. In instances where spermatorrhea was attributable to "natural phimosis" (a tight foreskin), "excess sebaceous matter" (not clearly defined but presumably accumulating because the penis was not washed regularly), or an "exuberant prepuce" (longer than he thought decent or proper), his preferred therapy was circumcision. Lallemand seems to have been the first physician to employ this procedure as a standard treatment for masturbation, spermatorrhea, and associated problems, and certainly the first to recommend it as a precautionary measure in children (213-44). He also seems to be the originator of an idea that would become an obsession with later advocates of routine circumcision—that the "secretions" beneath the foreskin caused irritation, which led to masturbation and other problems. Lallemand discusses this proposition in several contexts. First, he asserts that masturbation in cases where secretions had accumulated was usually "excited spontaneously, and it is likely enough that phimosis contributed to this result. Irritation of the glans . . . excites importunate erections and titillations, which attract the attention of children to the parts, and induce handling and friction. We may therefore attribute the spontaneous occurrence of masturbation in young children . . . to the presence of the sebaceous matter between the glans and the foreskin" (214). Second, Lallemand argues that the foreskin itself was a more significant source of irritation than the erectile tissue beneath, as demonstrated by the case of one patient with a very small penis, but an abundant (perhaps "exuberant") foreskin, who suffered from emissions while horse riding. He comments that the manifest sensitivity of the penis could not be traced to its "underdeveloped" erectile portion but to "some irritating cause" that must have induced "the abnormal sensitivity of the glans, and this irritation could only arise from the sebaceous matter on its surface being altered by too long retention."[78] Although there is a better explanation (the intense innervation of the foreskin itself, leading to acutely pleasurable sensations as it rolled over the glans), Lallemand believed his interpretation confirmed by the fact that "the simple excision of the prepuce suffice[d] to arrest the diurnal pollutions" (220). One could not want clearer evidence of the effect of circumcision in reducing penile responsiveness. Third, Lallemand suggests that in immature boys the foreskin itself is a cause of "premature" and thus pathological erections:

> The premature erections from which these patients suffered are certainly not attributable to the rudimentary condition of the genital organs. . . . [It] arose from simple local excitement of the penis; and this was not produced by the presence of semen, because . . . the testicles had not begun to secrete. The accumulation of sebaceous matter around the glans is the only sufficient explanation of this . . . irritation. . . . The remarkable facts produced by cleanliness and by excision of the prepuce leave no doubt on this subject. (220)

In other words, masturbation in prepubertal boys ceased when the irritable tissue that provoked it was cut off. Finally, Lallemand identified the dilemma built into the question of whether boys should be instructed to wash under their foreskin and clear away the offending secretions, since "causing children to practise ablution or friction of the parts . . . might, indeed, by drawing their attention, be dangerous" (221–22). Acton believed that strict cleanliness was enough, but his successors were not so confident that boys could be trusted both to keep themselves clean and to confine their manipulations strictly to that purpose if they did, and they eventually realized that the simplest solution to the dilemma was to excise the tissue that both trapped the secretions and offered the temptation to abuse. Lallemand advised that it was "wiser to perform circumcision than to trust to the patient's cleanliness, in order to guard against secretion . . . and to remove the parts beyond possibility of further irritation" (223), and by the early twentieth century this was the generally held conclusion.

In cases of spermatorrhea arising directly or indirectly from the foreskin, Lallemand recommended his usual treatments—cauterization and mineral baths, followed by circumcision if these were insufficient—but when the foreskin was noticeably long or tight it was "indispensable to commence the treatment by its removal." Contrary to some eighteenth-century authorities, Lallemand insisted that "simple division of the prepuce does not suffice . . . its entire removal is generally to be preferred" (223). As the U.S. surgeon Lewis Sayre was to discover in the 1870s,[79] Lallemand knew that disorders in many remote parts of a boy's body could be instigated by the condition of his genitals and that paralysis of the limbs might be caused by a narrow foreskin and at least partially cured by circumcision. In case LIII he recounted his treatment of a fifteen-year-old for paralysis of the lower limbs:

On examining the genital organs, I noticed that the prepuce was very narrow, and on pressing it to get rid of the sebaceous matter which presented at its orifice, the penis became erect. I learned from the parents that this boy had erections at the age of eight; and that, at nine years, he had been found attempting coitus. The boy admitted that the itching with which he was tormented led him to rub the genital organs, and thus induced manoeuvres which he had since continued.

Lallemand amputated the boy's prepuce and a week later cauterized the bladder and prostate, and a month after that he was able to report that the urine was transparent and that sensibility of the skin on his legs had returned. Sadly, recovery seems to have stalled at this point, and Lallemand "lost sight of the patient" (214–15). Lallemand further anticipated the conclusions of late nineteenth-century physicians by suggesting that circumcision need not be only a post hoc therapy but might be usefully employed as a preventive tactic, and even as a routine operation on children:

> In cases of superabundant secretion . . . it is more prudent to circumcise the patient than to trust to the most careful cleanliness; there is no comparison between this trifling operation and the importance of the involuntary discharges which may return with a return of the preputial irritation. . . . [T]he discontinuance of the practice of circumcising children is to be regretted; the operation is unnecessary in many cases, but it can never be injurious, and in a great proportion it would be exceedingly useful. (224)

Since children (other than those of Jewish or Muslim parents) had never been circumcised anywhere in Europe before the nineteenth century, it is difficult to know what Lallemand meant by the last sentence, although a similar regret was expressed by Dr. Copland in the 1850s. Perhaps they felt it was easier to revive an abandoned practice than to introduce a novel one.

Lallemand is an important figure in the rise of routine male circumcision. Building on the masturbation phobia of the eighteenth century, his theories turned normal male sexuality into a life-threatening disease that required constant watchfulness and drastic remedies; focused attention on the genitals (and the foreskin in particular) as the source of many illnesses, some real, some imaginary; and identified the hope of cure through painful and mutilating procedures on them. In his clinical practice he established several important precedents, some of which are still accepted today: that it was legitimate to alter boys' genitals, and even amputate parts of them, to treat or guard against health-threatening disorders; that in the case of minors, the parents would be considered the client and there was no need to consult the wishes of the actual patient;

and that there would be no question of criminal charges, or even social disapproval, arising from such intervention because the procedures were carried out with the consent of the legal guardian and in the belief that they would be of therapeutic or preventive value. Lallemand's medical discoveries exercised a profound influence on British sexual medicine throughout the nineteenth century, and the moral implications of his clinical practice are still asserted by defenders of routine circumcision today.[80]

Part II

Medico-Moral Politics in Victorian Britain

If the habit [masturbation] could be overcome, if the mind could be restored to its purity by any mutilation of the person, one would feel that no penalty would be too great to pay for such a boon.

CHARLES WEST, *Lectures on the Diseases of Women*, 1864

4 · The Shadow of Parson Malthus

Sexual Morals from the Georgians to the Edwardians

One of the greatest practical results of the discovery of Mr. Darwin of the descent of man from the animals which have gone before him is that by it the sexual instincts . . . are shown to be the most necessary as well as the most prevalent of all the instincts which have been evolved by the necessities of animal existence. . . . The sexual instinct has become . . . the great weapon of evolution. That it should by curbed, properly restrained and judiciously directed is now one of the great objects of civilization.

LAWSON TAIT, *Diseases of Women and Abdominal Surgery*, 1889

I had an instinctive objection to grown-ups getting to know about any unusual form of pleasure for fear it should be promptly condemned as immoral and forbidden.

LORD BERNERS (1883–1950), *First Childhood*

To be born, or at any rate bred, in a hand-bag, whether it had handles or not, seems to me to display a contempt for the ordinary decencies of family life that reminds one of the worst excesses of the French Revolution. And I presume you know what that unfortunate movement led to?

OSCAR WILDE, *The Importance of Being Earnest* (Lady Bracknell)

Although the masturbation phobia was a European phenomenon, it is a striking fact that circumcision was widely adopted only in Britain and other English-speaking countries. A full explanation for this exceptionalism would require a comparative study well beyond the scope of this book, but three points can be made: there was a higher level of sexual Puritanism, a more moralistic approach to prostitution and venereal disease, and a lower level of anti-Semitism in nineteenth-century Britain than in other European countries. Venereal disease is considered in chapter 12 and the contribution of the Jewish example to the acceptance of circumcision in chapter 11; in this chapter I attempt a brief outline of the part played by a code of sexual morals that became stricter as the century passed, reached its peak in the Edwardian era, and began to break down in the 1930s.

Because the word *Victorian* has long carried the connotation "sexually repressive," modern historians have sought to develop a more subtle and comprehensive picture, distinguishing what was prescribed from actual behavior and seeking to avoid stereotypes. Despite such efforts, it is apparent that many Victorians, especially among the middle and professional classes, really were sexually prudish and proud of it, and frequently contrasted their strict principles with Continental laxity. As Simon Szreter has observed, even a revisionist such as Peter Gay, seeking the sensual side of the bourgeois experience, ended up not so much demolishing the caricature of Victorian prudishness as producing "a more sophisticated and constructive understanding of it."[1] Twenty years ago Jeanne Peterson referred to claims that "Victorians were repressed about sex and obsessed about . . . masturbation" as "hoary old truths" and regretted that authorities like Acton were cited to "demonstrate that Victorian society was even more sexually repressed than anyone previously thought."[2] She was reflecting the revisionism of Peter Gay and her own discovery of a kindly doctor in the person of James Paget. Since then, however, the pendulum of opinion has swung again, and the detailed research of Simon Szreter, Peter Baldwin, and Hera Cook has demonstrated that middle-class Victorians who wanted to enjoy the comforts of a home graced by an angel and stuffed with the wonders of British trade and industry paid a heavy price in sexual denial. This was not because they had to forgo consumption in order to invest but because men had to climb the corporate or professional ladder, delay marriage, and then limit family size so that couples could consume at the level they desired.[3] In the past, discussion of Victorian sexuality tended to focus on the rather narrow question of whether wives enjoyed, or were meant to enjoy, sex.[4] The jury may still be out on that, but in the meantime the debate has moved on to broader issues in what Michael Mason has called Victorian antisensualism and Szreter has identified as a "culture of abstinence": their sincere spirituality, their faith in marriage, their campaigns against vice (prostitution, obscene literature, contraception, sex education), their suspicion of male sexuality, especially in juveniles, and their desire to have fewer children in order to lead less pressured lives. In a necessarily brief account of a vast literature, I hope to suggest how the Victorians' elevation of spiritual and consumerist pleasures at the expense of bodily ones made them receptive to measures aimed at bridling manifestations of libido.

The nineteenth century opened with a failed attempt to have adultery made a criminal offense, continued with campaigns to force the government to stamp out prostitution, and ended with the effective criminalization of mutual masturbation among males. Mason thus argues that the antisensualism popularly attributed to the Victorians was "widely and warmly embraced" by most sectors of society, from the radical working class to conservative Evangelicals, but that it was driven as much by secular and progressive forces, especially Benthamite utilitarians and campaigners for women's rights, as it was by old-time religion.[5] The strongest force of all was perhaps the medical profession, whose advice was deeply implicated in the transition from eighteenth-century permissiveness to Edwardian repressiveness—one of the swings in the moral pendulum noticed by Lawrence Stone and others. Surveying this oscillation, Stone identified a period of "moderate toleration" in the late sixteenth century, a period of repression from about 1570 to 1670, a phase of permissiveness from about 1670 to 1810, and a new wave of repression beginning in the 1770s and reaching its apogee in the mid-Victorian age.[6] Jeffrey Weeks has questioned this scenario, suggesting that the moral terrain was always contested, particularly until the 1870s, and that it was only in the 1880s that the forces of repression triumphed with the repeal of the Contagious Diseases Act and amendments to other legislation that (inter alia) raised the age of consent for heterosexuals, restricted the circulation of naughty books and pictures, banned nude bathing, and criminalized all sexual activity among males. It was thus in the late Victorian and Edwardian periods that repression reached its climax, simultaneous with the emergence of the first critiques of "Victorianism."[7] These insights have been confirmed by the research of Simon Szreter, who suggests that the Victorian age did not really come to an end until the 1960s; Peter Baldwin, who describes the British as significantly "more moral in sexual terms, prudish, indeed, than their continental neighbours"; and Hera Cook, who identifies the period from the 1860s to the 1950s as sexually inexpressive and detects "a broad shift toward a more prudish and respectable culture" in the late nineteenth century even among working-class women.[8] During this period, largely because there were no safe, effective, and acceptable forms of contraception, and thus no means of dissociating sex from reproduction, most people were increasingly ignorant of the facts of life and of the possibilities for pleasure offered by their bodies. The first cracks in "Victorian" sexual mores appeared in radical circles (such as the Bloomsbury group) before the First World War, but it was not until the 1930s that any significant loosening of the corsets occurred. By then, Cook writes, "books on physical sexuality and contraception were becoming more widely available, and such topics could be mentioned in newspapers. . . . Contraception was being used by all classes. Sexual ignorance was eroding, and a recognisably modern sexual culture began to emerge."[9] This phase of sexual repression matches the period during which circumcision enjoyed its vogue.

The antisensualism of the nineteenth century was the result of many factors, including a revival of religious belief and the rise of the medical profession, but four others are of particular interest here: the rise of anxiety (both medical and moral) about childhood sexuality and masturbation specifically; alarm at the "excesses" of the French Revolution; the warnings of Thomas Malthus about the danger of overpopulation and the consequent need for continence before marriage and moderation thereafter; and the middle class's desire to limit their families for economic reasons. In the eighteenth century positive attitudes toward sex rested on the assumption that it was about procreation: sexual intercourse was natural and enjoyable, and commendable because ordained by both Nature and God as the means to multiply the species. In a mercantilist age that believed in the need for an increasing population to provide the armies to fight for economic opportunities, reproduction was highly valued. When fear of overpopulation displaced that of depopulation, attitudes toward sexual activity changed sharply. Malthus asserted that while food production grew only arithmetically, human populations increased geometrically; because human sexual instincts were so inexorable, the only issue was how to curb them before the miserable consequences of overpopulation (famine, disease, and war) were felt. Although the argument was fallacious, it was highly influential at the time and rewrote the terms of sexual debate; public intellectuals were quick to emphasize the immorality of excessive procreation, especially among the poor, and hence of sexual indulgence except under stringent conditions: "What the young needed," write Porter and Hall, "was not sexual knowledge but sermons in temperance,"[10] and that is what they got from doctors as much as the clergy as the nineteenth century advanced.

Malthus was not the reactionary bigot of labor movement caricature, but he was determined to rebuke utopian schemes for human betterment inspired by the French Revolution, especially the blueprints of William Godwin and the Marquis de Condorcet. His original essay (1798) did not offer much sex, but in 1803 he added "moral restraint" as a third check on population growth, in addition to "misery" (illness and death) and "vice" (nonprocreative sex), thus setting the agenda for discussions of sexuality for much of the following century and spawning "left" and "right" trends. On the right were doctors like William Acton, with his insistence on absolute continence in the young and unmarried, and Jonathan Hutchinson with his professional opinion that contraception was both immoral and harmful to health. On the left were the neo-Malthusians, who advocated birth control as a means of raising working-class living standards, and at their radical fringe George Drysdale, with his passionate conviction that sexual abstinence caused physical ill health and mental misery, and his corresponding advocacy of premarital liaisons, plenty of sex within marriage, and contraception to guard against both pregnancy and venereal disease.[11] Malthus was not absolutely antisex: he defended the passions against Godwin's argument that they would decline as society became more civilized (a very Victorian view) and endorsed them as a spur to effort and a source of happiness. What was needed was not their extinction but their "regulation and direction" under the guidance of reason. But his definition of moral restraint was stringent—"a restraint from marriage from prudential motives, with a conduct strictly moral during the period of restraint." And he banned premarital sex entirely: "The interval between the age of puberty and . . . marriage must . . . be passed in strict chastity; because the law of chastity cannot be violated without producing evil. The effect of anything like a promiscuous intercourse which prevents the birth of children is evidently to weaken the best affections of the heart, and . . . degrade the female character."[12] Mason has stressed the presence of Malthus in Victorian sexual discourse,[13] but his possible influence on Acton and the nineteenth-century medical profession has not been sufficiently noted. The specter of overpopulation meshed nicely with the censorious fervor of the evangelical and other antivice movements, which had become a powerful force by the end of the eighteenth century: organizations such as the Methodists and Wilberforce's Vice Society were opposed to liberal politics, free thought, science, and democracy as much as sex, but that was also an important target. As Roy Porter concludes, "Bowdlerism, Grundyism, prudery, repression, anxiety and shame were summoned up to put sexuality back in its rightful place."[14]

The effects of the new mood were soon apparent in public and private life, and by 1815 the *Edinburgh Review* regretted that "our very advances in politeness have an undeniable tendency to repress all the extravagances of mirth or indulgence of humour which, at an earlier period, gave a variegated and amusing aspect to society."[15] In his autobiography the radical artisan Francis Place (1771-1854) reported an impressive increase in moral respectability from the mid-1790s, with the result that the attitudes and behavior normal in his youth had become unthinkable by 1815. He commented particularly on the decline in bad language,

bawdy songs, drinking, gambling, and whoring and on the disappearance of the "cock-and-hen clubs." These were establishments in which
young men and women gathered to drink and sing, gradually pairing off
for sex until only the unlucky remained; common in Place's youth, they
had vanished by the 1820s.[16] Place further claimed that while it soured
the propertied classes against Enlightenment ideas, the French Revolution turned the minds of working men from pleasure seeking to serious
reading and organization for social reform, leading to the "radical gen-
teelness" that became such a characteristic feature of left-wing politics.
The alarming events in France certainly turned the English against the
ideas of the Enlightenment, whether in the field of politics or sexual
morality. As the *Public Ledger* stated in 1816, "the French Revolution,
with all its constant horrors, was preceded by a total revolution in decency and morality, the virtuous qualities of mind being sapped . . . by
the baneful exhibition of pictures, representing vice in its most alluring
and varied forms."[17] Hume had said that reason was, and ought to be, the
slave of the passions, but in the puritan reaction of the early nineteenth
century it was increasingly enlisted to subdue them: under the new as-
ceticism, the body would be curbed by the mind.[18]

In the eighteenth century Samuel Johnson had been eccentric in his
statement that "man's chief virtue consists in resisting the impulses of
his nature,"[19] but this became the dominant outlook in the nineteenth;
as John Stuart Mill remarked, "nearly every respectable attribute of humanity is the result, not of instinct, but of victory over instinct."[20] The
Victorians pictured humans as divided between a lower (animal) side
and a higher (spiritual) side, and sought to ensure that the latter always
ruled the former; it was a dualistic outlook, which pictured the genitals
as primitive and unevolved, in contrast with the brain (meaning mind or
spirit), which had advanced toward higher things.[21] The image was probably consolidated by Darwin's demonstration that humans had evolved
from and were in fact animals, and it was an attempt to keep alive the
idea of a divine spark or soul as the distinguishing feature of our species.
Although a supporter of Darwinian theory, the influential physiologist
W. B. Carpenter made an important contribution to this understanding
in his metaphor of the rider controlling the horse,[22] and more generally
by popularizing the connection of mind and body and insisting on the
importance of will in maintaining the dominance of the former. This
dualism owed nothing to medical research but was merely a restatement
of the old Christian dichotomy of the flesh (body) and the spirit (soul).
The image of the horse rider goes back to the ancient Greeks, and specifically to Plato's *Phaedrus,* in which the soul is compared to a chariot driver
having to control two horses, one well behaved and obedient, the other

willful and impulsive. In this philosophy, the main thing that distinguished humans from animals was control of the passions: man was not a mere puppet, "pulled by suggesting strings," but possessed a will that guaranteed "the mind's power to act on its own."[23] In these comments from *Principles of Mental Physiology* (1874) Carpenter was reacting to Darwin's *Descent of Man* (1871), but he was also following the lead of David Noble, who in *The Human Mind* (1858) had written that the will marked man off from the lower animals: "Is it not by the agency of the will that our consciousness becomes its own object? Is it not by the same power that we . . . distinguish between virtue and vice?" Although man could not control his moods, in a healthy mind they are "more or less governable by voluntary effort."[24] William Acton's much derided claim that men could control their dreams if they tried was based on physiological principles like these.

In the respectable code, sexual temptation was pictured as a conflict between the higher part of human nature (soul or reason) and the lower part (body or appetite)—the first corresponding to civilization, the second to nature.[25] In sexual matters, humans were distinguished from animals by their capacity for love and their ability to keep lust under control. Carpenter defined love as "the combined operations of the reason, the imagination and the moral feelings" and argued that the "engraftment of psychical attachment upon the mere corporeal instinct" was the difference between "the sexual relations of man and those of the lower animals." A corollary was that "in proportion as the human being makes the temporary gratification of the mere sexual appetite his chief object, and overlooks the happiness arising from spiritual communion, which is not only purer and more permanent, and of which a renewal may be anticipated in another world—does he degrade himself to the level of the brutes that perish."[26] Such views were held by intellectuals across the religious and scientific spectrum. Self-control and chastity were "the basis of every good man's character," said Dr. William Pratt in 1872. "To get the body under, and to keep it in perfect subjection to a resolute and chaste will, is certainly the first duty of every one who aspires to anything here or hereafter."[27] An archbishop stated conventionally in 1894 that "the strongest hold which animalism has over the race lies in the sexual passion. The triumph over this passion . . . under the laws of reason is the supreme act of Spiritual power in man."[28]

Whether prostitution was "the greatest of our social evils," as the *Times* thought, or whether the "monster evil of the present" was syphilis, as Acton insisted, or sexual excess, as one of his reviewers countered,[29] Victorians tended to view sex as a nest of problems rather than a field of pleasures. G. Stanley Hall captured the attitude when he titled his chapter on sexuality in adolescence "Sexual Development: Its Dangers, and

Hygiene in Boys," as though sex meant peril, and dirt was a greater threat in spouts than funnels.[30] As Szreter comments, Victorians held "strongly negative . . . feelings towards sex, as something animal-like and base, associated with . . . dishonouring disease and with the . . . dirty parts of the body."[31] With increasing standards of hygiene but only slow development of the facilities to attain them, the Victorians increasingly saw the genitals as dirty and disgusting. "In this context of sin, dirt and disease," writes Cook, "a growing distrust and perception of physical sexual activity as repugnant was unsurprising."[32] In such an atmosphere we would expect the genitals to be not merely concealed but devalued, and any features of them that enhanced sexual pleasure (and seemed to serve no useful function like digestion or reproduction) would be regarded as not merely superfluous but as a menace both to health and socially approved behavior. As we shall see, doctors did categorize the foreskin in precisely these terms. Much of the demand for sexual self-control was a veiled reference to unmentionable vice, but it worked both ways: not only was will seen as necessary to restrain the impulse to self-gratification, but masturbation seen as psychologically harmful because it sapped a man's willpower and left him prey to other temptations. One of the reasons why masturbation was reprobated so violently was because of concern that it would lead to "habits of indulgence in sensual pleasure and thus cause the erosion of self-control. It was natural that a 'real man' would have a strong sexual drive, but a true man was one capable of exercising self-control."[33] A contributor to the *Journal of Psychological Medicine* in 1851 wrote that "many men lose their true manly character by unnatural stimulation of the reproductive organs."[34] Not that there was complete uniformity on the issue of nature versus civilization. To be consistent with his view of the sex drive as an animal urge, the surgeon and gynecologist Lawson Tait should have condemned masturbation by categorizing it as part of a natural eruption that had to be subdued by human reason and will. But when he noticed monkeys at the zoo masturbating, he did not conclude that this proved how natural it was but assumed they must have been corrupted by easy living: "Whether it may be practised by them in their native woods is not yet known, but I fancy that it is rather the result of their luxurious living, their freedom from the strain of earning an honest livelihood in [their] native circumstances. . . . idleness and luxury are always promotive of lust in monkeys as in men."[35] As so often with sexual issues in Victorian England, empirical observation tended to be interpreted in the light of received opinion.

Sexual restraint was thus central to the new definition of manliness embraced by the Victorian middle class. As John Tosh has argued, the expansion of urban industry, the demands of managing an empire, and the growth of evangelical religion led to a redefinition of middle-class identity, stressing "a punishing work ethic, independence from patronage, piety, high-mindedness, sobriety, chastity and dedication to family pursuits."[36] Tosh stresses the rise of patriarchy and sexual frustration in the late nineteenth century, which involved homosociality (men's bonding networks), the demand for chastity except in marriage, and the possibility that it led to deep psychological conflicts in many individuals: "Late Victorian manliness was a public, even military code, to be exercised among men. Relations with the other sex were taken for granted. . . . Purity was promoted as a call to cleanness—perfect manhood—rather than a moral obligation towards women."[37] One recalls Rupert Brooke's references to (un)cleanness, and the line from his poem "Peace" about the appeal of war: "as swimmers into cleanness leaping." It is widely agreed that the late Victorians reformulated manliness in terms of self-restraint and cleanliness, and Hyam argues that sexual moralism and the purity movement not only ensured ignorance of sexuality but helped to foster an entirely new concept of manhood: "by 1914 the whole British concept of masculinity—not least in the public schools—had been redefined . . . to mean not sexual prowess and maturity but sexual restraint and 'cleanness.' Real sexual activity receded so far into the background that, according to Larkin's famous poem, it was not rediscovered . . . 'until 1963.'"[38] The contradictory demands on middle- and upper-class men must have created considerable anxiety. On the one hand, writes Alan Hunt, masculinity was meant to be "outward looking," self-assertive, and self-confident; on the other hand a male was "beset by potential weakness, needing to keep his energy under careful management. He was a sexual being expected to manifest a strong but controllable sexual instinct, yet at risk from sexual indulgence."[39] The willingness with which so many men submitted to Acton's painful cauterization procedure when believing that they showed symptoms of spermatorrhea, and the alacrity with which they later agreed to let doctors circumcise their sons, is partly explained by the tension of these dilemmas.

The decline of the birthrate was another important strand in Victorian antisensualism. Between 1860 and 1940 the average number of live births per married woman declined from six to two, and the trend was most pronounced among middle-class and professional couples.[40] They sought to limit their family size in order to build up their economic and social position and accumulate the resources needed to display their rising status and educate their children properly, and all this meant late marriage (after the age of twenty-five, often after thirty) and fewer children. There has been much debate on the methods of contraception used, but Szreter has shown that by far the most important means was "attempted abstinence," meaning either coitus interruptus or complete abstention from intercourse in marriage.[41] Although strongly advocated by radicals, other forms of contraception—sponges, condoms, caps— were little used. There is thus a social basis for the high valuation that Victorians placed on chastity, and Stone's contention that it was mostly to do with the rise of evangelical religion must be revised.[42] Their anxiety to achieve a higher social and material position than their parents had enjoyed meant the need to establish their career and invest in the right symbols of success, and the consequent inability to afford so many children. Cook has shown that the gross reproduction rate (the number of daughters a woman has) remained constant at about two from the 1840s to the 1860s, declined sharply and steadily until the 1930s, then picked up again and rose until the arrival of the pill. If the fertility decline from the 1860s to the 1930s was the result mainly of abstinence, it indicates that the period was one of sexual restraint and that the 1930s marked a significant loosening of sexual practice and thus morals.[43] Another indictor of sexual attitudes is the level of illegitimate births, which declined steadily from 67 per thousand between 1846 and 1850 to a low point of 39.5 in 1901-5, then rose slightly to 43.5 in 1931-35 and to 47.5 in the early 1950s.[44] By this measure the period 1901-5 would be the height of the culture of abstinence and the early 1930s the beginning of its dissolution. None of this need have led to the acceptance of circumcision, but placing such a high premium on sexual restraint (the main means of birth control) generated interest in measures thought likely to reduce sexual interest and desire, and a tendency to regard sex and the genitals as relatively unimportant in the scale of values.[45] Anxiety about their children's success, however, might well have led middle-class parents to favor circumcision; since the future success of their sons depended on doing well at the right schools, and masturbation was held to damage both mental power and moral fiber, they might well have thought circumcision was a measure calculated to secure their sons' future. Drawing on U.S. sources, Nicola Beisel has argued that the moral crusades of the 1880s were directly related to anxieties that children would not equal or surpass their parents' achievements, and this situation would seem to be present in the English concern over masturbation at the public schools.[46]

A prominent feature of public life in the nineteenth century was the antivice crusade. In his study of such purity movements Edward Bristow identifies four peaks in antivice agitation: in the 1690s, in response to the license of the restoration, leading to works like *Onania;* around 1800 in reaction against the Enlightenment and the French Revolution; in the 1880s, involving attempts to curb prostitution, venereal disease, and extramarital sex of all descriptions; and in the early twentieth century in response to the panic over syphilis. Although Alan Hunt has provided a more sophisticated analysis in his *Governing Morals* (1999), he has not substantially redrawn the broad scenario set out here. The Society for the Suppression of Vice, established in 1802 and generally known as the Vice Society, focused on obscene publications, and its vigilantes were responsible for bringing many booksellers to court. Its first address to the public (prepared by a former anti-Jacobin pamphleteer) announced that since the "violation of religious principles" was the root of all wickedness, the society would campaign against Sabbath breaking as much as obscenity, as well as lower-class disorderliness like blood sports, taverns, and brothels. The society was particularly concerned with lewd publications because they were an aid to masturbation, and it worked closely with the police to prosecute distributors of such material, an activity facilitated after its great success in securing the passage of the Obscene Publications Act in 1857.[47] The society agitated for the suppression and then the regulation of prostitution and supported the Contagious Diseases Acts of the 1860s, but faded away in the 1880s as the purity scene was taken over by the Social Purity Alliance, the White Cross Movement (1883), and the National Vigilance Association (1885), with a focus on promoting male chastity rather than safe-ish sex.

There is now an extensive literature on the social purity or hygiene movement from the 1870s to the First World War, and the only point needing to be stressed here is its success in shifting the blame for prostitution and venereal disease from female depravity and economic need to male sexual desire, and hence the focus of control from quarantining prostitutes to bridling male lust. Alan Hunt has thus described the movement as "a medico-moral project" in which the reformers used the medical argument that sexual activity was physically harmful in order to bolster their case for "votes for women, chastity for men," as Christabel Pankhurst put it. The rather unexpected focus of a campaign that aimed to curb venereal disease putting so much of its effort into stopping juvenile masturbation thus becomes more explicable—although an expression like "the purity of the home" could be interpreted in many ways.[48] In a comparative study of approaches to syphilis and prostitution in Britain and European countries, Peter Baldwin has shown that moralism, aiming more at vice than disease, was a far more powerful force in Britain than on the Continent, meaning that state regulation of prostitution came only in the short-lived and limited form of the Contagious Diseases Acts (1860s to mid-1880s), whose main effect was to arouse demands to leave women alone and control male sexuality instead.[49] Michael Mason describes the Social Purity Alliance, which grew from this movement, as "a grotesque affair, a great bubble of extreme anti-sensualism whose only lasting achievement was to discredit sexual moralism." Perhaps this was true in the long run, but the movement commanded wide assent and was very successful for a while: in the 1870s prosecutions for publishing birth control literature (most famously of the freethinking Annie Besant and Charles Bradlaugh in 1877) had failed, but such efforts succeeded during the following decade.[50] They can hardly be regarded as "a hollow triumph" when respectable society and the medical profession remained opposed to the use of condoms for contraception, or even as protection against venereal disease, for another forty years. Although the authorities eventually distributed ointments and condoms to the troops in the First World War, it was in the teeth of much disapproval.[51] As late as 1920 the Federation of Medical Women warned that if effective prophylaxis became readily available, "promiscuous intercourse would be looked upon as free from the risk of infection and . . . conception . . . [and] a phase of society would be produced as vicious and degenerate as any of which history has record. . . . Moral degeneration and sex excess would rot the very foundations of society."[52] The Alliance had remarkable success in the 1880s, securing legislation that represented a kind of Clarendon Code in the sphere of sexual behavior, restricting the freedom of moral dissenters in much the same way that the Test, Five Mile, and Corporation acts had restricted the rights of religious dissenters in the vengeful days of the Restoration. This legislation was insufficient to protect women from coercion by men, but it did make life harder for libertines, including those who had no interest in seducing women. Henry Labouchere's motives in proposing his late night amendment to the Criminal Law Amendment bill in 1885 have never been fathomed,[53] but one little-remarked effect of making acts of gross indecency among men an offense was to criminalize group masturbation among boys. Any who practiced self-abuse with their mates were now not merely wrecking their health and damning their souls but risking two years hard as well.

Although *Victorian* was once a synonym for sexual repressiveness, it thus seems that *Edwardian* is a more appropriate word. As George Orwell (b. 1903) recalled with his usual concreteness:

> Society was ruled by narrow-minded, profoundly incurious people, predatory business men, dull quires, bishops, politicians who could quote Horace but had never heard of algebra. Science was faintly disreputable and religious belief obligatory. . . . There you were, in a world of pedants, clergymen and golfers, with your future employers exhorting you to "get on or get out," your parents systematically warping your sexual life, and your dull-witted schoolmasters sniggering over their Latin tags.[54]

The Edwardian period was marked by a polarization on moral questions, a revolt against Victorianism, and a corresponding reassertion of "old" values by conservatives.[55] Faced with the challenges of decadence, aestheticism, the satire of Shaw, the research of the Fabians, the plays of Ibsen, the battle for women's suffrage, fears about national decline, and the rise of German power, the establishment responded with greater efforts at the enforcement of restraint. Organizations devoted to spying on and regulating other people's conduct flourished with particular vigor between the turn of the century and the First World War, the most significant of which was the National Vigilance Association led by the Rev. James Marchant. He was the author of a series of *Aids to Purity*—booklets for the young that remained delicately vague as to details but left the impression that anything involving the naughty bits of the body was contrary to the laws of God and the rules of hygiene. In 1911 a manifesto issued by the National Council of Public Morals, signed by several professors and the editor of the *Lancet*, condemned contraception, the decline in the birthrate, pernicious literature, immorality, and drunkenness and averred that "the racial instinct" (Marchant's term for the sex drive) existed "not primarily for individual satisfaction, but for wholesome perpetuation of the human family." In 1909 the *Spectator* condemned H. G. Wells' novel *Ann Veronica* as "a poisonous book": "unless the citizens of the state put before themselves the principles of duty, self-sacrifice, self-control and continence, not merely in the matter of national defence, national preservation and national well-being, but also of the sex relationship, the life of the state must be short and precarious." A characteristic feature of the Edwardian period was strict censorship of plays, carried out beyond parliamentary, much less public, scrutiny in the antiquated recesses of the Lord Chamberlain's office by gentlemen whose personal taste set national standards. Its practice was entirely in accord with a remark of the official censor in 1892: "the essence of my office and its advantage . . . is that it is preventative and . . . secret."[56] The approving reference to prevention is a sign of the times, drawn straight from sanitarian discourse, and the justification is strikingly similar to many concurrent arguments for routine circumcision, all based on the same principles. Like the boy circumcised in infancy, the theater audience would never know they were missing something unless they had the opportunity to compare their abbreviated version with the complete and unabridged original. It was in this atmosphere that male circumcision achieved its greatest level of acceptance among the middle-class public.

However eagerly the doctors promoted the idea, it was the parents who decided whether their sons should be circumcised, and in practice that meant the father. The Victorian middle-class family has been characterized in many different ways since Ruskin praised it as "the place of Peace; the shelter not only from all injury, but from all terror, doubt and division . . . a vestal temple . . . watched over by household gods."[57] More critically, Stone has described it as embodying paternal authority; a quiet, deferential, and religious wife; remote and authoritarian parents; an emphasis on the training of children in obedience; and "the crushing of [their] sexual and autonomous drives."[58] Subsequent research has shown this assessment to be too sweeping and insensitive to variations between households and over time, but even a careful recent scholar such as John Tosh describes the middle-class and professional family as highly patriarchal: the father ruled the household, dominating both his wife and his children, especially his sons.[59] As Jeffrey Weeks has noted, the consolidation of the middle-class family presented paradoxes when it came to sexuality: it became both the privileged location for romantic emotion yet also the policeman of sexual behavior. Children's sexuality posed a particular difficulty and was treated with a mixture of denial and control. Stone comments that "in the psychology of sexual repression and its ever-attendant guilt, we may . . . find part of the explanation of the popularity of the myth of the innocent child and the savagery towards children in practice"; or as one of Saki's characters remarks, "people talk vaguely about the innocence of a little child, but they take mighty good care not to let it out of their sight for twenty minutes."[60] To preserve the image of the family as a refuge from strife and sensuality, children's sexuality had to be suppressed; the ideology was that they were asexual until puberty, and the inevitable proofs that they were not were regarded as signs of disease or depravity, to be treated as an illness or a crime. Although it is not clear that the age of puberty declined in the early nineteenth century,[61] it is true that the age of marriage rose in middle- and upper-class families, and with it the age at which young males left home to form their own households. They thus spent a longer period in the parental home under adult supervision: instead of leaving home at twelve or fourteen, they remained until their mid-twenties, the period when the sex drive is strongest but for which there was no sanctioned outlet. This tendency was strengthened by the need for youths to spend more years at school and university, as a more complex industrial society increased the demand for skilled professionals.

These demographic developments were given a medical interpretation in the light of nerve force theory.[62] Aristotle had stated that men could father children at sixteen, and Venette as soon as they were able to produce seed, usually around fourteen,[63] but by the 1850s Acton and others were declaring that boys were not even sexually mature until they were twenty-five and incapable of producing healthy sperm until then. From the 1830s to the Edwardian period it was a commonplace that children had to devote all their energies to physical growth and that excessive brainwork or other nervous strain could stunt development. Acton was only one of many who applied this principle to the "premature" exercise of the sexual powers: a contemporary wrote in 1851 that "too early development of the sexual function leads to disease—especially of the nervous system."[64] In 1874 one authority warned that intellectual precocity had much the same effects as premature deployment of the sexual organs, and that such children often died early from various obscure diseases because "the over-stimulated nervous system possesses little resistive power, and, exhaustion setting in, the disease is quickly fatal." As late as 1906 a writer on hygiene asserted that it was "a physiological fact" that neither "reproduction nor sexual function should be exercised until full bodily development is completed."[65] There was no agreement as to how long childhood lasted, and medical definitions tended to be far more conservative than those operative in the world commerce and industry. While doctors asserted they were not mature until twenty-five, many working-class boys already had jobs at twelve; they could join the navy at ten, and the telegraph lads who featured in the Cleveland Street scandal (1889) were all teenagers—though well developed if their clients are to be believed.[66] The concept of adolescence emerged toward the end of the century, but it was characterized as just another phase of incomplete development during which nerve force should be husbanded and the sexual powers kept on the leash. G. Stanley Hall claimed to have identified the specific element in ejaculate that made masturbation and early sexual activity so damaging, a substance called "spermin," described as "the highest and most complex of all things in the physical world," which played "an important role in the respiration of tissues" and the removal of waste products from cells. Hall added that the "dangers of uncleanliness and irritation" in adolescence were so great that "many primitive races have practised circumcision at this age as a preventive."[67] With similar concerns in mind, a "nerve expert" wrote in 1908 that "the child should be closely watched . . . and everything should be done to combat . . . nervous irritability or weakness. . . . Self-restraint and self-control are not only valuable moral qualities, but invaluable prophylactics against nervous disease."[68] These suggestions were little more than a medical interpretation of Malthus's demand for chastity before marriage. In the 1870s William Pratt was conscious of the problem, observing that "in a natural state of society" the union of the sexes would automatically follow the onset of puberty, and the male sexual appetite would find "legitimate gratification" in marriage. But since we lived in a "conventional society" in which early marriage was impossible, the question arose: "What are young men to do, tormented by an appetite which in many an ardent nature is a real demon?" Pratt deplored Malthus's rejection of early marriage and urged it as soon as feasible—around twenty in his view. Until that time boys just had to practice self-control.[69] With this tendency to infantilize children and adolescents, doctors contributed to the cult of the eternal boy, which became apparent in the Edwardian period. Acton's obsession with not arousing the sleeping dog of sexual interest and Edward Lyttelton's equivalent campaign to put the penis to sleep until marriage had its cultural counterpart in Rupert Brooke's reluctance to accept maturity and in his favorite play, *Peter Pan*, J. M. Barrie's unbelievably successful fantasy about the boy who would not grow up.[70]

One of the most difficult problems in an antisensual age is how much children should be taught about sex, and there were continual arguments about who was best fitted to provide sex education, how much boys should be told, and whether warnings against masturbation would only alert them to possibilities of which they had been ignorant. Then as now, sex education was a poison chalice that parents, teachers, doctors, and clergy kept tossing to each other.[71] The only point on which there was general agreement was the line to be taken: such instruction should be all about how harmful "premature" or "unnatural" sex was and why it must be avoided.[72] In 1885 the *British Medical Journal* deplored "the complete ignorance regarding the sexual organs and the sexual functions which is . . . fostered by ordinary education"; some men "even marry in complete sexual ignorance," and this condition is "extremely common among cultivated and refined women." The editorial hoped that the English would always show "delicacy of thought and expression" in relation to the reproductive function but felt that "the conspiracy of silence has gone too far." It advocated education in physiology at schools, beginning with the skeleton and ending naturally with the reproductive organs, in order both to dispel ignorance and to avoid arousing prurient curiosity and libidinous imaginings. It was particularly concerned to combat "the degrading error" that sexual activity was necessary for manliness or health.[73] Perhaps attempting to implement this program, a moderate among the purity campaigners was the Rev. Edward Lyttelton, a gentleman from the heart of the establishment, related to everybody from the Bishop of Southampton to the Chief of the General Staff. He wrote a number of books for teachers and clergy on sex education, including *Training of the Young in Laws of Sex* (1900). It was mainly about teaching boys, since Lyttelton accepted the prevailing wisdom that "animal desires" were "far stronger in the male than in the female" and that prostitution was the result of male lust, not of any strategy on the part of women.[74] The targets of his educational efforts were fornication and masturbation (both the group and the solitary variety), and their objective was to instill continence, self-control, self-sacrifice, and purity. He believed in the sexlessness of children, asserting that "childhood indulgence in bad habits is not natural and would never take place, normally, except from ignorance" (92)—a confused sentence that probably reflects his own uncertainty on this issue. If he meant that little boys played with themselves only because they had not been told it was wrong, this would mean that it was natural and that boys did it automatically unless instructed to the contrary. The reference to ignorance contradicts the widely held view that they were taught bad habits at school or even by wicked nurses, as well as his own statement that they picked up depraved ideas from other boys (8)—in other words, that the problem was not ignorance but learning the wrong thing. Whatever the source of the problem, Lyttelton hoped it could be overcome by teaching boys the right thing. Moving on to the medical side of the question, Lyttelton remarked that there was much divergence of opinion among doctors as to whether masturbation had harmful physical effects (96); he himself did not believe that it did any damage at all but preached against it on the grounds that it destroyed character and led to fornication and prostitutes. Boys should be taught that powerful sexual urges were God's way of developing their self-control: "measures should be taken to assist him to learn that no matter how imperious an appetite may be, it is given that it may be controlled, and that there is dignity in being master of the body. . . . The boy . . . will learn that the true beauty and honour of the body lie in the fact of its being a willing and obedient to spirit" (101). Above all, sex education should not be too explicit but surrounded with a halo of mystery and reverence, with a vague sense that sex was an expression of God's wonderful purpose in ordaining the miracle of love between two married people (85-86).

In a pamphlet directed at boys published around 1900 by the Australasian White Cross League (*A Talk to a Boy*), a remarkably similar line was taken by "A Doctor." The pamphlet was targeted at boys above ten years with the aim of giving them "very necessary information regarding the facts of life"—namely, "the very strange and wonderful facts about the beginning of life and the birth of children." The main fact was that "God has given to men and women the miraculous power to create life between them, and so be the means of bringing a new human being into the world." The remaining facts were that boys should not touch their own private parts or talk to each other about sexual matters; "A Doctor" was very insistent on both these points:

> There are private parts of your body through which the water and other fluids you drink pass out. These parts should never be touched except when you wish to pass water, or when you wash them. . . . If you touch

them without requiring to do so, you may bring bad health and sickness upon yourself, and so take away your strength that you will never grow into a big man. Many boys have ruined their lives completely by doing what I have just told you must never even think of doing.

If your private parts get itchy, you should not scratch or pull them, but tell your parents, who will know what to do to help you "get rid of these unpleasant feelings." If one of your friends tells you that "he touches his private parts and urges you to do the same," tell him what you have learned here and that he is doing himself "a terrible injury to his body and his mind," which will be "weak and stunted when he grows up." Just as importantly, boys should not "speak to other boys about what I am telling you here"; they should just get this leaflet and read it in private:

> Boys at school often learn something about these facts in a wrong way, and they tell what they know . . . to younger boys, who believe that they are hearing the truth. This secret and dirty-minded talk does boys a great deal of harm, and it is because I want to put a stop to such talk, as well as tell you the truth, that I am writing this letter.[75]

Don't believe your friends, believe me! Our doctor provided no details about what parents would do to help boys get rid of the itching, but purity pamphlets directed at parents rather than boys (such as Richard Arthur's *Training of Children in Purity*) were explicit with the medical commonplace that secret vice was often brought about by "local irritation" and that "the operation of circumcision" was then needed to "set matters right."[76] I have a letter from an Australian man who reports that when, as a little boy in the 1930s, he mentioned to his mother that his penis was itchy, she said she would fix it and quietly arranged for him to be circumcised.

In his insistence that boys should get their sex education from doctors like him, and not from other boys, the author of this sermon was indicating his awareness that there was a secret world of boy-lore about sex from which adults were excluded. The headmaster of Wellington College insisted that "there is no such thing as sex at College . . . and if there is I knock it hard on the head," but as late as the 1930s the old guard of housemasters there were obsessed with ensuring that the boys were kept constantly busy or under surveillance—entirely out of anxiety as to what they would get up to if they were left unpoliced for a few moments.[77] Another old boy recalled that despite the propaganda there was "a thriving sexual underworld" and reported that his housemaster "would have been shocked at the cheerfully cynical culture celebrating this form of sex [masturbation] amongst the boys of his house, [despite] the disciplinary system he enforced, with all its moral and religious overtones."[78] Such glimpses of the reality of young male dynamics, along with Walter's secret life, whether fact or fantasy, bear out the truth of the doctors' gloomy conviction that, despite a century of their best efforts, boys still picked up their wicked ways at school: masturbation "is a habit learned in a very large number of cases at an early age, and taught by one school-fellow to another," lamented Tuke's *Dictionary of Psychological Medicine* in the 1890s.[79] A contributor to the *Contemporary Review* in 1904 hailed the essence of the Jewish and Protestant religion as "obedience to divine rule, self-abnegation, moral rectitude and corporeal purity," but lamented that the typical schoolboy was sadly lacking in all these qualities, especially the last.[80] Most boys picked up the facts of life from other boys, and an important part of this knowledge was learning how to masturbate. John Addington Symonds (1840–93), who received the facts of life from "a dirty-minded school-fellow" when he was about nine, records that when he was a boy "a handsome lad . . . once masturbated in my presence . . . and wanted me to try the game"; when he got to Harrow he found the school full of obscene talk and "acts of onanism, mutual masturbation and sport of naked boys in bed together."[81] The fastidious Symonds did not approve, and whatever improvements in juvenile decorum there had been by the early twentieth century had not filtered down to the working classes. Harry Daley, the son of a fisherman, had his sexual initiation around 1910, when an older boy showed him how to do it, and he was soon "wanking merrily away" with his mates at every opportunity:

> We continued happily . . . for a long time, until the sort of people one finds on the fringes of church life . . . warned us that boys who played with themselves went mad and had to be locked away. This was a typical mean, dirty-minded trick, for they had been boys themselves and knew it was not true. In any case it didn't stop us. Henceforth we wanked and worried, whereas formerly we had experienced nothing but satisfaction and contentment.[82]

John Lehmann (b. 1907) reports that when he was about seven he learned about sex from a slightly older friend, who told him that his father's stable boy had taken him into a shed one day and shown him how to masturbate. He got the full facts of life from another friend at about age ten and a rather different version from his school headmaster a few years later: "he told us that because the male sexual climax involved, he supposed, a certain amount of pleasurable sensation, boys often tried to bring it about by themselves. He warned us grimly against the dangers of this habit, without specifying what the dangers were. . . . We left his office in sombre mood."[83] Similar stories are told by many of Havelock

Ellis's correspondents, J. R. Ackerley, and Tom Driberg, who reports that the only sex education he received from his parents was the advice that "you must never let anybody touch your private parts."[84] One of Ellis's case histories reported that when he was about twelve his father's young footman came into his room while he was in bed, felt for his penis, and masturbated him to his first orgasm. His initial resistance gave way in response to the "pleasant sensation," and afterward he could "hardly sleep from excitement. I felt I had been initiated into a great and delightful mystery."[85] In 1914 a survey of the source of sexual knowledge among 677 American college boys found that 544 learned it from their buddies, 33 from "girl associates," and 40 from servants, overheard talk, or observation of animals. The author of the survey commented indignantly that "91.5 per cent received their first permanent impressions about sex from unwholesome sources."[86] Alfred Kinsey similarly found that the main source of sex education for 60 percent of white college males and nearly 80 percent of noncollege males was a "same sex peer" and that only 2 percent had been given the facts of life by their father. Doctors trailed in at the rear with a derisory 0.3 percent.[87]

The general conclusion that may be drawn from this survey is that despite the efforts of the medico-clerical alliance to take over sex education, most boys got their knowledge of sex from other boys, usually at school or (in the case of upper-class boys) from servants. The poorer classes lived in close proximity with one another, brothers usually slept together, and children learned the facts of life by observation at an early age; in the country they soon got the message by watching farm animals. The content of boy-to-boy instruction included where babies came from, how to have sex with a girl, and what their cocks and balls were really for, but its central theme was how to enjoy their sexual capabilities. Boys showed each other the best techniques of masturbation and did it together as an entertaining and instructive experience. Writers of sexual autobiographies place learning to masturbate from and with other boys at the center of their youthful adventures in sex. The content of adult-to-boy sex education was quite different. It was about how *not* to have a good time: why boys should not touch their genitals, the dangers of sex, the perils of masturbation, the wickedness of doing it with other boys, the importance of restraint, the sober joys of eventual marriage. Of all these themes, the danger of masturbation was the most prominent: even sex education sessions that revealed nothing about intercourse were insistent on the ruin that would flow from "unnatural" activities. Medico-theological discourse sought to replace the informal network of instruction aimed at spreading pleasure with a medically rationalized moral code that denied it. Most significantly, doctors sought control over the circulation of information: sex education pamphlets in the Edwardian period instructed boys not to discuss their content with other boys. In their efforts to control the uses to which males put their bodies, sex educators wanted boys to have no sources of knowledge beyond what they provided, and not to question that information or even talk about it with anybody else; such information sharing would obviously permit comparisons, doubts, and criticism to emerge. Witting or otherwise, it was an attempt to impose a totalitarian system of thought control on sexual matters and was aimed at restricting sexual knowledge to the ideology of the harmfulness of premature sex, especially masturbation, thus curbing childhood and adolescent sexuality. It was not, of course, possible to restrict the flow of information as tightly as was desired, since boy-to-boy communication had always been underground and became more furtive as the propaganda intensified. A striking feature about eighteenth- and nineteenth-century sexual autobiographies is the prominence of the foreskin: it is central to boys' description of their penises, their experience of sex, and their enjoyment of masturbation. Learning to pull it back and manipulate it so as to be able to masturbate more effectively was a rite of passage from childhood to adolescence as significant as the first ejaculation. The doctors knew what the boys knew: that the foreskin made a difference to male erotic response, especially in solitary or group vice. It thus became the particular target of their campaign to curtail and regulate adolescent sexual activity.

5 · The Priests of the Body

Doctors and Disease in an Antisensual Age

As medical men, the priests of the body, and the teachers of the truths of medico-psychology and physiology, we can often help by our counsel. . . . We are the only persons who can judge . . . how much [an individual] ought to know and what risks he runs.

DR. THOMAS CLOUSTON, 1884

The primitive medicine man, thinking to make the body an intolerable habitat for the demon, exposed his patient to . . . alarming, painful or disgusting treatment. . . . Now there is abundant proof that . . . the efficacy of medicine was associated in thought with their disgustingness: the more repulsive they were, the more effectual.

HERBERT SPENCER, "Professional Institutions: Physician and Surgeon," 1895

Medicine, professedly founded on observation, is as sensitive to outside influences, political, religious, philosophical, imaginative, as is the barometer to changes in atmospheric density.

OLIVER WENDELL HOLMES

The Victorians took a lively interest in most natural, human, and divine phenomena, but perhaps nothing fascinated them more than health and disease. "No topic occupied the Victorian mind more than health," writes Bruce Haley; "Victorians worshipped the goddess Hygeia, sought out her laws, and disciplined themselves to obey them."[1] A growing demand for medical services by the increasingly health-conscious middle class led to a steady expansion of facilities for medical services, research, pub-

94

lication, and consultation and a steadily rising supply of doctors, both general and specialist, whose advice was eagerly sought and dutifully followed. The cause and cure of many diseases remained elusive, and the chronic invalid became a stock figure in Victorian discourse, eventually satirized by Oscar Wilde as Bunbury, the man who followed his doctor's orders so minutely that he expired on command. While clinical medicine made only a small contribution to improved health until the end of the century, the success of the sanitary movement in cleaning up the cities did much to reduce the death toll from "filth" diseases and had a major impact on adult mortality rates. Although it was an antisensual age, sex was written about in specialist publications with a wealth of explicit detail, freedom, and abundance never seen before; as Foucault has reminded us, while the practice of sexual libertinism declined, theories of sexual functioning and behavior became more elaborate. The specter of venereal disease haunted the Victorian imagination as grimly as that of AIDS in our own day and elicited many of the same moral and therapeutic responses; those experiencing a resurgent Judeo-Christian faith could not but see such physical affliction as sure evidence of divine punishment for moral transgression, though doctors were divided on this issue. Masturbation was reprobated with ever-increasing vigor and became central to nineteenth-century understandings of sexual pathology and bodily malfunction; both irregular sex and bodily disease were linked with dirt and seen as forms of disorder, requiring firm disciplinary measures, and there was much debate as to what was permissible. In this chapter I attempt to provide a broad picture of the nineteenth-century medical world and the moral codes that applied to medical and especially sexual matters. I consider the close links drawn between illness and dirty habits, both physical and moral, in the context of a resurgent but challenged Christianity; the development of theories of disease, especially the centrality of concepts of nervous disease in problematizing sexual activity and thus pathologizing sensitive ("irritable") parts of the sexual organs; the rise of the medical profession; and the consolidation of its power as the sole legitimate source of advice on matters of health. I conclude with some remarks on the relation of Victorian medical practices to modernity and scientific method.

Victorian England was marked by serious epidemic diseases and little improvement in health outcomes until the last twenty years of the era. The greater severity of disease in the nineteenth as compared with the eighteenth century was the result of poorer harvests; rapid urbanization as a consequence of industrialization, leading to overcrowded cities with inadequate infrastructure; and the arrival of new diseases like cholera, which thrived in such conditions, although epidemics of typhoid, typhus, and smallpox were also major killers.[2] Tuberculosis was the most serious single cause of disease and death, accounting for a third of all mortality for most of the period. Life expectancy had increased from thirty to forty years from the 1730s to the 1820s; stagnated until the 1870s as deaths from typhoid, cholera, typhus, tuberculosis, and diphtheria soared; and increased again to forty-eight years between the 1870s and 1900. According to Simon Szreter, the main factor in this development was the success of sanitary engineers and health officials in cleaning up the cities, providing uncontaminated water, regulating the food supply, and installing hygienic waste disposal (especially sewage) systems. In an analysis that emphasizes the vital role of public health, especially sanitary reform, in the decline of mortality after 1870s (as opposed to an older emphasis on improved nutrition), Szreter has pointed out that there was no contradiction between the simultaneous phenomena of rising wealth and falling health standards, as industrialization increased productivity while fostering urban squalor.[3] Infant mortality remained high throughout the century and was not affected by the general decline in mortality rates until the early twentieth century. From the 1850s to 1900 infant deaths remained constant at about 153 per thousand, representing a quarter of all deaths; each year 100,000 died before their first birthday. Such wastage naturally put a premium on the search for measures to improve infant health, but the single largest cause of death was gastric or intestinal infections leading to diarrhea and dehydration, usually caught from contaminated food (especially milk), water, utensils, toys, and the like that babies put in their mouth as they crawled around.[4] Such infections often produced convulsive symptoms, encouraging doctors to give the cause of death as "convulsions," sometimes blamed on nervous problems, masturbation, or irritation from a tight foreskin. Another significant killer was opium, widely administered in various cordial forms as a tranquillizer, a regimen that probably became more common as nurses and mothers were sternly warned against the previously common practice of tickling babies' genitals to soothe them to sleep. Doctors reported that infant victims of opium poisoning wasted away and "shrank up into little old men" or "wizened little monkeys"[5]—a condition not so different from the "marasmus" ascribed by Lallemand and others to the effects of masturbation.

At no time during the nineteenth century was there any systematic understanding of disease, and until the 1880s (when the work of the German bacteriologists became known) theories of disease were fluid. The implications of the new knowledge about germs took a long time to be appreciated and tended to be assimilated into existing conceptions of illness before being understood as a new paradigm.[6] Many different theories of disease causation contended, but few had much clinical significance because there was no effective cure for most afflictions. Most of the advances in bacteriology that led to the identification of the micro-organisms responsible for specific diseases occurred in France and Germany, and many British doctors evinced a stereotypical insularity in refusing to be impressed by Continental innovations. The ideas of Joseph Lister, once thought to represent the arrival of modern germ theory in Britain,[7] changed radically between the 1860s and the 1880s, as the discoveries of Louis Pasteur were supplemented by those of Robert Koch and the German school, and under the influence of surgical experience. What began as a germ theory of putrefaction, closely allied to the concept of zymotic disease, eventually became a germ theory of infection, recognizably modern in its understanding of disease transmission. Operationally, Listerism changed from a practice that sought to exclude air from wounds to one that emphasized cleanliness during operations.[8] Until this breakthrough the most important candidates were contagious, miasmatic, infectious, and nervous theories, but the concepts were often used interchangeably and inconsistently, even by supporters of germ theory.[9] In the 1850s William Farr, responsible for assigning causes of death in the new Registrar General's office, made an effort to classify disease by cause. Miasmatic diseases were spread through air or water and caused fever (smallpox, malaria); contagious diseases were communicated from person to person by contact, puncture, or inoculation (syphilis); dietetic diseases arose in the blood from poor diet or bad food; parasitic diseases were caused by animal or plant organisms invading the skin or internal organs.[10] By the 1870s classification had become more elaborate: T. L. Nichols identified five main schools of thought and their preferred treatments: nervous disorders—sedatives and antispasmodics; "solidist" theory—mercury "and similar chemicals"; humoral theory—bleeding and purging; chemical causation—alkalis and acids; and "mechanical" causation, or disease arising from "animalcular or mechanical irritation" (the closest to germ theory)—attempts to poison the enemy. Nichols himself stressed the role of filth, nerves, and sexual excess: "Uncleanly habits, wearing filthy clothes, the neglect of daily bathing, tend to clog the pores, prevent the throwing out of effete wastes and morbid matters."[11] All these categorizations remained descriptive rather than analytic, and it was left to the consumer to select the kind of treatment that appealed to him.

In an atmosphere of uncertainty and controversy the biggest division in the late nineteenth century was between pro- and anti-contagionists, and their major quarrel was over strategy, not theory. The contagionists advocated measures to quarantine infected from healthy populations, while the anti-contagionists (the sanitary reformers) urged eradication of the environmental conditions in which fevers thrived.[12] To understand the rise of circumcision as a preventive health strategy it is necessary to focus on the second of these approaches, which promoted the idea that there was a strong link between visible dirt and organic disease, and which won credibility through its success in improving urban health. Sanitary reform targeted dirt and overcrowding; reformers aimed to remove the conditions in which epidemic and zymotic poisons arose and spread. In the early 1860s sanitarian theory and practice were confirmed by Charles Murchison's theory of pythogenic disease, or diseases generated from "filth" (typically excrement but potentially any other bodily secretions or organic material). The theory remained unconfirmed because no one was able to isolate the element in the filth that caused the disease, but it seemed to work, since cleaning up the cities did remove the habitats in which the offending bacteria thrived.[13] At the same time, the vagueness of the concept of "filth" lent itself to an infinite range of corporeal and moral extensions, from dirty foreskins to dirty books.

In the 1840s Edwin Chadwick had popularized the idea of disease arising from or at least associated with bad smells: disease was caused by pathogenic miasmas arising from the decomposition of vegetable or animal wastes, particularly excrement.[14] The road to better health was constructed by purifying the atmosphere by "drainage, proper cleansing, [and] better ventilation"; in places where "the removal of the noxious agencies appears to be complete, such disease almost entirely disappears."[15] Chadwick's report was suffused with a class-conscious moralism that blamed the high incidence of disease among the poor as much on their bad habits and weak character as on their physical living conditions, but he was right about the harmfulness of ordure and the value of drains. The subsequent theory of zymotic disease was based on the research by the German chemist von Liebig on fermentation. William Farr proposed a disease process analogous to fermentation in which the rotting of organic matter produced pathogenic poisons, which might be chemical, seed-like, organic, or particular in nature; the possibility of spontaneous generation in such media was widely accepted until the 1880s.[16] The success of sanitary prescriptions may be seen in the fact that most of the decline in adult mortality in the late nineteenth century resulted from the fall in deaths due to water-borne (filth) diseases such as typhoid, cholera, and diarrhea and those connected with overcrowding and lack of ventilation (tuberculosis and typhus). Deaths from airborne diseases such as diphtheria, pneumonia, and influenza actually increased toward the end of the century, while those from degenerative or venereal conditions such as cancer, heart disease, and syphilis hardly changed.[17] These developments had an impact on the imagination, and drains became such a prominent topic that the internal workings of the human body were soon envisioned as a reticulated network. Theorists of autointoxication and the danger of constipation likened the intestines to a sewage system.[18]

With one significant exception, the major achievements of nineteenth-century health (apart from advances in surgery) were not the result of medical discoveries but of improvements in public health arising from better sanitation and isolation of tuberculosis sufferers[19]—though doctors were prominent in the movement, thus increasing the prestige of their profession. Perhaps the most famous example is John Snow, who in 1849 identified cholera's mode of transmission, and in 1854 proved his theories by locking the handle of the pump providing water from the local water company, thus ending the Soho cholera outbreak.[20] If all doctors had been as coolly inductive, and if the genitals had been regarded as neutrally as the digestive tract, circumcision as a preventive health measure might never have been heard of. The one disease that medicine was able to conquer by its own efforts, thanks to Edward Jenner's discovery of a safe method of vaccination, was smallpox, leading to a search for similar quick-fix tactics and great faith in the preventive approach.[21] "Prevention is better than cure" was the catchphrase as the success of the sanitary movement in improving urban health became evident, and in the 1890s no fewer than three institutes of preventive medicine were established, but it was really a case of making a virtue of necessity. In his many reports as medical officer to the Privy Council, Sir John Simon was influential in establishing the importance of preventive medicine, recognizing that once any zymotic agent had established itself in the body, the disease would run its course, and there was little anyone could do. In a situation in which there was no cure, prevention was the only option—if not by vaccination, then by cleanliness and other precautions.[22] By a process of imaginative extrapolation, preemptive amputation was eventually placed in this category: if diseases were caused by the accumulation of filth and mortality could be reduced by removing dirt from the urban environment, perhaps personal health could be improved by removing supposed dirt traps from the fabric of the human body. Many doctors spoke freely of the foreskin as a harbor of filth or a cesspool, and one later crusader for circumcision went so far as to claim that the operation conferred the same degree of immunity against tuberculosis as vaccination did against smallpox, with the implication that it should be equally compulsory.[23]

There was always a strong moral component in filth disease discourse, which tended to picture the most vulnerable categories of people as already weakened by "inheritance, ignorance, indifference and neglect of the laws of hygiene." Beyond dirt and overcrowding, it was factors like these that explained "the higher incidence of zymotic disease amongst the poor, the feckless, the dissolute, drunks, migrants and minorities," all eventually lumped together as "the Great Unwashed."[24] Although Malthus had asserted that disease was a manifestation of breaking the laws of nature, especially as regards dirt, not of divine displeasure,[25] the sanitary outlook was congenial to an older Judeo-Christian tradition, which held that epidemics were sent by God to punish wickedness, and it made heavy use of terms that originally had a primarily moral connotation: words such as *infectious* and *contagious* had a long history of association with (spiritual) impurity, defilement, and pollution.[26] By the 1860s utilitarian arguments for sanitary improvement, writes Margaret Pelling, "had been co-opted into a holistic religious and moral framework" that proved durable and flexible enough to survive and prosper with the rise of recognizably scientific concepts of disease.[27] Some class-conscious scholars have accordingly argued that the agenda of the sanitary reformers was as much political as hygienic, aiming at the insubordination of the laboring classes as much as the dirtiness of their homes and bodies. Frank Mort suggests that Victorian anxieties particularly centered on dirt and disordered hierarchies of social power,[28] while Joanne Townsend has commented that the Victorian understanding of hygiene, disease, and public health was a response to the "disorder brought by the Industrial Revolution. Public health movements were a way of gaining control over the physical environment and the bodies of . . . the working class." Following Mary Douglas (*Purity and Danger*), Townsend argues that "if the respectable middle class could eradicate dirt and contain disease, this would go some way toward establishing control over society, and transforming it into their own . . . ideal."[29]

The suggestion that the human body was pictured as analogous to an urban precinct, with its slums and dirty pockets needing the same sanitary makeover as the cities, is illuminating, but it is not clear that the primary targets of the sanitarians were the bodies of the working class. Fear of proletarian unrest might have been a factor in urban reform, especially slum rehabilitation, but drains and clean water supplies reached the suburbs of the rich long before they became available to the poor. A stronger case can be made that the sanitarians were more interested in disciplining the bodies of the middle and managerial class than those of the masses they were expected to direct. Alan Hunt has shown that the main target of the purity movement later in the century, particularly its antimasturbation propaganda, was the youth of the middle and professional classes, especially public school boys, not laboring lads at all,[30] and it is a fact that circumcision became significantly more common among the former groups. Although both Mort and Townsend exaggerate the danger of working-class revolt, the Victorians did draw close links between physical dirt, organic disease, and moral laxity. Chadwick's report was concerned that "the younger population, bred up under noxious physical conditions," was "inferior in physical organization and general health" to others and "less susceptible of moral influences, and the effects of education" than a healthy population. He painted a Hobbesian picture of the new race of barbarous aliens that seemed to be breeding in the rookeries: "these adverse circumstances tend to produce an adult population short-lived, improvident, reckless and intemperate, and with habitual avidity for sensual gratifications. . . . Defective town cleansing fosters habits of the most abject degradation and tends to the demoralization of large numbers of human beings, who subsist by means of what they find among the noxious filth accumulated in neglected streets and bye-places." Chadwick's solution—"the removal of noxious physical circumstances, and the promotion of civic, household and personal cleanliness"—and his key images—filth, neglected bye-places, removal—were all readily applicable to the human body.[31] Cleanliness became, in Townsend's words, "a key definer of respectability and thus a highly visible indication of class," but the middle class had access to running water, washing facilities, and soap long before such domestic innovations became available to the masses.

While the pro- and anti-Listerians struggled to understand the ways of germs and thus move medicine toward a scientific understanding of disease, the field of nervous illness remained firmly under the reign of old ideas. If anything, concepts of nervous or nerve-related disease became less scientific as the fanciful theories of James Cullen and John Brown were spun into wonderful new syndromes such as spinal irritation, reflex neuroses, neurasthenia, and masturbatory insanity. If one tendency of Victorian medicine was to seek materialist explanations for disease in the condition of cities and the agency of microorganisms, another was to value the power of mind over matter, whether expressed in the need to control animal passion by the moral sense or in the idea that organic disease could be caused by "nerves." There was scarcely any disorder that at one time or other was not blamed on imbalance in nerve force, and the prevention or cure of nervous disease became a major justification for operations on the genitals of both males and females. An important medical authority for these beliefs was W. B. Carpenter (1813–85), professor of physiology at University College London, and the foremost authority on human physiology for much of the century.[32] His *Principles of Human Physiology,* first published in 1842, went through numerous British and U.S. editions and remained the standard textbook for the next thirty years.[33] As a medical student, Jonathan Hutchinson studied it along with his Bible, and William Acton relied on it for many of his propositions about the danger of sexual excess, the power of the will, and the risks of rail travel for nervous equilibrium.[34] Carpenter's physiology is notable for its reticence on the penis, and for making no mention of the foreskin at all, thus contributing to the notion that it was a vestigial and functionless structure, but he has a whole chapter about the influence of the nervous system on organic functions, and several pages on the dangers of sexual excess and the moral (though not the medical) evils of masturbation. I have already noted the religious and philosophic origins of the horse-rider image he employs to illustrate how the nervous system influences organic functions, and within this perspective the nervous system not only controlled motor or contractile tissues but had a particular power over secretions, a fact that explained why sexual excess could lead to nervous exhaustion and thus physical illness.[35]

The Victorians took the concept of nerve force very seriously and relied on it to explain health problems that defied analysis and treatment. In 1867 Handfield Jones referred to the "mysterious interest" surrounding the nervous system and noted that "failure of nervous power is much more characteristic of disease of the present day than of that which prevailed thirty years ago"; he ascribed the trend to the conditions of modern life, but no doubt medical fashion was also a factor.[36] The idea of nerve force represented the application of old theories of bodily equilibrium in the light of recent discoveries about electricity and the second law of thermodynamics, which posited a steadily decreasing quantity of energy in the universe, and by extension that the energy of the human body was finite, nonrenewable, and in need of careful husbanding.[37] It was generally agreed that overexertion would drain a person's supply, leaving an exhausted system incapable of further effort and more susceptible to disease: hence doctors' constant exhortations to conserve nerve force by not overworking, overstudying, and the like—unless you were a male adolescent, in which case you were urged to play sports precisely so that you would have less energy left over for other games. Nerve force should certainly not be wasted on sexual adventurism. Humoral pathology "was largely discredited by the nineteenth century," writes Janet Oppenheim, "but doctors . . . had no equally satisfactory organising concept . . . until the germ theory of disease emerged," and it was not until the end of the century that this was widely understood.[38] While doctors and scientists argued about putrefaction and infection, old concepts of balance influenced the understanding of nervous disease until well after the bacteriological approach had come to dominate other areas. The notion of the nervous temperament was retained from the Galenic system and often used as an explanation for susceptibility to stress, depression, excitement, and such, and as late as 1886 Sir Andrew Clark held that this temperament was born of "a too rapid production and expenditure, together with irregular distribution, of nerve force."[39] Like theories of the harm done by masturbation, nerve force was often pictured in economic metaphors: as one health adviser put it in 1874, "man has a reserve of force: like the balance of a prudent firm at its bankers. If this is too far drawn upon a sudden demand becomes a very serious matter."[40] The spermatic economy discussed by Steven Marcus and others is an aspect of this "household budget" concept of energy.

Nerve force theory gave rise to many novel disease entities, three of which are particularly relevant to the increasing implication of the genitals in the generation of health problems: spinal irritation, reflex neuroses, and neurasthenia. Building on shaky concepts of irritation already popularized by John Brown, physicians of the 1820s invented spinal irritation, a pseudodisease involving acute sensitivity to sensation along the spine and the belief that peripheral symptoms were caused by invisible but real disorders in the spinal cord. The concept flourished until the 1870s in Britain, where James Paget took it seriously and even blamed it for many cases of masturbation, and yet longer in the United States, where William Hammond, a professor of mind in New York, published a whole book on the subject in 1886. Proposing an effect working in the opposite direction, he reported that the problem was often caused by sexual excesses and masturbation. Although the syndrome faded from the journals and consulting rooms in the 1880s, it did not wholly die but was incorporated into George Beard's brainchild of the 1870s, neurasthenia.[41] The hazy causation implicit in spinal irritation then gave rise to the opposite scenario: the idea that nervous connections regulated all bodily organs and members independent of human will and that disorder in an organ or body part could produce effects at distant locations which could be treated by procedures on the part thought to be exercising the effects. Reflex theory, as this body of knowledge was called, soon acquired what Edward Shorter calls a "breathtaking capacity to inspire meddlesomeness among doctors, and to suggest patients into preoccupation with fashionable organs that . . . had nothing to do with their symptoms."[42] In the female these sites often turned out to be the uterus or clitoris, and in the male the penis and particularly its foreskin; the distinguished orthopedic surgeon Lewis Sayre claimed to have proved that various forms of paralysis of the limbs in boys were often caused by a tight or adherent prepuce and could be cured by circumcision, a discovery that confirmed the assertions of Lallemand and contributed much to the rise of routine circumcision in both the United States and Britain.[43] Reflex theory reigned from the 1850s until the early Edwardian period, exercising a profound influence on how doctors treated both mental and physical disease. Its credibility was boosted by the work of Charles-Edward Brown-Sequard, whose widely read lectures on nervous processes in the *Lancet* (1858) inspired the London gynecologist Isaac Baker Brown with the idea that clitoridectomy might cure masturbation, epilepsy, hysteria, and other nervous complaints in women. As late as 1894 an "updated and modernised" edition of Quain's *Dictionary of Medicine* included an abstruse entry for reflex disorders, which were defined broadly as "a very varied group of affections" resulting from three essential factors, which seem to boil down to the proposition that irritation in one part of the body can be transmitted by the nerves to produce disorders in another. There were "multitudinous cases in which some sources of irritation . . . occasion, in various more or less obscure ways, through the intervention of the great encephalic centres, convulsions or fits." It was in this way that reflex paralysis of the limbs (as described by Sayre) was thought to occur.[44]

Neurasthenia was a coherent and respectable concept from the 1880s until the First World War. It was particularly associated with the American George Beard, who first published an article on nervous exhaustion in 1869 and then a book in 1880, but it owed much to the old idea of spinal irritation and existing theories of nerve force. In Beard's formulation, the brain, digestive system, and reproductive organs were all important nodes for reflex action, and illness could result from too little nerve force in any of these centers as a result of the nervous system becoming "dephosphorised."[45] The drain of nerve force through "over-use of any one of these centres sent fatigue and irritation ricocheting through the body, with physical ramifications in . . . the most unlikely places," writes Oppenheim.[46] Neurasthenia originated as a concept of nervous exhaustion but came to be understood in four senses: as a synonym for general nervousness and mood disorder; as the male equivalent of hysteria; as depression; and as fatigue, lassitude, or lack of energy, often caused by sexual excess.[47] Beard considered the foreskin to be a major factor in the generation of neurasthenic disorders, or sexual exhaustion—a special case of nervous exhaustion. Neurasthenia in general was the nervous equivalent of anemia and expressed itself in a wide variety of indistinct symptoms and arose from obscure causes, but the origins of sexual exhaustion were easier to pin down: phimosis and masturbation. Beard claimed that nearly all the cases of sexual neurasthenia that came his way had a history of early masturbation and involuntary emissions (spermatorrhea) and that in some of them there was an elongated prepuce or phimosis as well: "In a nervous person a redundant, elongated prepuce covering the gland [*sic*] and pressing upon it acts as an irritant to the whole system, and excites any number of nervous symptoms, even to melancholia and paralysis." In two-thirds of his nervous patients there was "a more or less abnormal condition of the prepuce." To remedy this situation circumcision must be performed to relieve the pressure on "the gland [*sic*] penis"; the operation "has been known to radically cure cases of nervous disease."[48] In a separate article titled "Circumcision as a Cure for Nervous Symptoms" (1882), Beard touted circumcision as an effective treatment for a swag of neurasthenic manifestations, including "morbid fears, fear of society, of solitude or travelling, of places of disease . . . mental depression, wakefulness, headache, impaired memory, deficient mental control."[49] If a simple snip could achieve all that, the clever doctors who had thought it up deserved the title of miracle workers, and their future status as a powerful force in society was assured.

The early nineteenth century was a decisive period for the development of the modern medical profession. Between 1790 and 1858 practitioners fought a successful battle to close their ranks to those they considered unqualified, to determine who could call himself a doctor, to gain a near monopoly over medical treatment, and to raise their social status from tradesmen to professional gentlemen on a par with lawyers and clergymen.[50] By the end of the century the profession had consolidated the business of medicine into the form still common today: the confidential encounter between doctor and patient, on a fee-for-service basis.[51] In 1800 the profession was sharply divided (in descending order of status) into physicians, surgeons, and apothecaries, all represented by associations that dated back to medieval times. This structure was challenged by the emergence of a new breed, the general practitioner, who specialized in meeting the needs of the expanding middle class. It was this group that founded the British Medical Association, outside the existing colleges, in 1832 and led the campaign for legal recognition that culminated in the Medical Registration Act of 1858. This act established the General Council of Medical Education (usually known as the General Medical Council) to govern admission to the profession, set skill requirements, and rule on professional ethics.[52] Such backing closed the profession to those the council considered unsuitable and allowed it to disbar those of whose behavior it disapproved, such as doctors who offered "secret remedies" or published works that had too explicit a sexual content or dealt with contraception.[53] In the process they raised the status of the formerly disreputable surgeons and humble apothecaries to the level of physicians, and the unified profession ensured steady upward mobility and rising incomes for its members.[54] Higher status brought a greater sense of self-importance, which in the first instance meant authority over customers, whose own standing correspondingly fell from that of clients with the privileges of those who paid the piper to that of patients who had little choice but to bow to their doctor's superior expertise. As Joanne Townsend has commented, by virtue of their expert knowledge doctors claimed far-reaching authority over the management of the lives of their patients, and if people wanted medical treatment they had to submit their own judgment or preferences to the recommendations of their physician.[55] It has even been suggested that patients "often welcomed imperious behaviour from physicians, who were accorded the status of Almighty Fathers intervening between the forces of life and death."[56] Not every practitioner went as far as a provincial GP in the United States who remarked that "something must be done ... to impress the patient with the fact that the doctor is boss,"[57] but Acton found it perfectly proper that men should ask his permission to marry and had no inhibitions in withholding it if he thought such a course unwise.[58] The physical examination was a development of the late Victorian period and one of the features that distinguishes modern from premodern medicine. In the past doctors were not allowed to examine patients' bodies, but the new rules gave them special privileges and new powers: "the right to ask intimate questions and ... to touch and penetrate the body"—actions that in any other context would certainly be offensive and probably constitute assault.[59] It is possible that the theory of masturbation-induced disease contributed to the institution of the physical, and especially the genital, examination: even before such physicals became routine, children showing signs of paralysis, rickets, whooping cough, and almost any other symptom were frequently subjected to genital examination in the belief that the problem could be caused by masturbation or preputial irritation.

Much of the profession's obsession with respectability, and its consequent sexual prudishness, arose from doctors' anxiety to demarcate themselves from the quacks—all those irregular or improperly qualified empirics who treated the desperate and the embarrassed, but particularly those who specialized in sexual medicine, such as venereal disease and cures for lost manhood. Before 1858 there was complete laissez-faire, and even the new act did not make unqualified practitioners illegal: it just meant they could not use a title for which they did not hold the appropriate license.[60] Mainstream physicians vehemently denounced the quacks at every opportunity, and above all for magnifying the anxieties of male patients about nervous diseases such as spermatorrhea, but the quacks were only trading on the fears already aroused by their own harping on the dangers of sexual excess.[61] As Spencer noticed, although many doctors avoided the sexual minefield entirely and regarded practitioners like Acton with suspicion, it was really a struggle for professional turf and perhaps a case of what Freud called the narcissism of minor differences.[62] As Herbert Spencer remarked, "along with incorporation of authorised medical men there has arisen jealousy of the unincorporated. Like the religious priesthood, the priesthood of medicine persecutes heretics and those who are without diplomas. There has long been . . . denunciation of unlicensed practitioners, as also of the 'counter-practice' carried on by chemists and druggists."[63] The physicians were in competition with the quacks for the growing middle-class demand for medical services, and they all held similar views on sex, especially masturbation, the widespread fear of which created a potentially lucrative market, if only the subject could be made more respectable.[64] Doctors scored a significant victory over the quacks with the passage of the Indecent Advertisements Act of 1889, which banned "any advertisement relating to syphilis, gonorrhoea, nervous debility or other complaint or infirmity arising from . . . sexual intercourse"; the measure was justified as a contribution to public decency, but it probably did not harm the doctors' claim to be the only legal source of advice in these areas.[65] Significant divisions in the profession remained, but sexual diseases proved to be of particular value to the efforts of surgeons to enhance their status vis-à-vis the physicians, who already enjoyed the prestige of the classically educated and socially connected but who were reluctant to defile themselves in this controversial area. Ellen Rosenman has shown that the spermatorrhea panic provided an opportunity for surgeons to offer surgical cures for sexual problems and pseudoproblems, thus validating their claim to expertise in a neglected but vital field of medicine. In her view, the rising importance of surgery in the late Victorian period was both a cause and a consequence of the efforts of this branch of the profession to strengthen its members' social and economic position: "The spermatorrhoea panic was one of a series of medical events . . . that helped transform the authority of the medical profession. . . . Surgeons certainly did not invent spermatorrhoea for the purpose of professional advancement . . . but in redefining their relationship to the body, it provided them with an ideal opportunity to enrich their cultural capital."[66] The events she lists are the cholera epidemics, the Contagious Diseases Acts of the 1860s, and the public health movement, to which one could add the invention of congenital phimosis and the introduction of surgical cures for childhood problems such as masturbation.

The profession's increasing exclusiveness manifested itself in resentment at efforts by nonmedical personnel to express opinions on medical matters. In 1866 one provincial fellow of the Royal College of Physicians (FRCP) commented that the gravity of medical subjects, especially ones involving sex, meant that discussion should be confined to "its proper place among other professional arcana," and he regretted that medical discourse was no longer conducted in Latin, "under the shelter of which our modest forefathers . . . shrouded such scientific details."[67] At the end of the century the *Lancet* expressed disapproval of Havelock Ellis's recourse to a popular publisher for the first volume of his *Studies in the Psychology of Sex*, made no protest at its seizure by the police, and commented that whatever the merits of his arguments, it was "important that such matters should not be discussed by the man in the street." The same issue included an editorial comment headed "Lay Criticism of Medical Affairs," which made the point that when this "man in the street" criticized scientific or technical matters he was "apt to do so in the light of his necessary ignorance, so that he falls inevitably into error" and was thus likely "not only to wrong himself but also to mislead others."[68] The increasing authoritarianism of the profession aroused some opposition, particularly among women who resented its assertion of power over the female body. In 1871 Mary Hume-Rothery attacked "medical despotism" as evidenced in the Contagious Diseases Acts, compulsory vaccination, humiliating gynecological examinations, and male control of childbirth; she compared doctors to "the priests of old" and complained that they had become "all-wise dictators in physical matters."[69] The popular novelist Ouida (Mary-Louise Ramee) likewise blasted them in a novel titled *The New Priesthood* (1893): "It is pitiful to see the public so cowed . . . that it dares not act for itself, and like an imbecile receives . . . any quackery which it is told by its medicine men will benefit its constitution. . . . Living flesh is the mere foolscap paper on which the physiologist writes with his knife, his caustic, or his red hot iron."[70] She might have been thinking of vivisection, but all these approaches were used to treat masturbation in both males and females.

If, as Thomas Laqueur has suggested, the aim of the nineteenth-century medical profession was to "substitute the physician for the priest as the moral arbiter of society," the convergence is consistent with the fact that its single most important source of recruitment were the sons of clergymen.[71] Many have noted the similarity between the doctor's consulting room and the priest's confessional, especially when shameful deeds were being admitted: "in the confessional of the consulting room, the truth on such subjects is oftenest heard," reported Acton.[72] In relation to these, "the well-known cycle of sin, confession, punishment or penance and redemption [was] carried out in medical rather than a religious setting," writes Arthur Gilbert. "In his new sacerdotal role, the physician was in a position to exercise tremendous moral as well as physical control over his supplicants."[73] To compare doctors to priests became a commonplace of Victorian discourse, sometimes with approval, sometimes in criticism. Recommending chastity as the only effective remedy for syphilis and condemning the chimerical doctors who reportedly prescribed visits to prostitutes as a cure for spermatorrhea and masturbation, the *Lancet* stated that the profession had weighty responsibilities: "Young men are looking to us as men looked to the old type of priests who combined moral and medical functions. If clerical teachers are for the moment in less authority, we are in more."[74]

In identifying the importance of being earnest, Oscar Wilde pinpointed one of the central features of the age he wished to satirize. Whether they were religious or freethinking, Whig or Tory, pro-Russian or pro-Turk, Victorians were above all serious, and none more so than the medical profession, which added anxiety to their makeup as they sought to distinguish themselves from the quacks and raise their status in the professional hierarchy. Sexual medicine was always a dangerous business for them, risking association with quackery and licentiousness; if they ventured into this territory they tended to take their cue from the moralism of the bishops, not the scientific and skeptical spirit of the philosophers of the previous century or the scientists of the present who were reshaping biology. In the field of sexual medicine, backward and unscientific understandings, heavily overlaid by religious and other moral sentiment, thus lingered far longer than they did in less controversial areas. As Scull and Favreau point out, anything that cast a shadow on their rectitude and probity threatened their social standing.[75] Such an attitude led naturally to a moralistic view of disease and a corresponding interest in the conduct, as much as the physiology, of their patients. As a provincial GP expressed it in the 1860s, "were it not for moral delinquency of some kind on the part of sufferers from disease or his forefathers, disease would not exist; but it does exist, and we, as medical practitioners, are called upon to make ourselves intimately acquainted with the moral as well as the physical infirmities of our fellow-creatures, and to treat them in such a manner as is best calculated to give tone to both."[76] Doctors had no hesitation in making pronouncements on the correct arrangements for domestic and national life, and in 1867 the *Medical Times and Gazette* devoted a lengthy editorial to what it termed "aberrations of the sexual instinct." These came in four main forms: (1) "sensual gratification without any union of the sexes, as in 'the besetting trials of our boys'"—that is, any nonprocreative sex, but masturbation especially; (2) temporary partnerships of the sexes, leading to incontinence and infanticide; (3) childless marriages; and (4) confounding of sex roles, such as women doing men's jobs and vice versa. It was a comprehensive list of pleasures and trends. The correct path of behavior was laid down in the Church of England marriage service, which stated that the purposes of the ordinance were the procreation of children, the avoidance of incontinence, and mutual support; unions not embodying these principles were "contrary to natural law." Observance of these rules was not just desirable for personal happiness but also for public order, since "the relations of the sexes are connected with religious and public policy"; any attempt "to disturb either is fraught with danger to the whole social fabric."[77]

Doctors might pronounce on moral issues, deplore the ignorance of sex among the middle-class young, and urge their instruction in suitably presented physiology,[78] but were physicians capable of providing it? Doctors themselves knew little about sexual physiology or anatomy, and as the Victorian passed into the Edwardian age they became, if anything, more resistant to learning. At the turn of the century Havelock Ellis commented that "our knowledge of the individual and racial variations of the external sex organs is still extremely imperfect,"[79] and in the first serious study of mammalian reproduction, Marshall's *Physiology of Reproduction* (1910), the author acknowledged that even the processes of erection were not fully understood.[80] Lesley Hall has commented that the book revealed that knowledge of sex was "scanty and in a state of flux," a professional inadequacy confirmed by the letters anxious men and women sent to Marie Stopes—"every one of them containing a pretty revelation of doctors' incompetence," she reported to Ellis.[81] In the Edwardian age the refusal to discuss sex reached such depths of petulance that a reviewer of Krafft-Ebbing's *Psychopathia Sexualis* could write that it was a "repulsive" book that "should convey solace by being put to the most ignominious use to which paper can be applied."[82]

The doctors' success in organizing themselves professionally was not matched by comparable advances in the cure of disease. Early in the century the *Lancet* recognized that medicine was still a trade like any other and deplored the "self-called 'experienced' practitioner . . . in whose mind a multitude of facts are mingled without order . . . with whom medicine is a trade, and not a science." It wished to create "men of science" and looked forward to the day when medicine had become "a science of observation."[83] That day was a long time coming, and it was not until well after interventions like circumcision had become firmly established in the therapeutic repertoire; as A. J. Youngson comments, "most doctors before 1850, and many as late as 1870 . . . simply did not observe or think scientifically."[84] Bleeding as treatment was still common in the 1850s, and uncertainty as to the origins and nature of gonorrhea persisted long after the identification of the guilty bacterium. For a start it was held to be a gender-specific disease, affecting mainly men, but not a very serious one. Acton believed that gonorrhea could arise simply from "mechanical causes" and agreed with another authority that it usually "arose simply from the continual irritation and excitement of the genital organs consequent upon their [the prostitutes'] mode of life."[85] The more orthodox position was similar to the explanation put forward by John Marten in 1709 and was essentially zymotic: that the disease was "generated by the decomposition of retained semen, especially after repeated indiscriminate intercourse without proper attention to cleanliness," as Erichsen's *Surgery* put it in 1877.[86] This theory allowed surgeons to account for the occasional appearance of gonorrheal symptoms in married (and presumably faithful) women, apparently as a result of the decomposition of her husband's semen or of her own discharges in conditions of poor hygiene. This scenario was very similar to the claim that "secretions" trapped under the foreskin decayed and putrefied, thus generating pathogenic poisons. Galenic/humoral theory and the nerve force paradigm coexisted with the debate over germs, and as late as 1863 one doctor was prescribing leeches as a treatment for gonorrhea.[87] If Conan Doyle's fond caricature from the 1890s is any guide, the old style of empirical practitioner took a long time to die out:

> Bleeding he would practise freely but for public opinion. Chloroform he regards as a dangerous innovation, and he always clicks with his tongue when it is mentioned. He has even been known to . . . refer to the stethoscope as "a newfangled French toy." . . . He always reads . . . his weekly medical paper so that he has a general idea as to the advance of modern science. He persists in looking upon it, however, as a . . . ludicrous experiment. The germ theory of disease set him chuckling for a long time, and his favourite joke in the sick room was to say, "Shut the door, or the germs will be getting in." As to the Darwinian theory, it struck him as being the crowning joke of the century. "The children in the nursery and the ancestors in the stable," he would cry, and laugh the tears out of his eyes.[88]

Conan Doyle was not describing a real person; his enduring point is that doctors are a conservative lot, slow to take up an idea but equally slow to abandon it.

Doyle also provides a useful checklist of the main achievements of nineteenth-century medicine: anesthesia (from the 1850s) and aseptic surgery (from the 1880s), leading to much lower death rates from surgical operations and other hospital treatment, but having little impact on the everyday diseases responsible for most of the mortality. English medicine lagged behind that of the French and Germans when it came to understanding bacterial causation of disease and appreciating the precautions needed to ensure a sterile operating environment.[89] Agreement that specific bacteria caused particular diseases did not immediately make it easier to cure them: although discoveries such as Salvarsan made headway against syphilis and the development of an antitoxin for diphtheria reduced child mortality after the 1890s, there was no reliable way of destroying bacteria within the body until the development of the first antibiotics in the 1930s. As the physician John Bristowe remarked in 1887, "the great aim of medical art is the cure of disease. Unfortunately, however, a direct cure . . . in the great majority of cases is totally impossible."[90] W. F. Bynum thus concludes that "the contribution of curative medicine to overall mortality figures before 1900 was probably very slight" and that "the mortality decline between 1850 and 1900 was the result of . . . prevention rather than therapy."[91] The establishment of circumcision as a valid procedure belongs firmly to an age when cure of disease was unlikely and prevention the only reliable option.

How modern and how scientific had Victorian medicine become by the 1880s? These questions are the subject of some debate, and a firm answer is not made easier by recent controversies over the nature of science itself. As we have seen, its modernity was undermined by the survival of ancient concepts of disease and methods of treatment, and its scientificity was likewise compromised by the continuing influence of religious morality, particularly in sexual medicine; priests no longer claimed sovereignty over the lungs or heart, but the genitals were a different matter. There is an old "triumphalist" view that the doctors' achievement of professional hegemony was the result of their success in harnessing science for the relief of sickness,[92] but this was overtaken in the 1960s with the more skeptical judgment that they were isolated from advances in European biomedical research, backward in physiology and germ theory, and did not, as Youngson phrases it, think scientifically. The popularity of mesmerism, phrenology, and other pseudosciences among medical practitioners until the 1850s also indicates a superstitious outlook.[93] This view has in turn been criticized as "whiggish," but even in one such critique S. E. D. Shortt does not deny that English understandings of infectious diseases were backward compared with those of the French and Germans, and he acknowledges the degree to which the study of physiology was compromised by prescientific concepts. Carpenter's work, for example, "combined moral with physiological instruction in an effort to preserve theological concepts of free will derived from William Paley's moral philosophy, which showed the beneficence of God's design" in the organization of life.[94] Peterson points out that it was not until the 1880s that scientific subjects such as physics and chemistry were included in the medical curriculum and that "a scientific orientation" was not a major consideration in the choice of a medical career.[95] A letter to the *Lancet* in 1878 commented that the British were slow to accept Listerism because they were suspicious of science: the Germans had "eagerly adopted" it because they were scientific; Scottish surgeons had incorporated it "a little grudgingly" because they were semiscientific; but the English had rejected it because they were "plodding and practical."[96] Both the *Lancet* and the *British Medical Journal* took a long time to show any support for Darwinism, and in 1873 J. L. Milton described Darwinism as "just one of those dangerous and reducing errors which . . . start into life when a man of great abilities gives up his mind to the illusions of a phantom"— such a contrast to his own cutting-edge ideas on spermatorrhea.[97] Darwin himself remarked in 1875 that "very many [medical] practitioners neither know nor care anything about the progress of knowledge."[98] They were, however, skilled—and this is what really counted—at harnessing the rhetoric of science in the cause of their professional advancement and as a visible sign of their skill. As Shortt argues, knowledge was not always necessary for social authority, and "by forcing the rhetoric of science into the social vocabulary of the period, physicians secured a vehicle for professional recognition"; they gained stature not because they could always act effectively but because "they could name, describe and explain."[99] A good bedside manner meant more than diagnosis or cure, since "efficacy was not the standard by which Victorian medical men . . . judged the status of an occupation," comments Peterson. "Prestige and authority derived from the social evaluation placed on the work itself."[100] Christopher Lawrence similarly argues that physicians employed the rhetoric of science to enhance their authority while remaining suspicious of and resistant to the application of scientific methods in practice.[101]

Although the arrival of "modern medicine" is generally dated from the 1870s, with the rise of Listerism and gradual acceptance of germ theory,[102] the nineteenth century might equally be described as the period in which old or traditional medicine declined as the one in which modern medicine arose. It was a long time before germ theory was understood, and early enthusiasm for the new paradigm led many to push it beyond its usefulness, producing ideas like autointoxication—the theory that the body poisoned itself and that cavities like the intestines or subpreputial space were meant to be sterile. Nerve force theory remained influential until the 1920s. Nineteenth-century medicine was thus characterized as much by the abandonment of old techniques as by the adoption of new ones, leading some observers not to praise advances but to bemoan stagnation. There was a sense of frustration in the late 1860s that methods of treatment were not keeping up with progress in knowledge of bodily processes and demands for a therapeutic breakthrough. As one practitioner put it in 1868, "as we review the rapid progress made . . . by physiology, pathology and other departments of medical science, and compare it with the slow advance of therapeutics, we experience . . . dissatisfaction with our present empirical methods of treatment, consisting in the mere tentative administration of drugs."[103] In 1873 E. W. Lane looked at the progress of medicine since the 1830s and concluded that most of the change had been in the abandonment of therapies formerly regarded as valuable. Apart from accidental discoveries like chloroform, "the most important improvements . . . [in] Old Medicine have been of a negative character—that is . . . a general abandonment . . . of certain heroic methods of dealing with patients." He listed bleeding and dosing with antimony, calomel, and mercury, but added that rejection of these techniques was a slow process and that "the Galenical notion of curing diseases by their contraries has held its ground bravely." Lane looked forward to the day when medicine stood on "a rational philosophy," blamed the survival of discredited therapies on the priestlike manner of the medical profession, and concluded that it would not become scientific until it had developed "a complete knowledge of the workings of [the human organism] in the state of health."[104] Those who were not satisfied with the "therapeutic nihilism" of a William Osler (professor of medicine at Oxford from 1905 to 1919), who considered that the task was diagnosis and prognosis rather than cure,[105] were eager to find magic weapons with which to break out of the impasse. They found them in the one area in which, thanks to anesthesia and antisepsis, medicine was making rapid advances—surgery.

In his study of the means used to repress masturbation in the nineteenth century, Thomas Szasz identified a paradox in the fact that surgical treatment of the habit became more widespread as belief in the theory of masturbatory insanity and its other harmful consequences declined. He explains this by suggesting that the phenomenon was related to "the development of surgical skills and aseptic operating techniques which allowed safe surgical mutilations," not to new medical indications.[106] This explanation is largely true of operations on the internal organs of women, especially hysterectomy and ovariectomy, and to circumcision in the United States after the invention of the Gomco clamp in the 1930s. It is also applicable to the sudden vogue for excision of other organs thought to be vestigial or functionless and assumed to be complicit in little-understood complaints, such as the appendix, the tonsils, and even the large intestine—denounced by Arbuthnot Lane as a "cesspool" that poisoned the system as energetically as the preputial sac.[107] But is the observation applicable to the more accessible foreskin, for which new reasons to cut were regularly generated? It is possible to make a case that circumcision was not classified as serious surgery at all. Because it was regarded as a simple matter, it was not reserved to qualified surgeons in the carve-up of professional responsibilities but usually left to GPs. Anesthesia was not commonly used—never on newborn infants and rarely on babies, though a few whiffs of chloroform, or even cocaine, was recommended to keep older children and sometimes toddlers quiet. Strict aseptic precautions did not become usual until around the time of the First World War, when it was realized that an alarming number of babies were being infected with syphilis, tuberculosis, and other diseases in the course of the operation.[108] It could therefore be argued that the major advances of nineteenth-century medicine were not relevant to circumcision and that it was thus a survival from the previous age of heroic surgery, when neither anesthesia nor asepsis had been heard of and the only chance for saving a person with a diseased or damaged appendage was by its amputation. But I think a better case can be made that although circumcision was not regarded as major surgery, it was still seen as a surgical procedure, and thus that it was looked upon as a realistic option once the possibilities of anesthesia and asepsis were available, even if they were not always used. Although the operation was often done by GPs, an advocate stated in 1950 that it was usually performed in hospitals by house surgeons.[109] Circumcision became acceptable in the 1860s, but it was not until the 1880s that it became common, and it is likely that the rapid progress of and general prestige of surgery were major factors in its rising incidence.

This very point was made by a correspondent to the *British Medical Journal* in 1950, who suggested that the rise of circumcision had "something to do with the astonishing advances and increased prestige of surgery," also seen in the "onslaughts on numberless juvenile tonsils, so that many a parent feels negligent if her child is not exposed to one or both of these procedures."[110] There can be little doubt as to the higher standing of surgery, compared with the other branches of medicine, by the turn of the century. In 1897 Malcolm Morris praised the progress of medicine generally but noted the more striking advance of surgery as compared with "physick." Surgeons had expanded their territory at the expense of physicians, including a takeover of the abdomen, to the great advantage of mankind.[111] In the early twentieth century, Geoffrey Keynes (b. 1887) decided to become a surgeon because he believed that more could be achieved by surgery than by the resources at the disposal of physicians and GPs. They could arrive at a diagnosis, but there were "few scientific drugs, and the doctor could only try to create the best circumstances in which natural processes could enable the patient to cure himself"; a surgeon, however, "proceeded to cure the patient by the skill of his own hands, a much more positive satisfaction."[112] Historians have confirmed these perceptions. Shryock comments that surgeons achieved "a popular recognition which was rarely bestowed upon their colleagues in physiology and anatomy," and Anne Digby has offered a similar argument.[113] There is also evidence that children were an important element in a surgeon's customer base. Digby points out that they were a sought-after element in a medical practice and could make up a third of a doctor's patients. Many hospitals specifically for children were established in late nineteenth-century London, including six in the 1860s and three in the 1870s.[114] They catered to the growth in children's surgery, much of it "concerned with the removal of adenoids, tonsils and foreskins," as Roger Cooter comments. He further argues that nearly two-thirds of in-patients at children's hospitals were surgical cases, and that an honorary appointment to such an institution could be an important career step for an aspiring consultant, offering "a training ground for entry into general surgical consultancy among fee-paying adults."[115] Increasing hospitalization of children gave doctors more opportunities to examine their genitals and thus to blame the frequently found "adherent prepuces" for whatever illnesses the boys were suffering from. The connection between the rise of surgery and the vogue for circumcision is emphasized by the fact that many of the most ardent crusaders for preventive circumcision—J. Cooper Forster, T. B. Curling, Jonathan Hutchinson, John Erichsen, E. Harding Freeland, and John Bland-Sutton—were all surgeons.

The influences of the public health movement and preventive medicine were also important. Although she makes no mention of circumcision, Lesley Hall has noted that the search for surgical solutions to masturbation peaked under the impact of the public health movement—and because "it was also the age of heroic surgery as antisepsis and anaesthesia enabled surgeons to go boldly where no scalpel had gone before." Such capability encouraged belief in "surgical cures for previously intractable conditions," leading to the "fantasy surgery" further discussed in chapters 1 and 11.[116] What was new about circumcision was not that it involved amputation but that it was the amputation of tissue in which there was no hint of injury or disease, merely a suspicion that it might cause disease later. To this extent its acceptance was the result of the rising status of preventive medicine in the last quarter of the century, and in his celebratory history of this movement Ernest Newman praised Listerism as leading to "preventive surgery" and identified circumcision as an instance of this: "Circumcision has been practised for some thousands of years, and became after long centuries a religious rite, but did that make it less an example of preventive surgery?"[117] Despite the validity of her general point, I would argue that Hall's dates for the peak of surgical solutions to masturbation (1850s-1870s) are too early; she is probably thinking of operations on women, but operations on boys were only beginning at that time and probably reached their peak between the 1890s and the 1920s.

The popularity of circumcision was also confirmed by important changes in surgical practice in the second half of the nineteenth century: the decline of "heroic surgery" and its supersession by a conservative approach. Before the development of anesthesia and asepsis permitted reasonably safe access to internal organs and tissues, most of the human body was beyond the reach of surgery. Mid-nineteenth-century medicine was thus characterized by an "amputational culture." Michael Worboys relates this to the dominant position of surgery as a mode of treatment: damaged parts were removed because there was no effective method of treating them conservatively or curing the problem.[118] The culture of British medicine was amputational because this was the normal—often the only—way to treat or prevent infection.[119] This style of medicine was referred to as the "heroic" approach, summed up in the saying that "a chance to cut is chance to cure."[120] "Heroic surgery" was a do or die tactic, justified by the patient's peril and the fact that although he might very well die if operated on, he would almost certainly die if left alone. The new surgery aimed to save rather than destroy, to cut only for purposes of removing malignancy or repairing damage, to do everything possible to save limbs and appendages, and to amputate only as a last resort.[121] The new approach was itself influenced by the preventive culture of the late nineteenth century and regarded it as acceptable to carry out preventive operations in order to check the development of pathological conditions, particularly in cases of cancer. A U.S. surgeon remarked in the 1870s that it had been discovered that "the true function of medicine is to prevent rather than cure disease. Surgery . . . has achieved some of its proudest triumphs in preventing pain and in saving life and limb."[122] This was often interpreted as a license for preemptive amputation of potentially harmful body parts, for as Christopher Lawrence sums up, conservative surgery was preservative: an operation today could correct an incipient malignancy, thus saving the patient "from heroic amputation tomorrow"; the new surgery sought to prevent excisions by small-scale but early corrective interventions.[123] Doctors took it for granted that men would prefer to lose their foreskin as an infant than their entire penis as an old man. It was this style of surgery that legitimized Freeland's demand for mass circumcision: "the universal practice of an operation which has for its object the wholesale removal of a certain healthy structure as a preventive measure."[124]

6 · A Source of Serious Mischief

William Acton and the Case against the Foreskin

The interval between the age of puberty and . . . marriage must . . . be passed in strict chastity.

THOMAS MALTHUS, *An Essay on the Principle of Population,* 1803

Sexual excesses are the monster evil of the present, no less than of former times. . . . Mr. Acton has done good service to society by grappling manfully with sexual vice, and we trust that others, whose position as men of science and teachers enable them to speak with authority, will assist in combating . . . the evils which it entails, and thus enable man to devote more enduring energies and more lofty aims to the advancement of his race, and to the service of his God.

British and Foreign Medico-Chirurgical Review, 1857

The prepuce often becomes a source of serious mischief. In the East, the . . . secretions between it and the glans [are] likely to cause irritation and its consequences; and this danger was perhaps the origin of circumcision. . . . I am fully convinced that the excessive sensibility induced by a narrow foreskin . . . is often the cause of emissions, masturbation, or undue excitement of the sexual desires.

WILLIAM ACTON, *The Functions and Disorders of the Reproductive Organs in Childhood, Youth, Adult Age and Advanced Life,* 1865

By the mid-nineteenth century British doctors were cautiously recommending circumcision as a treatment for masturbation, spermatorrhea, and venereal infections of the penis that caused phimosis in adults, and also as a possible treatment for an increasing list of nervous diseases, such as epilepsy, but the operation was not widely performed because few men could be persuaded to submit to it. Many doctors were reluctant to circumcise even in cases of pathological phimosis,[1] but the more adventurous were willing to follow the practical implications of Lallemand's condemnation of the foreskin as a source of mischief. If it was so much trouble in adulthood yet men were loath to part with it, why not remove it in infancy before it could do serious damage and while the boy was too young to object? The pioneers of circumcision as a preventive, rather than merely curative, procedure included T. B. Curling, James Copland, Jonathan Hutchinson, and J. Cooper Forster, and their efforts bore fruit in the late 1860s, when the medical profession as a whole determined that, unlike clitoridectomy, amputation of the foreskin, even without consent, was not a mutilation. In this chapter I consider the evolution of medical knowledge that led to this pronouncement, during the Baker Brown affair of 1866–67—a watershed in the history of British sexual medicine. I also consider the important contribution of William Acton to medical understandings of genital function, masturbation, childhood sexuality, and the problematization of the foreskin, and finally summarize the case made for preventive male circumcision in the 1850s and 1860s.

In order to make sense of the acceptance of circumcision it is necessary to trace changing conceptions of the differences and similarities between the male and female genitals. Using a one-sex model, traditional anatomy going back to Galen had viewed the genitals as mirror images: the female genitals were an inverted or inward-pointing edition of the male, in which the vagina (a hollow tube) corresponded to the penis, the ovaries to the testicles, and the uterus to the scrotum. In this scenario the foreskin was usually compared to the external female genitalia in their entirety, and more restrictedly to the labia minora; its function was to keep the rest of the penis warm and moist (heat being considered necessary for masculinity) and to provide pleasure to both parties during sexual activity. Galen likened the foreskin to the labia as a whole, proposing that if you turned the male genitals inside out, "the skin at the end of the penis, now called the prepuce, would become the female pudendum," and that if you performed the converse maneuver, "would not the neck [the cervix] . . . be made into the male member? And would not the female pudendum, being a skinlike growth upon this neck, be changed into the part called the prepuce?"[2] An Arabic author of the tenth century wrote that the vagina "possesses prolongations of skin called the lips," which were "the analogue of the prepuce in men and has as its function protection of the matrix [womb] against cold air." Da Carpi used the word *nymphae* to mean both the male foreskin and the labia minora, and in the sixteenth century Charles Estienne reiterated the Galenic paradigm: "what is inside woman likewise sticks out in males, but what is the foreskin in males is the pudendum in women."[3] This paradigm began to break down in the eighteenth century, when it became more common to liken the clitoris to the glans, and then to assume that because the former was the locus of pleasure in women, the latter must be the G-spot in men. But it was a halting and uneven process, and it was not until the nineteenth century that any serious comparisons of the clitoris with the penis appeared, and even then, as the debate over Baker Brown shows, medical opinions were divided. Thomas Laqueur correctly states that Jane Sharp, in her midwifery text (1671), affirms the Galenic paradigm (vagina corresponds to the penis), but that she contradicts herself two pages later by writing that "the clitoris is the female penis."[4] But she does not go so far: all she says is that the clitoris is capable of erection in a manner resembling the penis, writing that it will "stand up and fall as the Yard doth, and make women lustful and take delight in Copulation."[5] This was certainly not to view the clitoris as a female penis, and her perspective is shared by other texts of the period, such as those of Aristotle and Venette. Sharp also reiterated the traditional view that the female labia corresponded to the male foreskin.[6] As the two-sex model emerged in the eighteenth century, however, the old analogies broke down, and the foreskin tended to be seen as the male equivalent of the clitoral hood, which was not a feature mentioned much nor seen as playing any important role. The third edition of the *Encyclopaedia Britannica* (1797) explained that the "foreskin of the clitoris . . . bears a near resemblance and analogy to the praeputium of the male."[7] In his physiology textbooks W. B. Carpenter contributed to the emerging identification of the penis with the clitoris by describing both as "erectile tissue."[8] With the rise of anatomy it was the structure of organs that occupied the center of the medical stage, not how they functioned in real life. And since anatomists before the twentieth century were not able to identify nerve endings accurately, they were not able to see that the only part of the male genitals as densely innervated as the clitoris was the foreskin, particularly the triangular section on the underside of the penis containing the ridged bands.[9] In the new schema the foreskin seemed to have little anatomical significance and thus, it was assumed, no physiological function beyond facilitating masturbation—not an occupation that guaranteed survival in Victorian times.

By the 1850s English doctors were forgetting what their eighteenth-century predecessors had known. Under the influence of the masturbation phobia they regarded any manipulation of the genitals as harmful or wicked, yet under the influence of Lallemand they also came believe that the infant foreskin had to be drawn back regularly so that it could be cleaned underneath, as a precaution against irritation, handling, and the arousal of premature desire. They thus came to view the natural condition of the infant penis (tightly covered in a nonretractable and often adhesive sheath) as a pathological deformity requiring surgical correction. The term *congenital phimosis* came to be applied to any boy, no matter how young, whose foreskin could not easily be drawn back from the glans, and the condition was soon identified as the source of many diseases (from cancer to epilepsy) and a trigger for circumcision, whether signs of disease were present or not. At the same time, physiologists began to claim that the most sensitive, and therefore the most erotically important, part of the penis was not the foreskin but the glans, thus giving doctors the space in which to argue that the removal of the former would have no significant adverse effect on sexual functioning. Acton played an ambivalent role in the triumph of these misapprehensions. On the one hand, he was opposed to circumcision of children and only adopted it as a last resort in adults with serious infections or other problems necessitating surgery. He was also aware that the foreskin of infants and young boys was not normally retractable and thus that "phimosis" was natural in the young. At the same time, however, he regarded the foreskin as a source of moral mischief and physical problems and helped popularize the idea that since it served no useful function, it was a feature whose loss could not be regarded as a serious deprivation. Acton and his contemporaries were uncertain about the normal development of the prepuce: experience taught them that it should be tight and nonretractable in infants and young boys, but Lallemand told them that this condition led to masturbation and spermatorrhea and was therefore wrong. In the end they plumped for medical authority rather than traditional knowledge and their own observations, and in the new perspective adherent prepuces were soon observed everywhere.

The relative sensitivity of glans and foreskin is a more subjective and controversial question. Back in the days when circumcision was a Semitic peculiarity, da Carpi stated that the glans was "compact, hard and dull to sensation so that it may not be injured in coitus," while the job of the "soft skin" that surrounded it was to "furnish some delight in coitus and to guard the glans from external harm."[10] A similar view was expressed by Gabrielle Falloppio (1523–62), who gave directions for stretching inadequate foreskins to make sure that they covered the glans and condemned circumcision as contrary to the intent of nature and destructive of sexual enjoyment.[11] In the seventeenth century Giovanni Sinibaldi understood that the main source of sexual sensation in women was the clitoris and believed that its functional equivalent in the male was not the glans but the foreskin. He also considered that the male's foreskin contributed to women's enjoyment during sex, claiming that this

was why wives with circumcised husbands "most gladly accept the embraces of Christians."[12] The balance of opinion changed during the eighteenth century, and by the 1850s Acton could write that it was "generally
supposed" that the "chief source of sexual pleasure resides in the glans
penis."[13] The main authorities for this view were William Carpenter and
Georg Ludwig Kobelt. In his influential physiology texts, Carpenter
stated that in sexual intercourse it was the glans that increased in sensitivity as a result of erectile turgidity and that the male orgasm was
achieved "by the friction of the glans against the rugous walls of the
vagina."[14] Aristotle's image of the foreskin slipping back and forth has
dropped out of sight. On the genitals specifically, the standard nineteenth-
century work was Kobelt's *Die Mannlichen and Weiblichen Wollusts-Organe
des Menschen und verschiedene Saugetiere* (The male and female organs
of sexual arousal in man and some other mammals), first published in
1844.[15] Havelock Ellis wrote that Kobelt sought to show that "the female
organs are exactly analogous to the male" and commented that it was
only recently that the homology of the clitoris with the penis had come
to be appreciated.[16] This was certainly Kobelt's opinion: "The glans penis is the principal point of reunion of the sensitive nerves of the virile
organ, no other part which it regulates can be compared with it in this
respect. In respect of richness in nerves, the glans penis yields to no
other part, not even the organ of sense." Although he quoted this passage,[17] Acton was not convinced, citing the case of a patient who had lost
the whole of his glans but who reported that sexual intercourse felt no
different from before the accident (115), and specifically disagreeing with
Kobelt's claim that excision of the glans "would destroy all desire, as it is
the rendezvous of the sensitive nerves which excite venereal desires"
(166-67). He was probably as isolated on this question as James Paget on
the physical harmlessness of masturbation, and most doctors imbibed
the teachings of Carpenter and Kobelt. Under the influence of a vulgar
misreading of evolution it was then possible for a quack like Dr. Remondino to be taken seriously when he dismissed the foreskin as an an-
noying vestige from an earlier phase of human existence, the inevitable
disappearance of which should be accelerated by surgery. The loss of
medical knowledge represented by this opinion ensured that there were
few defenders of the foreskin when doctors began to agitate for its early
removal. Although the Baker Brown controversy produced many doctors eager to champion the integrity of the female genitals, not a single
voice was raised in support of the foreskin until the 1890s. Thomas
Laqueur has referred to the "general amnesia" surrounding the importance of the clitoris which descended on scientific circles around 1900
(epitomized in Freud's erroneous claims about the vaginal orgasm).[18] A

similar amnesia regarding the structure and function of the penis began to afflict the British medical profession in the 1840s, leading to equally erroneous claims about the greater sexual importance of the glans.

Although his name became associated with a peculiarly English rejection of sex, William Acton (1814–75) received most of his medical education in France. The second son of a Dorsetshire clergyman, he might have gone into the church himself had his elder brother not beaten him to it; instead he was apprenticed to the apothecary at St. Bartholomew's Hospital in 1831. Five years later he went to Paris, where he read all Lallemand's three volumes and studied the new venereology under Philippe Ricord, a specialist in the genitourinary organs who made important contributions to the understanding of syphilis and other venereal diseases. Returning to London in 1840, Acton became a member of the Royal College of Surgeons, thus acquiring a license to operate, and in 1842 a fellow of the Royal Medical and Chirurgical Society. He married in 1852 at the age of thirty-eight (fairly late even for a man of his time and class) and had at least four children.[19] After qualifying as a surgeon Acton took the then uncommon step of entering private practice as a specialist, and even more remarkably, one focused on venereal disease, and he employed the mercury treatment for syphilis refined by Ricord. From there it was a small step to the treatment of male sexual problems generally, particularly spermatorrhea, with the urethral cauterization technique devised by Lallemand. He made enough money from his medical practice to achieve that dream of every self-made Victorian man, acquisition of a rural estate, where he pursued the life of a country gentleman and died of heart disease at the age of sixty-one. Acton was a frequent contributor to medical journals and published three books: *A Practical Treatise on the Diseases of the Urinary and Generative Organs (in Both Sexes)* (1842, 2nd ed. 1851); *Prostitution Considered in Its Moral, Social and Sanitary Aspects* (1857, 2nd ed. 1870); and *The Functions and Disorders of the Reproductive Organs in Childhood, Youth, Adult Age and Advanced Life* (1857), a shorter work aimed more at the general public than the profession, which sold widely and went through six much revised editions before the author's death.[20] Beyond his medical practice Acton was prominent in public policy debates on prostitution and a supporter of the Contagious Diseases Act and of its extension from garrison towns to the general population; he also took a keen interest in the prosecution of unlicensed practitioners under the Medical Act of 1858 and was an activist with the Society for the Suppression of Vice. The achievement for which Acton was best known in his lifetime, and the main reason why historians study him today, was his popular manual on the male reproductive function, but the context in which the book makes the most sense is not solely a medical one: to appreciate fully its import we must recall that it was written by a clergyman's son and a member of the Vice Society who had probably read his Malthus, and who had certainly read and been shocked by George Drysdale's radical interpretation of his message in *Elements of Social Science.* The message of *Functions and Disorders,* that male chastity was physically healthful and morally desirable, was a direct reply to Drysdale's opposite view.[21]

No one could accuse Acton of trying to conceal his aims. The object of the book was to "enforce" a conviction of "the advantages of continence," a lesson that flowed inexorably from the "scientific facts" recounted (xiv). Or as Acton put it in the preface to the first edition, "the continent student will find reasons for continuing to live according to the dictates of conscience. The dissolute will be taught . . . the value of self-control. . . . The surgeon will learn . . . how to address himself to the audacious old libertine who, setting at naught religious principle and social customs, acts in open defiance of the laws of his country" (vii). There was evidently something for everyone, an interweaving of moral and medical argument which pervades the whole text. By *continence* Acton did not mean moderate sexual activity but "entire abstinence from sexual indulgence in any form."[22] Continence was not only avoiding masturbation and sexual congress but "controlling all sexual excitement" and exercising "complete control over the passions" (47). The "occasional" wet dream was thus not necessarily pathological, since it was "in this way that nature relieves herself," but masturbation was impermissible because no man could call himself chaste if he "by any unnatural means causes expulsion of semen" (47–48); there was no middle course. Strict continence should be observed by all young men until marriage, and he who does not marry "had better direct his thoughts to sexual matters as little as possible" (78). In support of these prescriptions Acton invokes religious feeling as "the greatest preservative of all" (81) and cites not medical authorities but the example of Saint Antony's resistance to temptation and a tract on Christian purity by a Catholic priest (62–65). The chapter on continence is the longest in the book (47–73) and is full of pious sentiments like these, yet it contains little strictly medical and few "scientific facts," a point that probably lay behind the comment of a reviewer that he "dissect[s] the moral and mental phenomena associated with these matters as fully as their medical relations."[23] The chapter on continence is really a sermon, packed with theological exhortation rather than medical advice, and the praise for continence in men looks remarkably like the traditional Christian valuation of virginity in women.

While Acton deploys arguments about the physical damage wrought by sexual excess as a backup, his primary objection is spiritual. He gives us the grisly description of the masturbating boy familiar to us from *Onania* onward—"the frame is stunted . . . the muscles underdeveloped . . . the complexion is sallow . . . [and] covered with spots of acne," and so on (48-49), but his objection to frequent sexual indulgence is more moral than medical:

> Man has other work to do, and to devote the whole energy of his nature to sexual indulgence is literally to . . . destroy those intellectual and moral capacities which distinguish him from the beast, and with the health of which such excessive indulgence is entirely incompatible. (119)

The last point enters only as an afterthought. Like Lallemand, Acton regarded sexual activity as acceptable only within the bonds of marriage and with a view to progeny:

> The moderate gratification of the sex passion in married life is generally followed by the happiest consequences for the individual. And no wonder, for he is but carrying out the imposing command of the Creator in the first book of Genesis . . . in the way appointed by the Almighty Himself. (102)

Acton denounced doctors who recommended sexual intercourse with prostitutes as a way of avoiding masturbation:

> Nothing could ever induce me to . . . recommend illicit sexual intercourse. Setting aside moral considerations, I feel fully convinced that no physiological or other motives can justify a medical man in suggesting . . . the breach of the Seventh Commandment. (79)

It is not at all certain that any doctors suggested traffic with prostitutes as a means of avoiding masturbation, but Drysdale advocated premarital sex for this reason, and he is probably Acton's target at this point. It is significant that Acton did not regard observance of the seventh commandment as a moral requirement, and the Protestant work ethic is not far behind his insistence that continence was indeed related to thrift: "The sighing, lackadaisical boy should be bidden to work . . . and win his wife before he can hope to taste any of the happiness or benefits of married life" (76). It was from a similar stance that Acton, like so many Victorians, urged the importance of will—a man's "intellect and moral nature"—to "thoroughly master [his] animal instincts" (65). He claimed to believe that men could so govern their thoughts as to keep lascivious ones at bay, and even guard themselves against erotic dreams, insisting that it was "not true" that patients cannot control their dreams: "The character is the same, sleeping or waking. It is not surprising that, if a man has allowed his thoughts during the day to rest on libidinous subjects, he finds his mind at night full of lascivious dreams," and he goes on to quote Tissot on the importance of self-control (178–79). Acton's final advice to men and boys—"to live a perfectly continent life, in thought, word and deed" (81)—recalls the General Confession from the Anglican communion service and was most famously taken up by Baden Powell, who copied it almost verbatim as the scouts' tenth law: "A scout is clean in thought, word and deed."[24]

Acton's discussion of masturbation is derived largely from Lallemand and Tissot, and he reproduces their uncertainty about how to define it and the process by which it causes physical damage. He defines it as "ejaculation produced by titillation and friction of the virile member with the hand," but he must have realized this was too narrow, since it excluded masturbation before puberty and nonstandard sexual activity with partners. He thus broadens the definition to include "emission attained by almost any other means than . . . the natural excitement arising from sexual intercourse" and then moves onto a discussion of how the practice arises in *young* boys (24). Even this does not seem to have satisfied him, for by the sixth edition of *Functions and Disorders* he has further broadened the scope of masturbation as "an habitual incontinence eminently productive of disease" (1903, 38). Like Lallemand, he considered that such disease arose both from the loss of semen and the shock of orgasm but was uncertain as to which was worse. In *Practical Treatise* he was "inclined to think that . . . the mischief arises in great part from the exhaustion of the nervous system, rather than from the mere evacuation of so much semen," a proposition supported by the fact that "many of the worst constitutional symptoms of spermatorrhoea may be seen in little children whose testicles do not . . . secrete semen, but who have learnt the early habit of tickling the genital organs."[25] In *Functions and Disorders* he explained that it was nervous shock that made masturbation as dangerous before puberty as afterward (26). In boys too young to emit semen, "friction of the organ is liable to produce that nervous spasm which is, in the adult, accompanied by ejaculation"; because this is often pleasurable, the habit may easily become confirmed (1903, 39). In older boys, masturbation occasioned "shocks from which the youth's nervous system will never rally" (90). Following Tissot, Acton considered that retention of semen was essential to normal development and that boys who masturbated or engaged in premature intercourse stunted their growth and became "pitiable wrecks" (48–49). He also advised that in order to stop masturbation, it was essential to check not just the emission but "the *secretion* of semen," particularly by fatiguing exercise, thus causing the secretion of semen to diminish and emissions eventually to disappear (32).[26] Although he remained undecided on this question, Acton followed the trend of nineteenth-century medical thinking that it was nervous irritation rather than seminal loss that did the most harm—a perspective from which an irritable structure like the foreskin became particularly suspect.

Acton's other major source for the harm of masturbation was Carpenter's physiology texts, which he quotes on the drain that sexual excess imposes on the nervous powers. Acton accepted the "hydraulic" concept of finite bodily forces whereby energy devoted to one activity denied it to others: physical activity reduced the energy available for the production of semen, so that its secretion diminished and sexual desire fell—the reason why he recommended strenuous games "just short of exhaustion" for adolescents.[27] Carpenter had written that the secretion of semen taxed "the corporeal powers" more heavily than was generally supposed, meaning that full "bodily vigour" required only "a very moderate indulgence in sexual intercourse." The nervous excitement of the act "produces a subsequent depression of corresponding amount," while "the too frequent repetition" has "consequences very injurious to the general health. This is still more the case with solitary indulgence."[28] Carpenter had doubts about whether it was appropriate to cite a moral tract on the virtues of purity in what was meant to be a work of scientific physiology, but that did not prevent him from doing so in a lengthy footnote. He justified himself on the ground that too many medical men developed "a laxity of thought and expression . . . that generally ends in a laxity of principle and of action."[29] Given the moralism of the medical profession as expressed in the *British Medical Journal* and the *Lancet,* it is hard to know what he means here, but he could be referring to the rumors that some doctors advised patients suffering from masturbatory urges or spermatorrhea to seek relief from prostitutes, or he could be making another dark allusion to Drysdale. Carpenter himself quotes from a clergyman's tract titled *Be Not Deceived* to explain why emissions within marriage are less debilitating than in illicit intercourse:

> When the appetite is naturally indulged, that is in marriage, the necessary energy is supplied by the nervous stimulus of its natural accompaniment [love] . . . which prevents the injury which would otherwise arise from the increased expenditure of animal power. . . . But when the appetite is irregularly indulged, that is in fornication . . . the energies become exhausted . . . [and] the mere gross animal gratification of lust is resorted to with unnatural frequency, and thus its powers become further exhausted.[30]

It was basically Tissot's explanation,[31] fortified with references to love. Carpenter also provided Acton with authority for his assertion that early death was a frequent result of "the excessive or premature enjoyment of the genital organs."[32]

Both his moralism and his pathological view of male sexuality are apparent in Acton's rules for married life. Because the effects of "marital excess" are similar to self-abuse (125), the adult "should be chary of exhausting those desires which nature has given him for the extension of the species" (234). It was only "excessive" intercourse that caused problems, and Acton makes some attempt to define this ubiquitous concept. Alas, it could only be recognized retrospectively: "An individual committed an excess when coitus was succeeded by languor, depression of spirits or malaise" (125). When a man married he might engage in intercourse so often that his health was permanently impaired, and when he eventually sought medical advice, he would be "thunderstruck at learning that his sufferings arise from such a cause" (122–23). Where Venette had asked how many times a man should caress his wife in a *night* (up to five he considered reasonable),[33] Acton cites Jeremy Taylor's *Rules and Exercise for Holy Living* as the authority for his opinion that "sexual congress ought not to take place more frequently than once in seven or ten days" (111), and he fortifies the bishop's teaching with the alarming discoveries of modern medicine. "So serious is the paroxysm of the nervous system produced by the sexual spasm that its immediate effect is not always unattended with danger, and men have died in the act just as insects perish as soon as the fecundating office has been performed. . . . They are [sometimes] found dead on the night of their wedding" (16–17). An act that might "destroy the weak" should be approached cautiously by the strong and should be repeated "rarely" and quickly—"some few minutes" only (115, 117–18). Since women generally take longer to reach orgasm than men, it is easy to see how adherence to such advice would have meant frustration on the wife's part, no doubt explaining why Acton felt called upon, in his best-known remark (133–34), to reassure husbands that since respectable women did not much like sex, there was no need for them to perform any more often than was safe. Acton tended to view impotence as a less serious problem than incontinence and regarded too many erections as markedly worse than not enough. Priapism was a "terrible and humiliating condition," fortunately rare, while satyriasis (an affliction in which erections were "morbidly frequent and persistent") was "one of the most awful visitations to which humanity can be subject" (160). Impotence was merely a "lamentable state of things" (138).

Although he did not frequently carry out the operation, Acton was a pivotal figure in the acceptance of routine circumcision of male infants and boys. In none of the many editions of his treatises did he advocate general circumcision, but his insistence on the necessity for sexlessness in children and abstinence in young men, coupled with his belief in the pathological irritability of the foreskin, prepared the ground in four ways. First, as we have seen, his construction of male sexuality as a nest of problems and danger, rather than a source of pleasure, made all sexual manifestations suspect and potentially pathological. Second, he gave authority to the notion that the foreskin performed no valuable functions but was a superfluous structure causing nothing but moral danger and physical problems:

> The prepuce . . . is an appendix to the genital organs the use and object of which I could never divine; in place of being of use it leads to a great deal of inconvenience, and the Jews have done well in circumcising their children, as it renders them free from one of the ills of humanity. The prepuce is a superfluous piece of skin and mucous membrane which serves no other purpose than acting as a reservoir for the collection of dirt, particularly when individuals are inattentive to cleanliness.[34]

Acton attributed these comments to Philippe Ricord in the course of a lecture, but a search of Ricord's publications has failed to find it, and the sentiment is not consistent with his other remarks about the foreskin.[35] Various versions of this quotation were in circulation from the 1870s onward and were much cited by advocates of routine circumcision. Third, by propagating the idea that prepubertal children should be asexual, he ensured that evidence to the contrary would be treated as signs of disease or deviance, to be cured or repressed rather than accepted as normal. Fourth, he completed the process of demonizing the foreskin and identified it as the principal source of the sexual problems discussed in his treatise. I consider the third and fourth of these points in more detail.

Nowhere is Acton's "dislocated awareness," as Marcus describes it,[36] more obvious than in his discussion of childhood sexuality. The first sentence of *Functions and Disorders* reads: "In a state of health no sexual idea should ever enter a child's mind"; this is because childhood should be "a period of purity and ignorant innocence" (17). Already we are in a world of moral prescription rather than empirical observation, but a couple of pages later Acton concedes that "in many instances . . . sexual feelings are excited at a very early age, and too often with the most deplorable consequences" (19). He asserts that it would be "well if the child's reproductive organs always remained in this quiescent state until puberty," but this was "unfortunately not the case" (18). Childhood "should be attended by a complete repose of the generative functions" (19), yet at an early age many boys experience erections and display "an almost ungovernable disposition to tickle and scratch the sexual organs"; what was worse, a "quasi-sexual power often accompanies these premature sexual inclinations" (19-21). In his discussion of child and adolescent sexuality it is apparent that Acton well understood that infants and young boys took up masturbation only too readily, hence the need for artificial means to stop it. It is also clear that he was perfectly, though uneasily, aware that what "should be" usually was not, and that many young boys were highly sexual and irresistibly drawn to explore every inch of their bodies. Had he been aiming primarily to widen the boundaries of knowledge he might have accepted this observation as a fact of life and built his theories of sexuality on an empirical foundation; that his reaction was to characterize these manifestations as pathological suggests that he was primarily a moralist whose aim was to stamp them out. Like any disease, he argues, sexual precocity had specific causes: hereditary predisposition; worms in the rectum; irritability of the bladder; irritation of the penis caused by "secretions" trapped under the foreskin; flogging on the buttocks; fondling of the penis by irresponsible nurses; and the example of other boys (20-23). Although he treats sexual precocity as though it was a physical disease, his approach is determined more by moral revulsion than a spirit of inquiry, or even healing, though the danger to health is added for those who are not swayed by his disapproval: "The premature development of the sexual inclination is . . . repugnant to all we associate with . . . childhood . . . [and] fraught with danger to his dawning manhood," he insists. The "dangerous propensity" to premature sexual interest must be "kept in check to preserve the boy's health and innocence" (19). A social construction of the natural is also apparent throughout Acton's discussion of male sexuality. He states that the impulse to masturbation and "premature" sexual congress in adolescent boys is "a natural instinct" (46), but immediately corrects himself to assert that it is not really natural: "Everything—the habits of the world—the keen appetite of youth . . . opportunity—all combine to urge him to give the rein to what seems a natural propensity. Such indulgence is, indeed, not natural, for man is not a mere animal, and the nobler parts of his nature cry out against this violation of their sanctity" (46). Acton appreciates that sexual desire is entirely natural, which is why elaborate artificial means must be employed to teach boys that "these new feelings, powers and delights must not be indulged in" (44–45). It is apparent that what he described as natural was really a cultural preference that had to be imposed by education or force.

With this objective in mind Acton subjects the foreskin to severe scrutiny. He was convinced that it was the major factor in the emergence of sexual precocity and complained that "the influence of the prepuce" on the development of bad habits had "not been sufficiently noted," pointing out that in young boys "the prepuce entirely covers the glans penis, keeping it in that constantly susceptible state which the contact of two folds of mucous membrane induces" (21). Medical opinion had also underestimated "the influence of a long prepuce in producing sexual precocity," but he was sure that "irritation of the glans penis arising from an unusually long prepuce or the collection of secretion under it is another exciting cause. . . . A long and narrow prepuce is . . . a much more common cause of . . . evil habits than parents or medical men have any idea of. The collection of smegma between the glans and the prepuce is almost certain to produce irritation." To prevent this, Acton recommended that boys be instructed "to draw back [their] foreskin and thoroughly cleanse the glans penis every day" (21). He realized that this routine might lead to the very manipulations it was intended to prevent but asserted that his precautions—parental watchfulness, cleanliness, fresh air, and tiring exercise—should usually be sufficient "to remove all ill effects arising from the existence of the prepuce." Yet he remained adamant that the foreskin itself was the root of such problems:

> That the prepuce in man . . . is the cause of much mischief, medical men are pretty well agreed. It affords an additional surface for the excitement of the reflex action, and . . . aggravates an instinct rather than supplies a want. In the unmarried, it additionally excites the sexual desires, which it is our object to repress. (22)

This was ominous enough, but Acton added an even more anxious footnote:

> To the sensitive, excitable, civilized individual, the prepuce often becomes a source of serious mischief. In the East, the . . . secretions between it and the glans [are] likely to cause irritation and its consequences; and this danger was perhaps the origin of circumcision. That the existence of the foreskin predisposes to many forms of syphilis, no one can doubt; and . . . I am fully convinced that the excessive sensibility induced by a narrow foreskin . . . is often the cause of emissions, masturbation, or undue excitement of the sexual desires. (22n)

Already the foreskin is to blame for syphilis, masturbation, the arousal of sexual desire, and the febrile excitability of modern man: why would any conscientious physician not want to cut if off? Although the washing routine was endorsed by the *London Medical Review*,[37] Acton himself must have had doubts about it, for in later editions of *Functions and Disorders* he advised against daily retraction and washing because "the withdrawal of the prepuce appears to promote erection, and to induce a gradual increase in the size of the penis" (1903, 1). To guard against such evils he suggested that daily washing was necessary only in instances where "the smegma is secreted early," but added that as boys grew older, "careful ablutions of the glans and prepuce every morning will be beneficial" (1903, 5). It remained important to teach boys "not to play with the external organs" (22)—a command difficult to reconcile with the necessity for daily washing.

Given Acton's suspicion of the foreskin it is surprising that he did not become an advocate of routine circumcision, an operation he always avoided if possible, "especially in young children" (1903, 7). In treating phimosis in adults he practiced the conservative technique of merely snipping the threads that prevented retraction and did not try to remove the whole structure (1903, 101), and even in cases of serious venereal infections of the penis he followed Ricord in holding that the surgeon "should first bear in mind, that he ought not to operate on the prepuce unless urgent symptoms demand it, particularly if the phymosis be habitual."[38] He followed the debate over whether general circumcision should be introduced, but he had found that men rarely submitted to circumcision, even when there was serious infection or scarring,[39] and thus concluded that the operation was "never likely to be introduced amongst us" (22). It does not seem to have occurred to Acton that fathers might allow things to be done to their children that they would never elect for themselves, and he was out of sympathy with the growing chorus in favor of the operation. Discussing control of "sexual precocity" in the third edition, he wrote that "cases in which an operation may be required on the prepuce are for the surgeon's decision" (22), but this had been deleted by the sixth edition, along with his baleful comment abut the susceptible state induced by the contact of two mucous membranes. By then he was critical of suggestions from "some persons that the universal performance of circumcision would be of no small benefit" in controlling masturbation and other premature sexual arousal, countering that this was merely a speculation, doubting that the idea would be accepted by the public, and insisting that his own precautions were enough to "remove all the ill-effects arising . . . from the retention of the prepuce" (1903, 7). How wrong Acton was on this point was demonstrated by the next generation of physicians, as they took up his strictures against the foreskin and developed them vigorously.

Why Acton did not follow the logic of his position is a puzzle. His reluctance is probably related to his age, generational cohort, and Christian religious convictions, which made it difficult for him to accept an operation that was still a distinctive marker of Jews and Muslims. Second, there was the influence of his teacher Ricord, whom Acton always revered. He not only never dreamed of preventive circumcision in boys but advised against it in most cases of phimosis and other problems arising from venereal infection. Third, there may have been physiological reasons. Unlike his younger colleagues, Acton seems to have appreciated that non-retractability was the foreskin's normal condition in childhood and rarely a problem requiring surgical correction. In later editions of *Functions and Disorders* Acton acknowledged that many boys had such tight or still adhesive foreskins that they could not draw them back without inflicting pain or injury, and perhaps disagreed with the theory of congenital phimosis introduced in the 1840s: "In childhood the penis is naturally small, with the foreskin pointed, and not only completely covering the glans, but even extending beyond it. The attempt to uncover the glans is attended with difficulty in consequence of a natural phymosis, and similarly the process of recovering the glans owing to a natural paraphymosis cannot be accomplished without resort to a degree of violence" (1903, 1). Behind these revisions lies the likelihood that neither Acton nor his contemporaries understood the normal development of the prepuce. They were not sure whether it was meant to be retractable in young boys and offered confused advice about whether it should be left alone, drawn back for cleaning purposes, or simply cut off. It is easy to see how the last option was an attractive tactic to disguise their ignorance. Acton also seems to have realized that the foreskin was desirable for optimum sexual performance (in appropriately moderate husbands only, of course). Acknowledging its contribution to erotic sensation in a positive light for once, he even suggested that in old age the prepuce might be necessary for copulation, for "without it there might be a difficulty in exciting the flagging powers" (23).[40] Why this should worry him, given his warning that old age should be a period of "entire continence" (238), is another puzzle but perhaps points to the existence of a secret war between his moral convictions and his scientific inclinations. Even though he did not appreciate the density of the foreskin's innervation, nor its role in facilitating erection and sexual activity, as a physiologist Acton appreciated its significance for sexual excitability, even though as a moralist he deplored its responsiveness and sought means to neutralize it. Whatever the answer, it was not a scruple that troubled many of his successors.

Of Acton's wide and enduring influence there can be little doubt. The pamphlets issued by the purity movement bristled with warnings about how masturbation would soften boys' muscles, stunt their growth, and destroy their powers of self-control; Sylvanus Stall quoted him, and Edward Lyttelton praised him as "the most eminent of all English authorities on the subject" (i.e., masturbation).[41] As late as 1918 Havelock Ellis referred to him as "the chief English authority on sexual matters."[42] Although his importance has been questioned by some scholars offended by Steven Marcus's rather nonacademic approach,[43] their argument for his lack of influence rests more on his passing references to women's indifference to sex than on his discussion of the male sexual function. Lesley Hall concludes that *Functions and Disorders* was widely read and much referred to; that his construction of male sexuality as a problem was very influential; and that his unforgiving stance on masturbation was more typical than the moderate position of Paget, who was himself the odd man out on this issue.[44] This assessment has been amplified and qualified by Ivan Crozier.[45] Although subsequent scholars have increased our knowledge and refined our understanding, no one has bettered Marcus's characterization of Acton as "a truly representative Victorian: earnest, morally austere yet liberally inclined, sincere, open-minded," determined to help his fellow man yet someone who created a world of fear, "resonant of danger, doom and disaster . . . hedged in with difficulty and pain," inhabited by men evincing "pitiable alienation . . . from their own sexuality."[46] The zeal with which Acton pressed Lallemand's cauterization procedure on men with sexual problems, and the readiness with which they accepted it, bespeaks a world in which male sexuality was regarded as a force to be suppressed rather than a potential to be cultivated.

A number of scholars have drawn attention to the inconsistency between Acton's pragmatic attitude toward prostitution (an unavoidable social phenomenon that should not be the target of suppression but regulated in the interests of public health) and his relentless condemnation of male incontinence.[47] This worldliness is in sharp contrast with the air of unreality surrounding his prescriptions for men: did he remain chaste until his marriage at thirty-eight? Acton was aware of undischarged sexual arousal as a troubling condition and even understood that it could cause "painful affections of the testes" and "many ailments" (77, 204), but his approach was to counsel that men should not have excited themselves in the first place, not that they should restore their equilibrium by sexual release:

> Patients [often] complain that . . . continence . . . produces a most irritable condition of the nervous system, so that the individual is unable to settle his mind to anything. . . . In such cases . . . sexual intercourse has enabled the student . . . to recommence his labours. . . . In all solemn earnestness I protest against such false treatment. It is better to live a continent life. The strictly continent suffer little or none of this irritability; but the incontinent, a soon as the seminal plethora occurs, are sure to suffer. (54–55)

Acton suggests that so long as a boy never yielded to sexual temptation, and thus did not turn on the seminal tap, he would never be troubled by desire; once the tap had been turned on, however, there was no shutting it off. Such a proposition seems highly improbable to us, but Acton had good authority for the assertion, and it became a recurrent theme of later commentary. Joseph Priestley had assured young men that there was no constitutional need for "carnal indulgence" and that if it were "not accelerated by an improper conduct of the mind," the "mutual inclination of the sexes" could be delayed indefinitely.[48] In Rousseau's *Emile* the tutor went further to suggest that any sexual desire was a product of the mind: "it is the imagination which stirs the senses. Desire is not a physical need; it is not a need at all."[49] Such assertions of the power of the rational mind over the animal body suited the antisensualism of the nineteenth century so much that J. S. Mill could think it probable that sexual desire "will become . . . completely under the control of reason."[50] Following Acton, other doctors offered a physiological basis for these views when making statements about the virtues of continence, many of them eagerly quoted by the social purity movement. W. J. Jacobson argued that it was only "incontinent men who are subject to this constant irritability of the sexual organs"; continent men "who keep themselves healthily occupied in mind and body, when attacked by imperious sexual desire, simply sally out and seek in exercise a change of surroundings." Jacobson even repeated Acton's teaching that physical exercise would lower the secretion of semen, thus reducing the incidence of wet dreams.[51] Another authority affirmed that the sexual organs could "lie dormant for years . . . and forgotten . . . until the time comes for matrimony."[52] The idea behind these pronouncements was that the penis should and could be put to sleep from infancy until marriage, and there was no shortage of doctors offering soporifics. If reason did not do the trick, there was always surgery.

By Acton's time circumcision of infants and boys was increasingly suggested as a cure or preventive of infantile phimosis, masturbation, epilepsy, retention of urine, and bed-wetting. In proposing the theory that a nonretractable foreskin in infancy was a pathological abnormality, Charles West and J. Cooper Forster were perhaps the originators of "congenital phimosis" as a disease condition. West claimed that a tight foreskin could cause many problems: "This congenital phimosis . . . [often causes] incontinence of urine in children, and is also an exciting cause of . . . masturbation owing to the discomfort and irritation which it constantly keeps up. In every case, therefore, where any difficulty attends the passing or the retention of urine , or where . . . masturbation is suspected, the penis ought to be examined, and circumcision performed if the preputial opening is too small."[53] The notion of congenital phimosis as a disease was further developed by Forster, yet what a strange disease it was, for he described it as a condition in which the boy was "in perfect health" but wants to urinate often and "frequently seizes the penis, as if it itched, and elongates the prepuce." Closer investigation revealed that the foreskin could not be withdrawn without "much pain to the patient," meaning that it was difficult for the doctor to examine the glans and meatus. Sometimes the prepuce became distended when the boy urinated—a phenomenon that had not worried Pierre Dionis but that was apparently no longer acceptable in polite households. Although Forster acknowledged that such boys were perfectly healthy, he had no hesitation in classifying the features he identified as a disease he called "urinary irritation arising from . . . congenital phimosis": "With a part so plentifully supplied with nerves . . . any undue irritation at the extremity of the penis . . . give[s] rise to symptoms connected with the bladder, and therefore the constant contact of the prepuce with the orifice of the urethra sufficiently accounts for the frequent desire to micturate. . . . The irritation and itching have their origins in the masses of filthy secretion poured out by the glandulae Tysoni." Urinary irritation was not a conventional organic disease but one of those "anomalous diseases of a purely sympathetic character" that arise simply from irritation. Just as the nagging of a tooth could produce "cephalic symptoms" that disappeared when the tooth was extracted, so irritation of the foreskin could produce symptoms of disease in the bladder, which might be alleviated in like manner. An alternative approach was to withdraw the prepuce and regularly wash away the secretions, but circumcision was a more reliable method not only as therapy but as an anticipation of future problems: "if this operation were more frequently performed upon young children, even when suffering from much less severe symptoms . . . it would do much to prevent . . . many of the diseases and troubles that occur in after-life." Forster asserted that "every surgeon" was aware of the advantages of circumcision in adults: "Who has not seen the annoyance of retained secretion, syphilitic sores under the prepuce, the swelling accompanying gonorrhoea &c as a result of congenital phymosis?" Anticipating Acton's characterization, he condemned the foreskin as "a source of evil" when it could not be uncovered and concluded his pioneering paper with a detailed description of how to perform the operation that would permanently solve these problems.[54]

It is important to understand the chain of reasoning here. In the past adults had left boys' foreskins alone, and the vast majority of them developed normally from adhesion to separation as the boys grew up. When masturbation became a worry it was proposed that the practice could be stopped by stringent cleanliness around the glans, an operation requiring the retraction of the foreskin: as Forster explained, the nurse must "carefully wash away the secretion which may form, which may easily be done by withdrawing the prepuce from the glans"; but since nearly all infants and most boys under five had foreskins that would not retract, or only with pain and difficulty, this was found to be impractical. Since masturbation was the main fear, doctors reached the logical conclusion that their prescription for subpreputial scrubbing was not erroneous, but that the adhesive foreskin was a congenital malformation, a "disorder" arising from "Nature having been too prolific in the supply of skin at the extremity of the penis." There was a simple method of dealing with that.

Forster's article attracted a warm commendation from the young Jonathan Hutchinson, later regarded as an expert on venereal disease but at that time a struggling GP in London's unfashionable East End and an editorial assistant at the *Medical Times and Gazette*.[55] In an influential article of his own, Hutchinson confessed that it had long been his own opinion that it was "the duty of the surgeon invariably to remove the prepuce of infants born with congenital phimosis"; in support of Forster's recommendation of "the more general practice of circumcision as a preventive of certain diseases of childhood," he contributed his own alarming discoveries about the greater vulnerability of normal penises to syphilis, as proved by the relative immunity of (circumcised) Jews to that disease. I discuss the argument that circumcision offered protection against syphilis in chapter 12; for now it is enough to note that Hutchinson regarded "congenital phimosis" in itself as a sufficient reason for a speedy amputation of the prepuce.[56]

Forster had referred to the "problem" of boys seizing their penis and stretching their foreskin. He might genuinely have regarded these manipulations as a response to itching, but many physicians in the 1850s would immediately have sniffed something far worse: masturbation. Lallemand and Acton had identified the foreskin as the major incitement to masturbation in boys before puberty, but the first English writers to insist on the connection and recommend circumcision were possibly T. B. Curling and James Copland. During a discussion of spermatorrhea, Curling wrote that "removal of an elongated prepuce has been attended with a good effect" in some cases, adding that "in lads addicted to masturbation this operation is very effectual. It at once breaks the habit, which, in many instances, is not afterwards renewed."[57] In his influential *Dictionary of Practical Medicine* Copland introduced the idea that "the neglect of circumcision in Christian countries" was a common cause of this vice and praised the descendants of Abraham and the "followers of Mahomet" for perpetuating "an enduring and healthy race" as one of the "beneficial results of circumcision." In treating cases of masturbation Copland argued that persons who lacked the willpower to restrain their immoral impulses were often really the victims of "physical conditions and local irritations," meaning that vicious behavior like masturbation was more the result of their physical makeup than a failure of reason and volition: "the occurrence of this vice is remarkably favoured by the physical condition of the male genitals, especially as regards the neglect of circumcision. I am convinced that the abrogation of this rite among Christians has been injurious to them, in religious, in moral, in physical, and in sanitary [*sic*] and constitutional points of view,—that circumcision is a most salutary rite."[58] In suggesting that masturbators were badly constructed rather than naughty, Copland laid out the poles of the debate about its control, which continued for the next century. Was it an ethical failing, requiring counseling and stronger will? Or was it a physical problem requiring medical (perhaps surgical) intervention? The position of the doves and hawks on the issue had been identified. At around the same time, the first reports of circumcision among Muslims and Jews began to appear in the medical journals, giving rise to the idea that what had once been thought of as purely a religious rite was also (perhaps more significantly) a meaningful part of the surgical repertoire.[59] As Copland warned, "he who devotes himself to self-pollution . . . should duly consider the severe denunciations and punishments which it provoked from the Jewish legislator."

An equally vehement advocate of circumcision as a treatment for masturbation was Athol W. Johnson, surgeon to the hospital for sick children. In a lengthy article published in 1860 he described the sad case of six-year-old George A—, formerly a healthy boy who was sickening inexplicably, and the stern methods employed to deal with his problem:

> It was soon noticed that his hand was frequently applied to his penis, which was often in a state of erection, and that the prepuce was somewhat elongated. . . . Suspicion arising on the part of his parents, a close watch was set upon him, when it was discovered that he was nightly in the habit of practising onanism. To put a stop to this, various means were adopted, including severe punishments by his father, after which he would promise to abstain, but during sleep he would get restless and excited, and on waking up would continue the practice. . . .
>
> His hands were then fastened out of bed, but he still effected his purpose by a peculiar convulsive or instinctive movement of the thighs. Repeated immersion in cold water at these times, and all other plans suggested having been employed ineffectually, as a last resource he was brought to the hospital. . . .

He was directed to sleep with his hands out of bed, and under the immediate surveillance of the night nurse. After the first night or two, the restlessness and movements were resumed, but of course immediately arrested. He was then placed on bromide of potassium, and afterward on belladonna. Perfect cleanliness was inculcated, especially with regard to any secretion between the foreskin and the glans; and bathing etc was ordered. At the same time he was informed that it would be necessary, on account of his health, to perform an operation, with the hope that the dread of this might prove effectual; but the nocturnal excitement still continued, and I have at last removed a portion of the foreskin, without placing him under chloroform. Since the operation he has been perfectly quiet, and he has now left the hospital, with instructions that he is to be brought back if any relapse occurs.

Johnson justified his approach by explaining how organic and intellectual functions in both boys and girls could be deranged through excitation of the nervous system arising from masturbation and why the utmost effort must be made to check the tendency before it became a habit. Surveillance, cleanliness, and the removal of local irritations were essential in infancy, and in childhood these should be supplemented by tiring exercise, keeping the hands outside the bedclothes "or actually fastened down," installation of a rubber shield, and administration of potassium bromide (for its "emasculating properties") and belladonna as a sedative. If these interventions failed it was necessary to break the habit "by inducing such a condition of the parts as will cause too much local suffering to allow of the practice being continued. For this purpose, if the prepuce is long, we may circumcise the male patient with present and probably future advantage; the operation should *not* be performed under chloroform, so that the pain experienced may be associated with the habit we wish to eradicate." Johnson was thinking mainly of boys, though he believed that masturbation was also common in girls. Noting that a Dr. Gros had advocated "complete or partial amputation of the clitoris" as the treatment most similar to circumcision, he considered that this would be called for only in extreme cases where "furious masturbation" was "associated with congenital malformation of the organ." Surgical intervention was called for less often in girls because "the practice seems to be more easily checked by surveillance than it is in males."[60] Johnson's report elicited an enthusiastic letter from Dr. Robert Fowler, seeking confirmation that circumcision would reduce the incidence of onanism; he could not recall even a suspected case among his Jewish clientele but regretted he could not say the same about Christian boys.[61] Another correspondent asked if Jewish boys were less prone to bed-wetting, citing a case in which a French doctor had circumcised a boy "for obstinate nocturnal incontinence," apparently with success.[62] Interest in the new therapy was growing.

Epilepsy was soon identified as another mysterious nervous malady induced by masturbation and curable by circumcision. Men had sometimes been treated for epilepsy by castration,[63] but by the 1860s it was suggested that the real cause was nervous irritation induced by either masturbation or the secretions trapped by congenital phimosis. N. Heckford, a surgeon at London Hospital, argued that masturbation could provoke epilepsy and other nervous diseases via "excitement of the cerebrospinal and vaso-motor systems," leading to "nervous prostration" and debility. He felt it was not widely realized that masturbation was practiced by young children and even infants, and cited the case of a fifteen-month-old boy suffering from a deformity that caused his legs to remain crossed. It was noticed that his penis was often erect from friction on the thighs and that he had "congenital phymosis" but seemed to have no trouble urinating. He was circumcised by Mr. Hutchinson, and the masturbation ceased "for a time at least," though his subsequent history was unknown. Heckford himself circumcised five boys aged from six to thirteen years and suffering from epilepsy or chorea induced by masturbation. The mother of an eight-year-old reported that he "was constantly 'pulling his privates about', and that she frequently punished him" with little success, but eight months after the operation the chorea had vanished, his health "had greatly improved, and he had been completely cured of his former bad habit." Heckford could not claim the same results with the other boys but concluded that "the partial success of the . . . treatment" was "sufficient to warrant a repetition . . . in similar cases." The value of circumcision in these situations was that it both broke the habit of masturbation and, in children with phimosis, prevented the accumulation of irritating secretions. For good results, however, it was necessary "to remove the prepuce freely [i.e., cut tightly], and to delay as long as possible the process of healing."[64] A couple of years later it was reported that congenital phimosis had been observed in eleven out of twenty-five epilepsy cases admitted to the London Infirmary for Epilepsy and Paralysis, naturally raising the possibility of a reliable association. The author of the report regretted that so many doctors neglected to examine the genitals in nervous cases, thereby overlooking the possible effects of congenital phimosis, and emphasized that "this malformation has considerable pathological importance." In such cases there was "always an accumulation of sebum between the prepuce and the gland [sic]. . . . This irritation often leads to great sexual excitement about the period of puberty, and to masturbation, with all its consequent evil effects; frequent emissions of semen at night may also be traced to the same cause. A variety of cerebral symptoms may then be induced . . . which, where they depend only upon this condition, may be entirely removed by circumcision." Although epileptic fits were probably not the direct consequence of phimosis, it was always legitimate to perform the operation in these cases, since "all sources of irritation should, on principle, be removed in convulsive disorders." Several patients at the infirmary had been circumcised without any cessation of their fits, but the supervising physician reported that "it generally seemed" as if the disorder "yielded more readily to the remedies employed than it had done before."[65] That, apparently, was enough.

7 · A Compromising and Unpublishable Mutilation

Clitoridectomy and Circumcision in the 1860s

But in the cutting away of this small bit, I warn that we should proceed scrupulously, if indeed the woman ought to be eager for bearing children in wedlock; if ever it happens that the quite pleasant little tag of love is removed also from there, and as a result the woman comes back to intercourse less cheerfully, she will engage in the office of procreation more coldly and more sluggishly; from this cause indeed barrenness often arises.

GIOVANNI SINIBALDI, *Geneanthropeiae,* as quoted in the *British Medical Journal,* May 1866

Clitoridectomy is neither more nor less than circumcision of the female; and as certainly as that no man who has been circumcised has been injured in his natural functions, so it is equally certain that no woman who has undergone the operation . . . has lost one particle of the natural function of her organs.

ISAAC BAKER BROWN, 1867

By the time of the Baker Brown scandal the medical profession had accepted circumcision of boys as a useful treatment for phimosis, nervous complaints such as epilepsy and urinary complaints, and most importantly, masturbation.[1] Clitoridectomy was also being recommended by some European doctors for masturbation in girls, but English authorities were not convinced that girls were so wedded to the habit that such a drastic approach was needed. The outcome of the controversy over Baker Brown's operations was to confirm these understandings, thereby protecting the genitals of girls while declaring open season on those of boys. To understand the rise of male circumcision in Britain and the failure of attempts to introduce widespread clitoridectomy it is necessary to set aside the common prejudice that nineteenth-century medicine sought to repress female sexuality in the interests of patriarchal dominance or that Victorian men were anticlitoris because they had no interest in the pleasure of their partners. Despite, or perhaps because of, women's generally subordinate position, the truth is more complex: while women's sexual enjoyment (only in marriage, of course) was regarded as morally proper and physically beneficial,[2] men's sexual desires were increasingly condemned as lustful urges, dangerous to themselves and others, which had somehow to be reined in.

Unlike male circumcision, clitoridectomy was an exotic procedure about which English doctors knew little. Their main source of information at midcentury was a single article by W. F. Daniell, "On the Circumcision of Females in Western Africa" (1847), which combined a functionalist anthropological perspective on the customs of savage tribes with a stereotypically Victorian recoil from sexual depravity. On the one hand Daniell felt it was reasonable to assume that in the past the procedures "constituted no unimportant branch of medical hygiene, and that probably . . . fragmentary data may more explicitly unfold the use and purport of this singular custom—one among many that has been faithfully preserved by the African races through the lapse of centuries." This reading was similar to the theories about the materialist (hygienic) origin of male, particularly Judaic, circumcision that were emerging at the same time. On the other hand, "social life in most of the pagan towns . . . is darkened by scenes of the grossest demoralisation. . . . An illicit and promiscuous sexual intercourse is constantly carried on by nearly all classes of slave subjects, who, not fettered by any moral obligations, and solely intent on the gratification of their passions, give them an unrestrained rein long before the age of puberty." That was just the sort of sexual disorder the Victorian middle class dreaded: while male circumcision was associated with chaste and industrious Jews, the female version conjured up images of primitive debauchery.[3]

Although several European authorities had recommended clitoridectomy to treat nymphomania,[4] they had few English followers. One was Samuel Atwell, who wrote in 1844 that "an enlarged clitoris" was sometimes marked "by exquisite sensibility of its mucous membrane," which often "gives rise to sexual passion and subdues every feeling of modesty." The result was headaches, attacks of hysteria, and loss of mental discipline, and Atwell recommended extirpation of the organ in these instances.[5] English doctors tended to be skeptical, but one cited a comment in Thomas's *Practice of Physic* that "as the clitoris is the seat of pleasure . . . nymphomania might possibly be cured by extirpating the organ."[6] He also referred to the case of a young French woman whose constant masturbation had so sapped her strength that her parents took her to a Dr. Dubois, who removed the organ and reported complete success in curing her habit.[7] Comparisons between the male and female anatomies were central to the debate over clitoridectomy, but it was widely assumed that the foreskin and clitoris had similar a function and played the same vital role in masturbation. Doctors did not write in Atwell's terms about the penis, but it is exactly how they characterized the foreskin. Sander Gilman has noted that the German authority Hermann Rohleder advocated circumcision for male masturbators and burning of the clitoris with acid for female, and comments that "circumcision and clitoridectomy were seen as analogous medical procedures."[8]

The Baker Brown affair is often cited as evidence of the Victorian medical profession's hostility to women's sexual enjoyment, but its deeper lessons lie in the other direction.[9] Brown's disgrace showed that the profession appreciated the significance of women's sexuality for happy and fruitful marriages, with the result that they were largely spared the sort of operations on their external genitalia that became commonplace on boys.[10] Assumptions about women's natural purity and relative lack of interest in sex had their obverse in the view of men as wild beasts who needed to be tamed. These attitudes helped establish the principle that while clitoridectomy, even as a treatment for masturbation, was an outrageous mutilation, amputation of the foreskin was unobjectionable; there was a double standard, but in this area it operated to women's advantage. Despite this, it is remarkable how close the British medical profession came to endorsing clitoridectomy. Had the controversy blown up a few years later, after Richard Burton's revelations about the sophistication of ancient Muslim civilization, female circumcision might have seemed less barbaric and more acceptable, for as he wrote in the notes to his translation of *A Thousand and One Nights,* "female circumcision . . . is the proper complement of male circumcision, evening up the sensitiveness of the genitories by reducing it equally in both sexes: an uncircumcised woman has the venereal orgasm much sooner and oftener than a circumcised man, and frequent coitus would be injurious to her health."[11] Brown was part of a widespread movement to apply the logic of nervous disease theory and the lessons of male circumcision to the part of women's genitals most resembling the foreskin in function, and in the early years of his activities (1858–65) he attracted considerable interest and support. Scores of medical men flocked to watch him operate at the London Surgical Home, and many were keen to try the same techniques in their own practice. It was only after the publication of his book in 1866 that the determined opposition of a few members of the Obstetrical Society turned professional opinion around, and with a rapidity that left Brown all but speechless. He had thought it was enough to insist that clitoridectomy was merely female circumcision; since circumcision was already accepted as a legitimate treatment for nervous complaints in men, it followed that the medical profession must endorse the equivalent operation in women. To his surprise and dismay, they declared that it was not equivalent at all.

Isaac Baker Brown (1812–73) became one of London's leading obstetric surgeons. After qualifying in 1834, he entered general practice before specializing in gynecology, became an accoucheur of some repute, and helped to found St. Mary's Hospital. He occupied various surgical posts in other London hospitals, pioneered several tricky operations on the female reproductive organs, and published a textbook on women's diseases in 1856.[12] He belonged to prestigious medical societies and enjoyed fame as an operator: in the words of an obituary, the publication of his textbook *Surgical Diseases of Women* "established his celebrity as an operator at once bold, ingenious and successful. . . . His operating theatre was one of the most attractive to the professional visitor in all London, admiration being invariably evoked by his brilliant dexterity and the power he displayed by the use of his left hand when operating on the female perineum."[13] He was firmly ensconced at the respectable end of the medical spectrum, bearing no taint of quackish practices—not, that is, until he encountered Dr. Brown-Sequard's "Lectures on the Physiology and Pathology of the Central Nervous System" in 1858.[14] After reading these Brown was struck by "the great mischief which might be caused in the system generally, and in the nervous centres especially, by peripheral excitement." Sequard's research threw new light on hysterical and other mysterious nervous afflictions in women, leading Brown to the conclusion that the most obstinate cases "depended on peripheral excitement of the pudic nerve." He put the theory to the test by "removing the cause of the excitement" and was so impressed with the results that he left St. Mary's and established a small private clinic, the London Surgical Home, where he specialized in the procedure so coyly alluded to. Brown's greater respectability compared with Acton is nowhere better illustrated than in his refusal to use the term *masturbation,* although that is what he meant by peripheral irritation.[15] The first fruits of his reading were apparent in the second edition (1861) of his textbook, *On Some Diseases of Women Admitting of Surgical Treatment,* to which he added a new section on the hypertrophy and irritation of the clitoris, conditions he believed to be "more frequent . . . than most medical men suspect" and that were mostly brought about by self-abuse: "The deplorable effects of this baneful habit both on the physical and mental health have been less considered in the case of females than of men, and yet they are of equal gravity, and probably as prevalent." Fortunately, a rapid cure was easily achieved by the excision of the offending tissue.[16] Brown was doing his best to demonize the clitoris in the same way that Lallemand, Copland, and Acton had demonized the foreskin.

All went well for a few years: many other members of the Obstetrical Society came to see Brown in action, and the Home gained a reputation for successful treatments of uterine prolapse, tumors, and other real diseases. It was only when he sought permanent fame by compiling a book based on his experience there that his medico-commercial enterprise came unstuck. In early 1866 Brown published a compendium of his cases,[17] preceded by a theoretical introduction in which he explained that he was applying the theories of nervous disease already being advanced as a rationale for male circumcision, especially in cases of masturbation, to women, and treating them in analogous manner by amputating the clitoris. He was convinced that "a large number of affections peculiar to females depended on loss of nervous power . . . produced by peripheral irritation, arising originally in some branches of the pudic nerve, more particularly the incident nerve supplying the clitoris, and sometimes the small branches which supply the vagina, perineum and anus." Brown insisted that there was nothing new in this. In addition to Sequard's lectures he cited Handfield Jones's *Functional Nervous Disorders,* from which he had learned that "a nervous centre may be more or less completely paralysed, without having undergone organic change, in consequence of some enfeebling morbid influence," and that "the general exhaustion induced by excess of venery . . . show[s] how excessive consumption of nerve force in one part weakens it also in others." Jones was referring to intercourse as much as other forms of excitement, but Brown was particularly interested in diseases "arising from a loss of nerve tone caused by continual abnormal irritation of the nerve centre," and we know what he meant by that. He laid out a seven-stage process of degeneration, beginning with hysteria and ending with mania and death, commenting that the "severity of the functional affections . . . depended on the amount and length of irritation and the consequent amount of loss of nerve power," and he cited the case of a thirty-two-year-old male to prove that "complete paralysis" followed by death was indeed the climax of "excessive venereal indulgence."[18] All this was perfectly orthodox by contemporary Victorian medical standards.

Brown claimed that other doctors agreed that a cure in these cases required the neutralization of the offending nerve but that they were undecided as to the best method. Some used cautery (either hot metal or silver nitrate), but he felt his treatment was both more effective and more humane. He acknowledged that the innovatory nature of his approach had provoked criticism, but he denied that his operation "unsex[ed] the female, prevent[ed] the normal excitement consequent upon marital intercourse, or . . . cause[d] sterility," and he insisted on its moral value: the object of the treatment was "cure of a disease that is rapidly tending to lower the moral tone . . . dictated by the loftiest and most moral considerations." He warned that nervous irritation could "unhinge" the mind from "that steadiness which is essential to enable it to keep the passions under control of the will; to enable . . . the moral tone to overcome abnormal excitement." He thus agreed with Dr. Copland that it was perfectly legitimate for surgery to come to the aid of moral exhortation, for was it not likely that cases treated by "spiritual advisers as controllable at the will of the individual may be . . . cases of physical illness amenable to medical and surgical treatment?" As with boys, the problem behind female masturbation was anatomical.[19]

The initial response to Brown's book was cautiously favorable, and there were guarded but positive reviews in the *Lancet* and the *British Medical Journal*. The reviewers' main reservations were whether Brown had enough evidence to prove his case, whether milder treatments (such as caustics) might be sufficient, and whether moral influences might be more effective than surgery. A surprising convert was the *Church Times*, which greeted the book with glowing enthusiasm for offering "a remedy for some of the most distressing cases of illness which [the clergy] discover among their parishioners."[20] The *British Medical Journal* was more skeptical but not affronted, doubting the efficacy but not the propriety of the operation, since it had "long been an established fact that onanism practised to the extent supposed by Mr Brown will occasion all the various nervous disorders named." The reviewer suggested that Brown's cases showed that the operation often had good results but suspected that he had exaggerated his achievements and wanted further information before endorsement could be given.[21] The *Lancet* responded similarly: "If it can be clearly shown that [these] diseases . . . are due to irritation of the clitoridian branch of the pudic nerve, and that the operation . . . effectually and forever removes the irritation, all persons will agree that it should be performed . . . after other methods of treatment have been found to no avail." The reviewer's hesitation was over whether Brown had established these vital points.[22]

Brown's thesis was the subject of a discussion at a meeting of the Obstetrical Society on 5 December 1866, when Dr. T. Hawkes Tanner read a paper with the explicit title "On Excision of the Clitoris as a Cure for Hysteria etc." Like the reviewers, Tanner questioned not the legitimacy of the operation but its effectiveness, arguing that clitoridectomy was unlikely to prove "of permanent value" as a cure for epilepsy and similar afflictions for four main reasons. First, although removal of the clitoris was "analogous to circumcision in the male," the latter had additional advantages, but since castration could not cure epilepsy or insanity, neither could circumcision. Second, even if these diseases were caused by peripheral irritation of the pudic nerve, removal of the clitoris left other branches of this nerve intact. Third (and here Tanner quoted the article by Daniell), the African nations that practiced clitoridectomy still presented "scenes of female licentiousness and debauchery." Fourth, he himself had excised the clitoris in three cases and had been "disappointed in the results." In the discussion that followed there was a good deal of argument over Tanner's analogy between circumcision and clitoridectomy. Dr. Routh agreed that it was "a kind of extended circumcision," yet differed from Tanner in believing that the operation was often successful. He cited the cases of "an idiot girl who . . . improved so as to read the Bible and converse and . . . was now in service," and of lady who used to have seven fits daily but was now entirely free of them. Routh insisted that it was correct to perform clitoridectomy in cases in which caustics and blistering had failed and that it was not an invalid procedure merely because it was not always successful. Dr. Tyler Smith, by contrast, in opposing clitoridectomy felt obliged to emphasize that it was not in the least like circumcision: "The prepuce was a very unimportant structure as compared with the clitoris. As regarded sensation, the clitoris was the analogue of the male penis, and was the organ of sexual sensibility in the female. . . . [Its removal] in cases of hysteria and self-abuse could not be justified. We might as well think of removing the penis in cases of masturbation in the male." Dr. Greenhalgh supported Tyler Smith with the contention that "the frequency and evil effects of self-abuse in the female had been greatly exaggerated"; he believed that the practice arose not from the condition of the genitals but from lack of moral control. Greenhalgh became one of the leaders of the reaction against clitoridectomy, and his opinion that women did not masturbate enough to justify such a drastic response became one of the chief arguments of Brown's critics. If the operation were effective in nervous diseases it was justifiable, but he considered it based on a "false theory as to the cause of these conditions," for "although self-abuse was temporarily checked by loss of blood [and] soreness of the parts . . . ultimately the irritation and the habit returned with increased intensity." Brown's own contribution to the debate consisted mainly of references to cases in which his operation had cured women of whatever had ailed them, from paralysis of the limbs to incontinence of urine. He particularly rejected Tyler Smith's observations and emphasized that "his operation did not alter sexual excitement on marriage . . . not only had many of his patients borne children after clitoridectomy, but he had now five cases in which, from having disliked marital intercourse and preferred self-abuse, the state of things had been entirely changed after the operation." At this meeting Brown had both supporters and opponents, but the discussion was conducted in a spirit of professional interest and scientific inquiry. As Dr. Rogers summed up, it was clear that the operation had produced "great good" in some cases and failed in others, but that was no reason for denouncing it; the Society was "bound to inquire into the facts in a calm and dispassionate manner."[23] It was a very different atmosphere that prevailed when the Society met to consider a motion for Brown's expulsion only four months later.

A less gentlemanly debate raged in the correspondence columns of the medical journals, but the central concerns there were similar: Was clitoridectomy the equivalent of male circumcision? Was it effective? Did the operation destroy all sexual feeling, or did it merely reduce excitability to the point where masturbation was no longer worth the effort? One of the first responses was from Thomas Littleton, of Saltash, who offered the observations of Sinibaldi as a warning against "such a serious mutilation" and asked whether Brown would "resort to an analogous deprivation in cases of the same diseases similarly induced in the male," on the principle that what was sauce for the goose was sauce for the gander. What analogy Littleton had in mind he did not spell out, but unless Saltash was very far behind the times he must have known that circumcision was already being performed on males in these cases, and it follows that he must have assumed that the clitoris corresponded to the whole penis.[24] A different view was put forth by an anonymous Fellow of the Royal Society who doubted the "old opinion" that the clitoris was the chief source of female pleasure and thus that its removal would cure nymphomania. He had no objection to the operation and seems to have viewed it in the same light as doctors were coming to regard male circumcision: "The operation is . . . devoid of danger—its removal of little consequence. . . . Why then should such importance be attached to a harmless operative procedure upon so rudimentary an organ?"[25] Another correspondent took the opposite line, insisting on the importance of the clitoris and regretting that so few women seemed alive to its potential: "I am sorry that females have not as much knowledge of the clitoris as we have, for if that were the case I am sure there were very few who would consent to part with it, and when questioned about it afterwards say, 'Oh, I have only had a little knot removed.' Verily they know not the nature of that little 'knot.'" He thought it perfectly proper for doctors to educate patients as to the sexual function of body parts about whose potential they were ignorant and considered that medical practitioners had "scarcely more right to remove a woman's clitoris than . . . to deprive a man of his penis."[26] The *Lancet* weighed in authoritatively with the bold claim that "everyone must admit that the clitoris is the anatomical homologue of the penis,"[27] but that is exactly what Brown's party was not admitting. Dr. Routh came back with anatomical evidence that clitoridectomy was indeed no more than circumcision, claiming that "during the venereal orgasm it is not the clitoris or the crura alone which become erected, though, like the glans penis, the clitoris may be the most sensitive part, but the entire erectile system becomes turgid. . . . Until you can remove all these parts . . . with the clitoris you have not removed the analogue of the penis."[28] Routh embodied the new understandings that the penis was what became tumescent and that its most sensitive region was the glans. He was supported by a Dr. Shettle, who wrote that it was not correct "to regard the clitoris simply as the homologue of the penis" because "the vast difference in the construction of the organs of generation in the two sexes" meant that while cutting off the penis would be fatal to reproduction, no such outcome would result from clitoridectomy.[29]

The battle over the medical legitimacy of clitoridectomy was thus fought around the questions of whether the clitoris was the female equivalent of the penis and whether its removal was the equivalent of circumcision: amputating part of the penis was acceptable, cutting off the entire organ was going too far. Such a debate would have been impossible under the old one-sex model in which the penis was seen as the analogue of the vagina and the foreskin of the labia. This schema had broken down, but traces of it remained in the doctors' determination to seek similarities between the male and female genitals; only Dr. Shettle was sufficiently up to date to suggest that the two ensembles were so different that it was a misconceived quest. The theoretical acceptance of circumcision as a cure for masturbation and nervous diseases in men is shown by the arguments of Brown and his supporters: to secure legitimacy for their operation they had to convince their colleagues that clitoridectomy was the female version of what had already been accepted as useful in young males. His opponents had to defeat this argument, and in doing so they promoted the misleading propositions that the foreskin was expendable and that the clitoris was the analogue of the penis; even fanatics were not going to recommend amputation of that. But although the medical arguments revolved around the question of equivalence, this was not the issue that generated the bulk of the opposition to Brown, nor was defeat on this point the decisive factor in his ruin. Arguments about the effectiveness of the operation and its impact on sexual enjoyment were recruited to serve a more urgent anxiety: its ethical standing and moral propriety.

Although doubts on these grounds had been raised as soon as the reviews of his book alerted doctors outside London to what Brown was doing,[30] it was not until autumn that the winds of opinion began to blow strongly against him. When two prominent figures who had previously supported his procedures turned against him, disowning their own past as much as his present, the trickle of objections grew to a flood. The first of these was Charles West, a leading gynecologist with his own skeleton in the cupboard: as the author of a standard text, *Lectures on the Diseases of Women* (1864), he had made the suddenly embarrassing comment that "if the habit [masturbation] could be overcome, if the mind could be restored to its purity by any mutilation of the person, one would feel that no penalty would be too great to pay for such a boon."[31] Brown triumphantly quoted this passage in his confident reply to critics in November, when he denied their three main complaints: that the operation "unsexed a woman" and was thus a mutilation; that masturbation could be successfully treated by moral persuasion; and that recognition of the frequency of the habit might alert the pure-minded to undreamed of possibilities. On the first point he reported that a number of his patients had become pregnant following the operation, thus proving that the clitoris was "not an essential part of the generative system." He also pounced on the obvious contradiction in West's position: if, as he had observed in his textbook, "the seat of sexual pleasure is by no means confined to the clitoris," how could he call its removal a mutilation? On the second point he reasserted his conviction that it was perfectly proper for the surgeon to come to the aid of the counselor to enforce moral conduct:

> Who has not met with a case of masturbation, in the male or female, in which no amount of moral reasoning has sufficed to put a stop to the habit? I myself have met with cases in which . . . years of restraint, moral and physical . . . [and] the endeavours of the patients themselves have not sufficed to overcome the habit. Are we then to forbid that "surgery shall come to the rescue, and cure what morals should have prevented," but . . . are so often impotent to stop?[32]

Such provocation goaded West into a powerful counterattack in which he asserted that Brown had misrepresented his true position by selective quotation and raised eight points against his operation.

What is particularly interesting about West's charge sheet is that although his arguments about the harm of masturbation applied as much to boys as to girls, he qualified them so as to quarantine clitoridectomy from circumcision. His fundamental point was that masturbation was so "much rarer in girls and women than in our own sex" that drastic responses like clitoridectomy were unnecessary. More controversially he added that "the injurious physical effects of habitual masturbation [were] the same as those of excessive sexual intercourse" and that he had never seen "convulsions, epilepsy or idiocy induced by masturbation in any child of either sex." He then argued that removing the clitoris to treat nervous diseases was too rarely successful to warrant its frequent performance and claimed that Brown's alleged cures were not permanent. Turning to the moral side of the question, he deplored "attempts to excite the attention of non-medical persons . . . to self-abuse in the female sex" as "likely to injure society and bring discredit upon the medical profession," and finally he criticized Brown for operating without informed consent: "The removal of the clitoris without the cognisance of the patient and her friends [i.e., relatives], without a full explanation, and without the concurrence of some other practitioner . . . is in the highest degree improper."[33] West thus displayed his own unorthodoxy as an adherent of the Paget line that masturbation caused no more physical damage than any other means of procuring orgasm, another point on which Brown taxed him, describing his view as "extraordinary": "It follows that Dr West must also believe that the physical effects of moderate masturbation to be the same as those of moderate intercourse. . . . [He] will not find many converts in the profession to this opinion. Nor would it be for the welfare of society that such a belief should prevail; the fear of the injurious physical effects of masturbation has . . . a most wholesome deterring influence."[34] Brown waxed indignant as the voice of orthodox social authority because he knew West was vulnerable on this issue. Had his more moderate views been accepted as applying to boys as well as girls there would have been a much fiercer debate on the introduction of male circumcision than actually occurred.

Brown's second major opponent was Dr. Robert Greenhalgh, but he had been a supporter and seems to have changed his line only after the discussion of Dr. Tanner's paper had revealed how few allies Brown had and the medical journals had come out strongly against him. Both the *Lancet* and the *British Medical Journal* noted that "the current of opinion certainly ran strongly against" him at that meeting, and in the New Year a correspondent "rejoiced" that he had so little support.[35] The published record of the meeting at which Dr. Tanner's paper was discussed shows Greenhalgh making a strong attack on grounds similar to Dr. West's: the frequency of masturbation in the female had been exaggerated, and cases of self-abuse, epilepsy, and so forth were not cured by clitoridectomy. Greenhalgh reiterated these points and added fresh ones in subsequent letters that left Brown floundering. Not only did women masturbate less than boys, but the idea that they did so at all was "founded on the most unwarrantable assumptions respecting practices to which it is calumniously pretended the women of England are largely addicted."[36]

Brown's offense was to falsely tax "our wives and daughters" with addiction to "filthy habits." Second, Brown gave "offensive publicity" to vicious habits, thus corrupting the innocent. Third, the operation was ineffective. Fourth, it was "fraught with considerable danger to the morals of the public and the high tone of the profession"—the issue that loomed largest in the formal charges. As Greenhalgh added, "the profession . . . are bound to repudiate as strongly as they can practices fatal to their good name." Still following West's lead, he also raised the issue of informed consent, claiming (almost certainly with justification) that Brown had often operated without telling the patient what he was going to do or what it meant. Despite all this, Greenhalgh concluded that if the operation were capable of achieving the benefits claimed, it deserved support: "if insanity, epilepsy, catalepsy and hysteria in females . . . could be made to yield to the knife . . . Mr Brown would have no warmer supporter than myself."[37] It was a big if.

All this was quite a turnaround. According to Brown, Greenhalgh had been very interested in his operations and had paid no fewer than nineteen visits to the London Surgical Home between 1861 and 1865, and he had actually referred a patient for "removal of the clitoris" in May 1865. Even more interestingly, Brown claimed that Greenhalgh had spoken in his favor in the discussion of Dr. Tanner's paper but had sent a quite different report of his remarks to be published in the medical journals.[38] If these allegations are true, they strongly suggest that Greenhalgh became anxious to jump ship once he saw which way the wind was blowing. Its direction was made very clear in editorials in the medical journals in December, all of which were strongly critical of Brown.[39] The *British Medical Journal* was the least hostile. It did not seriously question the ethics of the operation but noted that it rarely checked self-abuse or cured the diseases for which it was indicated. Brown was criticized for exaggerating the incidence of masturbation in women, casting a stigma on the moral character of his patients, and performing the operation too frequently. *BMJ* regretted that "very little was [being] urged on scientific grounds for or against" and advised the profession to consider the points at issue calmly and reach "a judicial decision as to the practical value of the operation" by means of a committee.[40] The *Lancet* took a stronger line. It denied that "irritation of the pudic nerve" produced the dire results Brown claimed and thus that excision of the clitoris could cure women of nervous complaints: although the clitoris was "a principal organ in the large system of erectile and excitable structures," there were "others of scarcely inferior importance." It agreed with Dr. West that hysteria, epilepsy, and insanity in women were not caused by masturbation, and with Dr. Barnes that insane women masturbated only after disease had degraded their mind. The *Lancet* also raised the issue of informed consent and concluded that acceptance of the operation would have serious implications for medical ethics: "are we prepared for a revolution in those principles which, for the public good, have governed medical men in the practice of their profession since the days of Hippocrates?"[41]

The *Medical Times and Gazette* took the most vehement line and introduced a new element into the debate. The arguments of West and Greenhalgh, as well as the *British Medical Journal* and *Lancet* editorials, could easily be read to imply rejection of all mutilating operations of dubious value, including male circumcision, but the *Gazette* did not want to send doctors down that path. Perhaps reflecting the influence of Hutchinson, it made the rejection of clitoridectomy conditional upon the acceptance of circumcision. With all the authority it could muster, it pronounced that clitoridectomy was "infinitely more severe than mere circumcision"; any woman so treated, even if she did have children, must be "maimed and imperfect" and "reduced to the state of the *mulier frigida* of Heberden."[42] Even though there was lively disagreement on this point, the editorial claimed that "all anatomists and physiologists will agree" that the clitoris was "the true representative of the penis" and thus "the chief organ and centre of sexual satisfaction in the female." The editorial then contradicted this position by agreeing that the operation was often ineffective because in some women sexual sensation was "so widely distributed that clitoridectomy neither cures the patient of masturbation nor destroys her aptitude for coitus." The operation did not cure "the most debased cases." The *Gazette* went on to assert that clitoridectomy was justified only when the organ was diseased and that no operation of any sort was permissible "without full knowledge and consent of patient and friends"; it concluded with a warning about the risk to the reputation of the profession if such a proceeding were sanctioned: "A kindred mode of practice . . . exists already in Asia and Africa, but it would tend to reduce our profession to contempt in this country to make the mutilation of women a recognised operation. Already foreigners are not stinting in their condemnation of our tolerance in this matter. . . . better that girls and women should suffer from malpractices than that this degradation of our profession should flourish."[43] It could hardly have been serious in its opinion that the reputation of the medical profession was more important than whether women masturbated, but the outburst indicates the depth of the crisis into which the fraternity felt Brown had plunged them. The reference to Asian and African practices confirms the point that female circumcision was associated with barbarism and licentiousness. Once the medical journals had delivered their verdict, influential fence-sitters were quick to join the anti-Brown tide. Holmes

Coote, an authority on venereal disease, quickly dissociated himself with the observations that self-abuse was rare in women and much easier to treat in them than in males.[44] More damagingly, Henry Maudsley, perhaps Britain's leading expert on madness and promoter of the theory of masturbatory insanity, denied that self-abuse was a frequent cause of insanity in women. This was a double blow, since Brown had cited his opinion (in a lecture to the Harveian Society in October 1866) that there was no cause of insanity more common than self-abuse.[45] Maudsley clarified his position with the deadly qualification that he had been referring only to men; masturbation among women, even those in mental institutions, was rare—he had encountered only two cases in every fifty.[46] As the scissors released the clitoris, they closed more tightly on the foreskin.

The hostile reaction evident in the medical journals convinced many doctors who had been interested in or who had actually carried out clitoridectomies that they had better play it safe. There were more of these than you might think. A provincial GP who visited the London Surgical Home in March 1866 saw between forty and fifty "middle aged practitioners" watching Brown at work, suggesting a high degree of collegiate interest in and not a lot of disapproval of what he was doing. Their lack of objection convinced this observer that the operation must have curative value.[47] Greenhalgh named five other former supporters who had severed their connections with the Home since the outbreak of the controversy.[48] Defending his clinic's procedures, the registrar, Dr. Granville Bantock, pointed out that many eminent practitioners used silver nitrate or actual cautery on the clitoris to deaden the nerves and asked how this differed from "extirpation of the organ."[49] Brown was dismayed at all the backtracking, and at the meeting of the Obstetrical Society at which he was expelled he accused many of his colleagues of having secretly performed clitoridectomies, suggesting that they were now trying to make him the scapegoat for their own offenses.[50] By then he had few supporters left, and the result (expulsion by a vote of 194 to 38) was a foregone conclusion. The surprising thing is that 38 fellows were willing to stand up—though not speak—in his favor. Speaker after speaker rose to denounce his activities as underhanded, unethical, and immoral; his lame and halting reply, so different from the patrician self-confidence he had evinced in his letters to the journals, shows how far the desertion of his friends and the impotence of his central argument had disoriented him. He had been sure that all he had to do was repeat that clitoridectomy was circumcision in the female and the profession would endorse its extension from males to females without demur; when the fellows refused to allow, or even listen to, the comparison, he was left all but speechless: "Clitoridectomy is nothing more nor less than circumcision (*cries of Oh!*

Oh!) You may say 'oh! oh!', but I maintain that clitoridectomy is neither more nor less than circumcision *(loud laughter, hisses and groans)"* (402). What stirred his colleagues up the most was neither the effectiveness of the procedure nor the validity of the physiology on which it was based, but its implications for professional ethics and their respectability. Brown and his supporters had repeatedly called on the Obstetrical Society to set up a committee to investigate the value of the operation in an impartial spirit, "care being taken to divest the scientific question of all extraneous matter," as Dr. Shettle put it, but that is exactly what the Society did not want to do, and their conduct confirmed the complaint of Dr. Bantock that "the moral aspect of the question has been too much harped upon to the exclusion of the scientific."[51] If it could be shown that clitoridectomy was scientific, that presumably was the end of the debate.

Brown's disgrace represented more than the rejection of clitoridectomy as a legitimate medical procedure. It was a statement of values by the profession on male honor, medical ethics, female (and by implication male) sexuality, and the proper relations between doctor and client. It confirmed that the client was as much the guardian (that is, the parents or husband) of the patient as it was the patient herself and in this way kept the road clear for operations on the genitals of boys who had not given their consent; Brown's opponents were careful to define their objections in terms that would not rule out circumcision. As summed up by the *Medical Times and Gazette,* the decisive charges against Brown were four. First, he had performed clitoridectomy "on married women without the knowledge and consent of their husbands, and upon both married and unmarried women without their own knowledge of the nature of the operation." Second, he had operated "without the concurrence of the patient's ordinary medical attendant," thus violating professional etiquette. Third, there was a rather confused issue over whether Brown had seriously offered to submit his theories to the evaluation of the Obstetrical Society. Fourth, there was his "want of credibility as to matters of fact and detail."[52] In historical perspective we can see that his downfall was more particularly related to contemporary beliefs about (1) the nature and significance of female sexual desire; (2) the relevance of chivalry; (3) the dialectics of consent; (4) the public standing of the profession; and (5) the menace of quackery.

Despite the revisionism of Peter Gay and others, there is a lingering view that Victorian middle class women did not or were not meant to enjoy sex. Thomas Laqueur writes that sexual pleasure lost its place in nineteenth-century medical science and that doctors were interested only in whether conception occurred.[53] This comment might be applicable to the attitude of many advocates of male circumcision, but the outcome of the Baker Brown affair confirms the truth of Michael Mason's judgment that the Victorians did not doubt that women enjoyed sex and considered their orgasm important, but also that they believed that women's desires were less pressing than men's and took longer to arouse.[54] A leading gynecologist, Lawson Tait, stated that because the female is "the vehicle for the maturation of the ovum, and for the receptacle of the fertilizing influence of the male," she represents "the passive factor." The female thus requires "only enough of sexual passion . . . to indicate to the male the stage at which his share may be effectually performed. To the male . . . a constant tendency to aggression is necessary that he may be in readiness at the time required. . . . In the human race the sexual instinct is very powerful in man, and comparatively weak in women." It was thus "not surprising that masturbation is very common amongst boys and comparatively rare amongst girls."[55] In 1862 a review of *Functions and Disorders* had rejected Acton's comment that "venereal pleasure is almost entirely on the side of the male" as contrary to experience, asserting that "the female does participate fully in the sexual passion."[56] The psychologist D. Hack Tuke was confident that physicians would repudiate "Pope's slander" that women were libertines at heart, though he acknowledged that "religious and moral principles alone give strength to the female mind"; when these were weakened by (mental) disease, "the subterranean fires become active."[57] Because women were less interested in sex than men and less easily excited, it was important not to do anything that would dampen their enthusiasm yet further; if they did not enjoy sex, or at least not find it too unpleasant, they would not respond eagerly to the embraces of their husbands, leading to problems for both their satisfaction and procreation. A husband who failed to find sexual fulfillment in marriage might well console himself with masturbation or prostitutes. The fellows of the Obstetrical Society were representative middle-class men, and they manifestly did not want their wives to exhibit a just-lie-back-and-think-of-Britain passivity in the marriage bed but to respond passionately to their advances. Although most Victorians would not have known what the clitoris was, Walter's erotic daydreams suggest that men prided themselves on their ability to please their partners as much as the average male today: in empathizing with the present and future husbands of Brown's patients, the fellows were thinking of themselves. Part of the reason for this concern, particularly among doctors, was the persistence of the old belief that a woman had to experience orgasm (thus releasing her seed) in order to conceive.[58] Although this idea was disproved by the discovery of spontaneous ovulation in the 1830s, the new knowledge took a long time to spread, and Copland's *Dictionary of Practical Medicine* stated baldly that orgasm was necessary for conception "in most cases."[59] This was Dr. Littleton's point when he cautioned that the quote from Sinibaldi should "deter us from such a serious mutilation." If clitoridectomy was going to produce frigid and barren wives, that was too high a price to pay for whatever vices it discouraged and whatever diseases it cured.

There is strong evidence, too, that surgeons did not like performing clitoridectomies, which they found a difficult and often messy operation. Unlike the temptingly obvious and all too vulnerable foreskin, the clitoris is an elusive knot of tissue, often difficult to identify among the folds of its hood and the labia, and consequently less easily isolated for surgical purposes. Because it was a delicate operation, even doctors who deplored Brown's activities paid tribute to his surgical skill: John Pickop was very impressed with his "coolness and dexterity as an operator," and Greenhalgh admitted that he had observed "surgical operations of considerable difficulty executed with conspicuous success"; even Charles West made a similar comment.[60] But it could still be a bloody business: at the meeting that debated Brown's expulsion Dr. Oldham gave such a gruesome description of his modus operandi that his horrified listeners howled him down with cries of "Enough!" (408). In addition to being repelled by the process, it is likely that the fellows did not care for the result: imagining themselves in the husband's position, they preferred to have sex with a woman whose genitals had not been surgically reduced or interfered with by another man. A bride was expected to be a virgin in those days, but how virginal could she be if a surgeon had already known her so intimately? (Many doctors also objected to the use of the speculum in examinations for much the same reason.)[61] None of the doctors placed themselves in the woman's position with respect to male circumcision and asked whether she would wish to marry and have sex with a "mutilated" or "imperfect person" (407) or wondered whether her satisfaction might be affected by the alteration of his penis.[62] Nor did they sympathize with the position of a boy whose partially flayed organ bore testimony to the disgraceful practices for which he had been treated or care whether he might be reluctant to reveal the stigma of his shame to potential partners. If one reason the obstetricians cared about women was because they imagined themselves as their sexual partners, on this assumption they would be indifferent to boys because they were not interested in having sex with men and thus did not face the prospect of intimate contact with whatever scarred mess the surgeon had left behind. As the admission of Dr. Spratling suggests, many nineteenth-century physicians seem to have relished performing circumcisions, and it is possible that some of them got quite a thrill from the exercise of such priestly power over another man's sexual and reproductive capacity.[63]

Both the chivalry of the doctors and their claim to expertise-based authority are revealed in Mr. Haden's declaration, in moving Brown's expulsion, that obstetricians were "the guardians of their [women's] interests and . . . the custodians of their honour (*hear, hear*). We are in fact the stronger and they the weaker. They are obliged to believe what we tell them" (396). The *British Medical Journal* agreed, affirming both the chivalrous code and the profession's assertion of unquestionable authority. Women were "at the mercy of the obstetric practitioner. They depend on his probity. They rely on his judgement. If he tells them that they must, in order to preserve their reason, their health or their life, undergo an operation, they can hardly gainsay him." Obstetricians were not only the "guardians of life" but of "female honour and purity," and thus they had the duty to protect women from both the imputation of filthy habits and the knives of overeager surgeons (387–88). Closely related to chivalry was the doctors' concern with informed consent. West provoked a sensation at the meeting when the letter he sent accused Brown of operating "without the knowledge or consent of the patient" (409), but the objection rested nearly as much on the lack of concurrence from husband and family. Dr. Tyler Smith claimed to have encountered "families where the husband is annoyed and the wife made wretched for life" and described the gloomy implications of the operation for the prospects of unmarried women: "Should any proposal of marriage come to them the young women or their parents are obliged to tell the parties proposing that they have been mutilated and thus . . . to expose themselves to the possibility of being treated as imperfect persons" (407). The *Medical Times and Gazette* suggested that operating without consent was not merely a violation of medical ethics but probably a breach of the law. It also stressed the importance of informed consent not only of the woman but of those on whom she was dependent as wife or daughter: "As a woman's character affects theirs, they have the right to decide whether a female relative shall undergo this operation, with the disgrace it involves."[64] Just as the double standard on sexual desire made doctors reluctant to believe that the chaster sex was much given to self-abuse, so women's subordinate position in Victorian society helped protect them from the scissors and the cautery iron. Men, being free agents, and boys, having to learn to be little soldiers, could not expect such solicitude.

It is unlikely these considerations would have prevailed had the fellows not feared for the good name of the profession and its standing in society. As Dr. Barnes put it, the "expressions of public and professional opinion" already aired in the medical journals and newspapers "threw the matter upon our honour, therefore we could not resist it." Because Brown's activities "had become a matter of public scandal," the Council of the Obstetrical Society was compelled "in vindication of the honour of the Society to bring it forward"; in order "to have the Society held in the slightest respect, we must act in this matter" (400). Behind these appeals to the importance of professional honor lay concern that if doctors were going to accuse middle-class women of self-abuse, their husbands and fathers would not send them along for consultations. As the *Medical Times and Gazette* summed it up, clitoridectomy must be rejected if the profession were to have "free and familiar access to families." It voiced the fear that had brought hundreds of fellows from remote corners of England to a draughty meeting hall in central London: "if the clitoridectomical theory and practice were established, no parent who sent a daughter to any medical man . . . could be sure that she might not return tainted with filthy inquiries, or branded by filthy suspicions—a thing incompatible with the honour of the profession and . . . the frank intercourse between practitioner and patient that happily exists now."[65] The *Medical Times and Gazette* was not so vulgar as to mention fees, but the resulting loss of business was the specter behind this consideration.

Clients might even be driven to the quacks. Brown's penchant for quackish self-advertising (manifest in the garish presentation of his book) had been criticized by the *British Medical Journal* reviewer, and even earlier,[66] but Mr. Haden made the charge of quackery central to his case for Brown's expulsion from the Society. Warning that "inroads of quackery" would lower the profession's standing in public opinion, he pointed out that it came in two forms: first, it was the pretense of diagnosing a nonexistent disease; second it was the pretense of curing a real disease "by means which have no foundation in philosophy or fact," an impropriety made worse if the cure is of "a secret, unpublishable, compromising character." Brown had made promises to ignorant and naïve clergymen that a class of hitherto incurable diseases could be fixed by a simple surgical operation, yet he had been forced to admit that he had never even operated on, let alone cured, a women of proven unsound mind (397–98). An equally serious aspect of Brown's quackery was that he had addressed himself to the public rather than his peers and touted his business through circulars and advertisements; as Dr. Barnes exclaimed indignantly, "he had used means to excite the attention of nonmedical personnel . . . to the subject of Self-Abuse in the Female Sex" (398). This had been one of Dr. West's original charges and was a violation of the *British Medical Journal*'s injunction that if such a "dirty subject" had to be discussed at all, it must be "handled with an absolute purity of expression and . . . in strictly technical language," not aired before mixed audiences.[67] Brown's disregard of both medical ethics and professional etiquette meant that he had to go.

It is thus apparent that the opposition to Brown was more on moral than scientific grounds. He had consistently argued that clitoridectomy was the equivalent of amputating the foreskin and that it no more eliminated women's capacity for sexual pleasure than it rendered men incapable of orgasm, merely that it reduced excitability and thus discouraged masturbation. In seeking to apply the new theories that organic and mental disease could arise from nervous irritation, Brown was more consistent in his adherence to Victorian medical-scientific standards than were his opponents. But as the *British Medical Journal* had warned, although the Obstetrical Society owed a duty to science, it owed "another duty to professional honour and public morality";[68] in this case scientific considerations had to give precedence to moral considerations. Even at the level of science the arguments of both sides were riven by a fundamental contradiction. Brown's opponents maintained that clitoridectomy was ineffective because the clitoris was not the only source of sexual excitement and nervous irritation, yet also that its excision deprived a woman of all sexual pleasure. Although he taxed Dr. West with this illogic,[69] Brown was caught in the same dilemma: he argued both that the operation was effective *and* that it did not deprive a woman of all sexual pleasure, which was the same contradiction. Each side wanted it both ways, and neither was willing to admit its ignorance on the vital question of what role the various elements of the external genitalia played in sexual response. Doctors tended to conflate sexual pleasure and sexual desire, and did not know how the latter arose. Following Kobelt's identification of the source of male capabilities in the glans and accepting the analogy of penis and clitoris, they feared that excision of the latter would eliminate female desire just as the removal of the glans would eliminate it in men.[70] But so long as a male kept the glans and was thus capable of erection and ejaculation, he had not been deprived of anything that mattered, even if removal of the foreskin meant that there was little erotic sensation until orgasm—a common complaint of circumcised men.[71] This is still the position of many doctors in circumcising cultures,[72] but such a view is little different from Brown's confidence that so long as a woman was capable of intercourse and becoming pregnant, she had not been injured in her reproductive functions.

The doctors' ignorance of the relative contribution of glans and foreskin to the generation of sexual pleasure in males was greater than their uncertainties about the clitoris, but that did not stop them from rejecting the analogy of circumcision and clitoridectomy: no one disputed Brown's assertion that a male who had been circumcised had "not been injured in his natural functions." The *Medical Times and Gazette* phrased its own rejection of clitoridectomy in terms that actually required the acceptance of "mere circumcision": "Instead of taking away a loose fold of skin it removes a rudimentary organ of exquisite sensitiveness, well supplied with blood vessels and nerves, and the operation is . . . occasionally attended with serious bleeding; in these respects it differs widely from circumcision."[73] This is a remarkable statement, overturning millennia of Western medical thinking and implying that the foreskin was neither sensitive nor "well supplied with blood vessels and nerves"—that it was a mere fold of skin. The *Medical Times and Gazette* could cite no research in support of these claims, and its breezy contention that circumcision was never "attended with serious bleeding" was equally speculative. In fact, as Hutchinson himself was later to admit, the operation often resulted in serious hemorrhage and infection, regularly causing death.[74] Brown's unwitting attempt to legitimize clitoridectomy by comparing it to circumcision gave the champions of the latter the opening they needed, allowing them to promote the surgery they favored at the same time as they condemned the one they disliked. The same editorial further attacked clitoridectomy as unethical because it was wrong to amputate a body part showing no signs of disease and contrary to medical science to amputate something merely because it was subject to irritation: "Intense itching is a common malady, but . . . to cut off part of the body because it itches is monstrous." Yet the *Medical Times and Gazette* supported the excision of normal foreskins as a precautionary measure, and it had endorsed Forster's contention that itching certainly was a sufficient reason for circumcising boys who were in "perfect health." Pace Dr. Littleton, the sauce withheld from the goose was to be administered to the gander.

The Baker Brown affair was the closest Victorian England came to a debate on male circumcision, whose role was to provide the standard of harmlessness by which the infamy of clitoridectomy was measured. The outcome of the debate was a double standard on genital mutilation that has persisted to this day, at least in Anglophone countries, where cosmetic alterations on the genitals of girls are regarded as abominations that must be stopped by law, while circumcision of boys is seen as a harmless adjustment and even continues to be performed for cultural, family, or "hygiene" reasons. Looking back on the controversy, Charles West recalled his condemnation of claims about "the frequency of masturbation in the female sex, and the removal of the clitoris as its cure." He commented that "all right-minded men" were compelled to reject both the operation and its leading proponent, but that "happily we need not now dwell further on the subject, for all practitioners are agreed that the only indication for removal of the clitoris is furnished by the disease of the organ itself."[75] This outcome was not applauded by all. Lawson Tait regretted Brown's disgrace and attributed it to the machinations of one of his rivals (probably Greenhalgh). He also considered it a "disaster" that, as result of the affair, "clitoridectomy was absolutely discarded"; although he remained "certain that in many cases it would be useful," he had never heard of it performed after 1867.[76] The attempt to demonize the clitoris had failed, but at the cost of entrenching the legitimacy of male circumcision: the happy outcome enjoyed by girls was not to be shared by boys.

Part III

The Demonization of the Foreskin

It is not alone the tight-constricted, glans-deforming, onanism-producing, cancer-generating prepuce that is . . . at the bottom of the ills and ailments . . . that may affect man through its presence. The loose, pendulous prepuce, or even the prepuce in the evolutionary stage of disappearance, that only loosely covers one-half of the glans, is as dangerous as his long and constricted counterpart.

P. C. REMONDINO, *History of Circumcision*, 1891

8 · One of the Most Grievous Diseases of Humanity

Spermatorrhea in British Medical Practice

It [spermatorrhea] is one of the most grievous diseases of humanity, but one in which an immensity might be done, which is not done, for its prevention and cure.

GEORGE DRYSDALE, *The Elements of Social Science, or Physical, Sexual and Natural Religion,* 1855

The secretion of the testicles is the hope of the future of the race, and yet if wrongfully used it is so potent that it may figuratively be classed with the secretions of the poison fangs of venomous reptiles.

"A doctor," ca. 1913

You might find some white matter exuding from your private parts. Don't worry about it. It's only a sort of disease like measles.

English housemaster, ca. 1920

Diseases desperate grown,
By desperate appliances are relieved.

Hamlet, 4.2.9–10

During the nineteenth century, attitudes toward the male foreskin soured: it was transformed from "the best of your property" to "a useless bit of flesh" and a threat to masculine health. It is hard to think of any body part whose standing fell so far and so rapidly, nor one that came to be regarded with such suspicion and treated with such savage hostility; even today, in countries with a past history of routine circumcision, doctors seem to regard the foreskin as guilty until proven innocent.[1] As Chris Cold and John Taylor point out, the prepuce has been a feature of the external genitals of all primate species for 65 million years, and the species in which it has developed most luxuriantly is precisely the one that has been most successful in the struggle for existence; yet since Victorian times it has been "the most vilified normal anatomical structure of the human body."[2] The demonization of the foreskin was a paradoxical process by which its anatomical and physiological significance was belittled at the same time as its role in the generation of illness was inflated. As the credibility of nerve force theory declined, and with it belief in the idea that preputial irritation could cause organic illness, germ theory was recruited to explain why the foreskin was still pathogenic and needing to be excised in the interests of health. In this and the following chapters I consider the contours of this process, as well as the specific areas in which the foreskin was thought to cause or contribute to disease, and thus the situations in which early circumcision was indicated, particularly spermatorrhea, infectious diseases, syphilis, and a crop of even less likely afflictions. I also consider the popularity of circumcision as a cure for or preventive of masturbation, and the problem of "congenital phimosis"—how a normal condition in childhood and a minor matter (if a problem at all) among a few adults came to be regarded as an abnormality responsible for an ever-expanding list of medical complaints and a strikingly unscientific vocabulary, such as the description of the foreskin by G. N. Weiss (in 1997!) as a cesspool. The origins of this designation lie in the link Victorian doctors drew between filth and disease and the success of the sanitary reformers in reducing adult mortality rates from "filth diseases." The prestige that cleanliness enjoyed by the end of the century arose from the conviction that dirt (including harmless bodily secretions) meant disease, and in a moral context that held sexual activity itself to be dirty. The result was that the uncut penis came to be regarded as more unclean than the teeth or fingernails, or even the anus. The case for prophylactic circumcision was boosted by the realization that many diseases could not be cured, only prevented; by the development of hygienics as a branch of medicine, with its slogan "Prevention is better than cure"; by the emergence of "fantasy surgery" as a legitimate medical approach; by a devaluation of the role of the foreskin in the bodily system to the point where it was regarded as an inconvenience at best and a menace at worst; and by the sanitarians' discovery of a hygienic rationale in the ancient rites of Islamic and Judaic religion. The rising philo-Semitism of the late nineteenth century was matched by growing acceptance of a Semitic practice that formerly had been regarded as unchristian and unmanly.

The doctors' willingness to excise a healthy foreskin grew along with their ignorance of its possible functions. In 1907 one doctor expressed disappointment that an advocate of automatic circumcision had not discussed the physiological functions of the foreskin; it was found in all mammals, he remarked, yet no information seemed to be available: "I have consulted physiological works in vain; they are all silent." Considering how frequently circumcision was recommended, "one would like to know what function the prepuce possibly subserves, if any."[3] Actually, that was just what most doctors did not want to know. Even those who recognized some of the contribution of the foreskin to normal sexual function, such as J. Bland-Sutton, were keen advocates of its removal; he actually pointed out that the "lubricating matter" provided by the "desquamating epithelium of the glans and corresponding surface of the prepuce" facilitated the "gliding of the prepuce over the glans."[4] By then there had been neurological research establishing that the glans was not particularly sensitive, or sensitive only in a protopathic sense, and that the pleasure-sensing nerves of the penis were concentrated in the part that circumcision removed.[5] But it made no difference: the general view by his time was that the foreskin was a relic like the appendix—a mere pouch for the collection of bacteria, which ought to be extracted before it got infected; circumcision was not the amputation of part of the penis but its liberation from an alien oppressor. In 1871 M. J. Moses stated that the purpose of circumcision was "to liberate the glans from its close mucous covering," and in 1900 the *Medical Press* commented that "no obvious advantage attaches to the retention of this appendage which, like the vermiform appendix, appears to serve no useful purpose in the economy of nature."[6] So devalued had the foreskin become, and so contemptuous were medical attitudes toward it by the turn of the century, that when a thirteen-year-old boy was attacked by a dog that bit his penis in such a way as to partially sever the foreskin, all the doctors did was "complete the operation begun by the dog." The account of the incident showed more amusement than sympathy.[7] In 1916 a doctor reacted with indignant surprise to the suggestion that "one function of the foreskin is to moisten the glans so that it can be lubricated for entrance and then to retract" during intercourse. "No I do not agree with that," he replied tartly; then he added mysteriously, "the Jews have been removing it for thousands of years."[8]

Since no one was making any effort to study it, the idea of the foreskin as a functionless vestige gained credence largely by default. Carpenter overlooked it entirely in the slight attention he gave to the penis in his works on human physiology, and a similar turning of a blind eye was exhibited by Michael Foster, the first professor of physiology at Cambridge. Foster's textbook (1877) was decently reticent about the genitals but held that the glans of the penis was the center of nervous sensation; he was completely silent about the foreskin.[9] By the 1880s, reflecting the increasing practice of circumcision, even the boundaries of the penis had been pruned back: the eighteenth-century conception of a unitary structure (consisting, in Lallemand's terms, of an erectile and a nonerectile portion) was replaced by the idea that only the erectile part was the penis; the rest was extraneous. As Dr. Kellogg expressed it, "the organ is protected by a loose covering of integument, which folds over the end."[10] In 1907 Bland-Sutton stated that the function of the prepuce was to "serve as a sheath for the protection of the delicate nerve-endings . . . in the skin covering the glans penis which are concerned with sexual sensation."[11] At least these views recognized that the covering had a certain limited utility, but the more important point was that they pictured the foreskin not as an integral part of the penis but as a separate anatomical feature, as superfluous as an umbrella sheath. Crusaders like P. C. Remondino (1846-1926), author of a tub-thumping diatribe against the foreskin called *History of Circumcision from the Earliest Times to the Present: Moral and Physical Reasons for Its Performance* (1891), were quick to exploit the opening and assert that in this civilized age the penis did not need the protection it had required in the far-off days when men were naked savages. As he put it, "always careful that nothing should interfere with the procreative functions," nature had provided primitive man "with a sheath or prepuce wherein he carried his procreative organ safely out of harm's way, in wild steeple-chases through thorny briars and bramble-brakes or . . . when not able to climb a tree of his own choice, he was . . . forced up the sides of some rough-barked or thorny tree. This leathery pouch also protected him from . . . the bites of ants or other vermin."[12] That was in the days before underpants, but modern man no longer required such "necessaries of a long past age." Remondino tried to give an evolutionary gloss to his attack on the foreskin, asserting that it was atrophying along with the "climbing muscle" that our ancestors once used to shimmy up trees.[13] The problem he could not solve intellectually was why the foreskin was taking so long to disappear, despite the fact that, unlike other vestiges (most of which were harmless), it was "from the time of birth a source of annoyance, danger, suffering and death" and seemed "in bulk out of all proportion to the organ it is intended to cover." Evolution could evidently not be relied on to do its duty and thus required some assistance from culture. Turning from pseudoscience to outright ideology, Remondino went on to praise "the fathers of the Hebrew race, inspired by a wisdom that could be nothing less than of divine origin [who] forestalled the process of evolution by establishing the rite of circumcision" (9-10). Anxious to appear in touch with the march of science, Remondino returned repeatedly to his evolutionary analogy (206-7, 244-46), but there is irony in the fact that his attempt to associate even a crude and anti-Darwinian version of evolution (involving progress toward a desired goal rather than undirected descent by modification) undermined the argument of the sanitarians. The very conditions in which he declared the prepuce necessary as a protection against burrs and beasties were those in which others said ancient tribes were adopting circumcision to improve hygiene in hot climates: to guard the penis against irritation by desert sand or from invasion by waterborne parasites. Many tribes that practiced circumcision, such as the Aboriginals of central Australia, lived in precisely the primordial conditions described by Remondino as necessitating retention of the foreskin. Despite his rhetorical references to Darwinism, he had so little faith in the power of evolution to abolish the appendage he hated that he relied on the intervention of priests and surgeons and the attractiveness of the excised tissue to those seeking to establish a lucrative market in skin grafts (206-7).

Remondino was an extremist even by the standards of the 1890s. His book is largely a paean to the beauties of ritual circumcision, and the medical element is full of the wildest claims about the connection between the foreskin and disease, expressed in colorful Victorian rhetoric:

> The prepuce seems to exercise a malign influence in the most distant and apparently unconnected manner; where, like some of the evil genii or sprites in the Arabian tales, it can reach from afar the object of its malignity ... making him a victim to all manner of ills, sufferings and tribulations; unfitting him for marriage or the cares of business; making him miserable and an object of continual scolding and punishment in childhood, through its worriments and nocturnal enuresis; later on, beginning to affect him with all kinds of physical distortions and ailments, nocturnal pollutions, and other conditions calculated to weaken him physically, mentally, and morally; to land him, perchance, in jail or even in a lunatic asylum. (254-55)

Those who retained their foreskins ought to pay higher insurance premiums, since "a circumcised labourer in a powder-mill or a circumcised brakeman or locomotive engineer runs actually less risk than an uncircumcised tailor or watchmaker" (290). Circumcision was touted as the cure-all and prevent-all of the century: going one better than Baker Brown, who had been forced to back down from his claim that he had cured cases of insanity in women by means of clitoridectomy, Remondino asserted without a blush that he had restored a lunatic to sanity by circumcising him, and that soon after the operation he had left the asylum a normal man (272-73). No one has sung the praises of circumcision with quite the barnstorming fervor that he brought to his mission, but his uncertain status in Britain is suggested by a reviewer in the *British Medical Journal*, who commented that some of his loftier flights seemed "excessive and strained." Yet even the reviewer conceded that Remondino's views were "worth putting on record as the opinion of a man who has given a great deal of time and trouble to his subject."[14]

The loss of medical knowledge represented by these views made it very hard for those who wanted to oppose circumcision to argue effectively against its advocates, who simply asserted that the foreskin was a mere flap of skin that served no useful function and hence that its removal was no deprivation. Not that many defenders were stepping forward. While the Baker Brown controversy produced many champions of the clitoris, not a single voice was raised in support of the foreskin until Herbert Snow published his booklet in 1890, and that shared so much anatomical ground with his opponents (particularly in accepting that "congenital phimosis" was a pathological malformation) that its arguments were crippled from the start. Since doctors were cutting off foreskins long before they understood anything about the anatomy and function of the penis, they could not have known whether the excision was harmful, beneficial, or neutral. Circumcision was introduced incrementally, with a certain stealth, and there was debate about neither its efficacy nor its ethical standing, quite unlike the scrutiny of clitoridectomy in the Baker Brown affair. The claims made for its advantages were not subjected to empirical verification, no experimental trials were conducted before the procedure became widely performed, and there was no follow-up on the subsequent lives of those operated on to determine whether they turned out to be happier and healthier than those left alone. The "advantages of circumcision" became accepted as medical lore by dint of mere repetition. By the First World War the onus was being placed on the opponents of circumcision to prove that it was harmful, not on its advocates to prove that it was beneficial. Remondino had written that "all attempts to find reasons for its [the foreskin's] existence that are of real benefit to man have so far proved unsatisfactory, and, unlike the reasons for its removal, are . . . founded on speculation" (218). Abraham Wolbarst replied to those who criticized circumcision as "a fetish surviving from ancient times" with the argument that it was up to them to prove that the operation was not desirable: "If there is any objection to circumcision it should be based on valid, scientific grounds."[15] It was naturally as hard to prove the harm of circumcision as it would have been to prove (as opposed to merely assert) its advantages. Like the supporters of Baker Brown, Wolbarst assumed that if circumcision was "scientific," there could be no valid objection to its automatic and universal performance, without the need to bother with consent.

When Remondino published his history, doctors were fond of priding themselves on their scientificity, and he was confident that the case against the foreskin flowed inexorably from the advance of medical knowledge. Spermatorrhea had never enjoyed secure standing as a proven disease entity, and by the 1890s it was so out of favor that Remondino did not even mention it among the benefits of circumcision. Yet even before masturbation, spermatorrhea was identified as an affliction from which men could be saved by circumcision, and as the work of Lallemand became better known in England there was no lack of surgeons stepping forward to apply his remedies.

Understanding of spermatorrhea as an episode in the history of sexual disease has come a long way since Jeanne Peterson dismissed it as "a fiction of Victorian medical quackery."[16] Fictional it might have been, but a phenomenon that inspired such deep anxiety among the male public, and commanded such wide acceptance among the medical profession, demands deeper analysis. In his illuminating studies of Victorian sexuality Michael Mason has explored the status of spermatorrhea in British medicine and drawn particular attention to its contradictory constellation of symptoms: nocturnal emissions, premature ejaculation, diurnal emissions—yet also impotence. He identifies the ambiguous status of the disease but concludes that there was "a body of widely read literature from quacks and less finicky medical popularisers" that successfully packaged all these symptoms, along with unspecified urethral discharges arising from infection, as a single disease susceptible to a single set of cures.[17] Lesley Hall and Roy Porter have situated spermatorrhea among the various moral and medical discourses of Victorian England,[18] and Ivan Crozier has further enriched our understanding of its context in his consideration of William Acton among a web of contemporary authorities on male sexual problems, from the skeptical F. B. Courtenay to the quackish Richard Dawson.[19] More recently Ellen Rosenman has surveyed "the spermatorrhea panic" and sought to answer such vital questions as "What led doctors to imagine this disease and patients to produce such symptoms? Why did both doctors and patients respond with such extraordinary and brutal interventions?"[20] Although spermatorrhea was "a pathological category of the shakiest sort," writes Mason, it possessed "a terrible power to depress and frighten men of all ages" and appeared to be endorsed by the medical hierarchy.[21] As Courtenay commented, there was no category of disease that provoked "more intense mental anxiety" or more deeply embittered a man's social relations than those that affected "his generative system or copulative powers."[22] It was the depth of this anxiety that explains why men were willing to submit to cauterization and even castration, and later to subject their sons to circumcision as a precaution.

The invention of spermatorrhea was an extension of theories about masturbation, but whereas emissions as a result of the latter were sinfully deliberate, those from the former were mystifyingly involuntary. Eighteenth-century doctors had already identified a form of uncontrollable seminal loss not easily distinguishable from urethral discharges arising from venereal disease. John Marten listed seminal loss and other discharges among his varieties of gonorrhea and identified youthful masturbation as the most common cause,[23] and Robert James described a "benign gonorrhoea" in which "the retaining vessels of the organs of generation are so extremely relaxed as to permit the seminal juices to pass off upon the slightest stimulus." James did not explain why this condition should be a problem but hastened to say that where it is accompanied by "continual weeping or gleet," the outcome is a form of impotence "which scarcely ever admits of a perfect cure." On causation, however, he was more assured: venereal dreams; horse riding; irritation of the seminal vesicles; or "weakness in tone of the seminal organs" caused by "frequent embraces," nocturnal pollutions, or masturbation. How often James actually saw men suffering from the effects of constant seminal loss is an interesting question, since his account of the symptoms is drawn not from clinical experience but from a description of "gonorrhea" by Aretaeus, a Greek physician of the second century.[24] Although James was eloquent on the sin of masturbation, he did not identify it as the most important cause of spermatorrhea and thus did not see its prevention as the first step toward curing the condition. His own treatments were firmly in the eighteenth-century mold: various medicines and recipes, baths, cold embrocations on the genitals, purges, and bleeding. A generation later John Hunter had little more to offer except the new term *seminal weakness,* defined as "secretion and emission of the semen without erections." Hunter noted that the condition came in many forms and that the cause was usually sexual excitement, either mental (as in lascivious dreams or thoughts) or physical (as in "friction on the glans" from walking or horse riding). The only treatments he mentions were laudanum and washing the genitals in cold water, but his observation that involuntary emissions could be provoked by the friction of the foreskin over the glans raised the possibility of a surgical cure that would render the penis less susceptible to tactile stimulus.[25]

A variety of ideas about seminal loss had been around for a long time, but it was Lallemand who consolidated them into syndrome that became recognized as a new disease. Although, as Mason observes, Lallemand's work today reads like the ravings of a madman, he was a respected medical scientist in his day; at a time when most pathology relied on syndromes and lacked knowledge of real processes, "the grotesque constellations of sexual history and symptoms" that made up his cases "were not obviously unscientific." An English translation of *Les pertes seminales* was published in 1847, and "spermatorrhoea was on the British medical agenda for the rest of the century."[26] Lallemand's teachings received a mixed, though on balance favorable, reception in England and were popularized through articles in the leading medical journals. Although not every doctor was convinced that it was a real disease, the mainstream profession took it seriously at least until the 1870s, many doctors until the 1890s, and they all vied with the quacks in offering treatments; no discussion of the subject was complete without a ritual anathema hurled at the empirics who duped and fleeced the public with their spurious nostrums. As Crozier notes, the main object of sexual medicine in the early nineteenth century was to find an effective cure for spermatorrhea,[27] and there was no shortage of practitioners contending for the lucrative honor. Their favored technique was cauterization of the urethra with silver nitrate.

The origins of urethral cauterization as a treatment for spermatorrhea are obscure, but it seems to have been taken over from a similar treatment for gonorrhea. Irrigation had been recommended by medieval Arab physicians and Maimonides, and around 1818 Richard Carmichael (1779–1849) had the idea that a more powerful agent might be found in silver nitrate.[28] Acton believed the treatment was discovered by army surgeons, who found it useful against ophthalmia at Chelsea Hospital in 1814, though William Buchan was prescribing frequent injections of white vitriol (zinc sulphate) before the 1790s.[29] These were dangerous techniques, risking more damage to the urethral tract than to the bacteria, but they seem to have worked in some cases, or at least stopped the discharge for a while. The treatment was vigorously taken up by Ricord and his followers in the United States and Britain, especially Acton, and in 1843 G. B. Childs claimed that it "always destroys the virulence of the disease."[30]

Throughout the period there was much confusion between discharges arising from normal excretion of seminal or prostatic fluid and those from gonorrhea as we would understand it or any other infection of the urethral tract, and no reliable way of telling them apart.[31] One believer in spermatorrhea confessed in the 1850s: "The character of the secretion varies . . . from a transparent mucus to the greenish-yellow appearance of pus [closely resembling] . . . the discharge of gonorrhoea. So close . . .

is this resemblance, and so alike are the attendant symptoms, that on the history of the case alone can we rely for a distinction."[32] In an environment in which all discharges from the penis except urine were suspect and masturbation reprobated, it seems safe to conclude that spermatorrhea was the invention of surgeons who could not distinguish between emissions of seminal or prostatic fluid and discharges of pus or other matter produced by infections or other disorders of the urinary tract. The strongest evidence for this is simply that the identical treatment was proposed for each condition: Acton used cauterization of the urethra with silver nitrate for both gonorrhea and spermatorrhea, the only difference being slightly different instruments—a syringe for the former, a more elaborate sound-like device for the latter, both illustrated in his treatise on the diseases of the generative organs.[33] The incidence of gonorrhea and other urethral infections in the nineteenth century is not known, but a survey in 1882 found that 75 percent of males in one doctor's practice had experienced one attack, 40 percent two, and 15 percent three or more.[34] If so many British men had contracted the disease at some time, it is possible that many of those who sought treatment for spermatorrhea were really suffering from gonorrhea but did not want to admit what it implied; a diagnosis of spermatorrhea allowed them to seek treatment without confessing their patronage of prostitutes or other promiscuous sex, and the silver nitrate (which could have had no effect on seminal loss) might have had a temporary effect in cases of such infections, allowing Acton to claim his many cures with some degree of justification.

It was probably in the 1830s that cauterization was first used as a treatment for spermatorrhea. In 1842 Benjamin Phillips reported that he had introduced the technique in 1831, after reading about it in French, and that his own experience had confirmed the views set out in Lallemand's treatise. He recommended the method and provided instructions on how to perform it.[35] Phillips considered that seminal emissions were either voluntary (caused by masturbation or intercourse) or involuntary (caused by other factors) and that cauterization was ineffective in the first instance "unless the patient has sufficient determination to abstain from the practice." In a subsequent article he focused more specifically on masturbation as the principal cause of spermatorrhea, reporting that of 109 cases that had come to his attention, 84 were in patients aged twenty-two years or less and 97 both admitted to the habit and blamed it for their sexual problems.[36] As the decade passed, however, Phillips became increasingly skeptical, pointing out that silver nitrate cauterization had been "energetically tried here" but that the results had been pain, bloody discharges, urinary retention, inflammation of the prepuce, and bladder trouble; "even when the plan succeeded, it sometimes left . . .

irritability of the canal."[37] The following year Phillips questioned the soundness of Lallemand's entire edifice, doubted whether involuntary emissions were harmful at all, saw masturbation as the real problem, and advised patients to marry, though he continued to apply the caustic treatment in severe cases of irritation.[38]

Had this disillusion been general, spermatorrhea might have sunk from sight by midcentury, but it was given a new lease on life in the 1850s by a fresh band of enthusiasts led by Acton, T. B. Curling, Marris Wilson, John Milton, and the rather shadier Richard Dawson, whose *Essay on Spermatorrhoea and Urinary Deposits* had first been published in 1848. In 1852 yet another convert, Henry Thompson, praised Lallemand for pioneering the application of silver nitrate, a treatment now acknowledged "among the most valuable remedies for what were, before his time, some of the most intractable . . . and neglected affections it was the lot of the surgeon to . . . notice." But Thompson had certain reservations about Lallemand's instrument and had designed one of his own, an illustration of which was printed with his article.[39] Wilson complicated diagnosis by explaining that spermatorrhea could be either an excessive discharge of seminal fluid or, in its later form, a deficient discharge and that only an expert could tell which was which.[40] He also revealed how seriously the public was taking the doctors' warnings and what anxiety had been created in reporting the case of one man plagued by the disease "brought on by evil habits acquired at school." Having tried every known means of cure the man eventually sought castration and arranged to have one and then the other testicle removed; even this did not seem to be sufficient, since discharges resumed when the wound had healed, though "they did eventually disappear."[41] In a series of articles titled "On the Nature and Treatment of Spermatorrhoea" and published in the *Lancet* during 1854, Milton deplored the neglect of this serious problem by the mainstream medical profession and praised recent contributions by Lallemand, Curling, Phillips, and Acton. Cauterization remained controversial, and Milton defended its use by denying that it was infallible and insisting that it was always safe: "Many circumstances tend to counteract the beneficial effects of the caustic, such as want of self-control to check bad habits and the thoughts dwelling on impure subjects, occupations and modes of living detrimental to health. But [Curling] says 'cauterisation has rarely failed to give more or less relief. . . . Of its safety there can be no doubt.'" An important issue on which Milton differed from Lallemand was on his policy of "excising the prepuce in every case where accumulations of sebaceous matter behind it coincide with spermatorrhoea." He granted that "where there is also contraction of the prepuce, so that the glans cannot be uncovered without pain; or where a

firm, constructing ring has formed underneath the mucous membrane
... the remedy is circumcision; but where the prepuce passes freely over
the glans, plenty of soap and water every morning and the use of zinc or
tannin ... lotion will almost always effect a cure."[42]

As the century advanced, enthusiasm for circumcision was related to
whether a surgeon believed it was the loss of semen or the nervous shock
that did the most harm; it was thus the moderates on spermatorrhea
who turned out to be more receptive to circumcision than the old guard
of quacks. Milton's own therapeutic regime featured doses of quinine,
bathing the scrotum and perineum in saltwater, gymnastic exercise,
"checking erections" with camphor, and applying a blister to the perineum or penis. Where the patient indulged in self-pollution or excessive
connection, the best approach was to apply "some irritative ointment" to
the penis and thereby make it too sore to touch.[43] Milton is known today
as the inventor of various spiked penis rings, chastity cages, and electric
alarms that rang a bell in the event of an erection, intended to be worn
at night to prevent both nocturnal emissions and willful manipulation.[44]
By the time he had consolidated a lifetime's experience in the seventh
edition of *Spermatorrhoea: Its Causes and Consequences* (1872), he was so pessimistic about the possibility of cure that he doubted whether any male
could have a healthy sex life: erections were a threat and emissions debilitating, yet continence could itself lead to impotence: anyone who
negotiated that tightrope successfully was not likely to come knocking at
his surgery. Milton seems to have dimly apprehended that since spermatorrhea was little more than a rude name for the male sexual function, the only permanent cure was the excision of all the secreting organs: not just the testes, but the prostate, seminal vesicle, and Cowper's
gland as well. Even the fanatics around the Orificial Surgery Society in
early twentieth-century United States were not prepared to go that far.[45]

Blistering the penis was a common tactic against masturbation also
used by Richard Dawson, who directed one patient suspected of the
practice to rub "unguent.antimon.potassio-tartrat" on his penis "till the
usual eruption was brought out"; the part became "so sore that he could
scarcely endure the slightest touch," and further indulgence was prevented. Dawson followed Lallemand in warning that phimosis was a
frequent cause of spermatorrhea and reported that the problem could be
overcome by relieving the tightness and exposing the glans.[46] Whether
this was by means of circumcision is not made clear, but as shown by the
sad case related by Dr. Chambers (see below), he certainly performed circumcisions on men who believed that they were suffering from phimosis; although he does not discuss circumcision explicitly in his book, it
is likely that he urged the operation during consultations. Despite his

radical views on contraception, women's rights, and the joy of sex, George Drysdale was also a fervent disciple of Lallemand and particularly identified "a long foreskin, or a congenital phymosis" as a predisposing cause of spermatorrhea: "unless great attention be paid to cleanliness, the sebaceous matter collects around the base of the glans, becomes acrid and causes irritation. In many of M. Lallemand's cases there was a long foreskin." Where its length "favours irritation, he practises circumcision."[47]

Lallemand's most important English disciple was William Acton, who specialized in treating spermatorrhea with his new techniques and probably made the bulk of his substantial fortune from men who sought help with this condition. Acton exhibited his own syringe for injecting silver nitrate to the Westminster Medical Society in 1841; unlike previous designs, it was made of glass so that the practitioner could observe the quantity of fluid injected.[48] In his early work, *A Practical Treatise on the Diseases of the Urinary and Generative Organs*, the discussion of spermatorrhea consists largely of quotations from Lallemand, translated from the French original. Acton defined spermatorrhea as "emissions of spermatic fluid taking place without the will of the patient, and in sufficient quantities and at such short intervals as to produce local and constitutional disturbance." This was scarcely an advance on the master, although Acton is obviously trying to give a more precise meaning to the word *excessive*, and his list of causes is equally derivative, though he tried to classify them at a more abstract level: (1) erotic thoughts; (2) direct causes, including hemorrhoids, worms, a long prepuce, and accumulation of secretions under the foreskin; (3) gonorrhea; and (4) "venereal excess." As we have seen, Acton was uncertain about whether it was the drain of semen or the depletion of nervous power caused by orgasm that was most damaging but tended to favor the latter position: "when the constitution becomes shattered . . . the mischief arises . . . from the exhaustion on the nervous system, rather than from the mere evacuation of so much semen," he wrote. Evidence was provided by boys incapable of secreting semen yet who exhibited the "worst constitutional symptoms of spermatorrhoea" because they had picked up "the evil habit of tickling the genital organs."[49] This emphasis was consistent with the rising prominence of nerve-based theories of disease in the mid-Victorian period, as well as the intensifying condemnation of masturbation, defined in boys before puberty as no more than tickling.

In his better known *Functions and Disorders*, Acton is uncharacteristically defensive about spermatorrhea, acknowledging its ambiguous status in British medicine and conceding that the seriousness of the problem was often exaggerated by quacks, leading others to deny its reality. Of that Acton was in no doubt, yet here he defined spermatorrhea as "enervation produced, at least primarily, by the loss of semen." The most common causes of spermatorrhea were masturbation, venereal excess, or too much study, and the symptoms were loss of semen (in wet dreams, or when urinating or defecating), non- or imperfect erection, irritation of the genitals, and "clergyman's throat"—not a kinky sex position popular among country vicars but a persistent sore throat that might prove a trial to those who had to deliver a weekly sermon.[50] For the benefit of skeptics, Acton explains that it was well known that "affections of the throat" were closely associated with disturbances of the genital organs: "That sexual intercourse has the singular effect of producing dryness of the throat has long been known. Masturbation or . . . nocturnal emissions have the same effect." He himself had treated two such cases.[51] The *London Medical Review* did not comment on this application of the theory, but it generally applauded Acton's discussion of spermatorrhea and endorsed his belief in the curative effects of cauterization. It did, however, consider that he had exaggerated the incidence of the disease by not emphasizing the distinction between genuine discharges of semen (containing sperm) and the mere exudation of urethral mucous. On this point the review quoted a comment by John Hunter, who seems to have been as skeptical of the firming belief in seminal weakness as of the dogma that masturbation was physically harmful. He had pointed out that the glands feeding the urethra constantly secreted a "slimy mucous, similar to the white of an egg," often found on underclothes, especially after "lascivious thoughts." He emphasized that the discharge was entirely harmless, though terrifying to those who imagined they were suffering from gonorrhea—to the great profit of the quacks.[52] If more nineteenth-century doctors had studied their Hunter, fewer would have believed in the harm of masturbation and spermatorrhea.

In treating spermatorrhea Acton followed the prescriptions of Lallemand: moderation in sexual activity; various potions and diets designed to calm the blood; and the cauterization procedure already described. He gives precise details on how to perform this excruciating maneuver but assures readers that he has never seen ill consequences from it, though his text is also innocent of testimonials to its benefits.[53] One of the distorting features of the medical works available to the historian today is that the voice of the physician comes across loud and clear, but we rarely hear from his patients: they are just case histories narrated by their adviser, not individuals with their own story. A glimpse into their world is offered by George Drysdale and John Addington Symonds. Drysdale sought treatment for his own spermatorrhea (brought on, he was sure, by masturbation) and allowed "a medical friend" to cauterize him, with no effect except pain and the production of a stricture of the urethra. He sought further treatment from Lallemand himself, with equally disappointing results, although he reported benefit from following the master's advice to travel and find a mistress. Despite constant spermatorrhea, Drysdale reported that "his muscular development remained good, and in outward appearance he seemed in vigorous health"—a fact that would seem to be inconsistent with the condition being a disease, but Lallemand assured him that such superficial signs of vigor were common in victims "whose nervous system was shattered by the disease . . . and who might even be reduced to the verge of idiocy."[54] The voice of medical authority was evidently more powerful than the testimony of experience. Symonds, who consulted Acton about his sexual difficulties in 1864, tells us that he had a nervous hereditary disposition and from puberty had been subject to "excessive involuntary losses of semen,"[55] showing that he had learned somewhere that such effusions were harmful, but that he did not masturbate more than once a week and then, having been warned by his father, gave it up entirely in his midteens. He then experienced frequent nocturnal emissions, which were treated with doses of strychnine and quinine.[56] Symonds had always been attracted to young men, a preference not altered by his marriage, and the couple soon stopped having sex together. He had a strong sex drive, however, and was aware that doing "what nature prompted" would probably cure his physical symptoms and mental anguish, but he was uninterested in women, was held back by moral scruple from men, and was afraid to masturbate, with the result that he was sexually frustrated and possibly suffering from what we would call "blue balls." In this condition, at age twenty-four, he consulted Acton and "allowed him to cauterize me through the urethra." Symonds might have hoped that this would stop his involuntary emissions, but what he really wanted, and what he probably thought the treatment was designed to achieve, was the wiping out of sexual desire: "I had treated the purely sexual appetite (that which drew me fatally to the male) as a beast to be suppressed and curbed, and latterly to be downtrampled by the help of surgeons and their cautery of sexual organs."[57] The patient grasped that the real object of cauterization was not to restore sexual functioning but to deactivate it. As it turned out, the treatment had no effect at all—not on Symond's emissions, or his sex drive, or his anxieties; some years later, however, he started having regular sex with partners to whom he was attracted, and according to Ellis his neurotic symptoms and physical problems soon disappeared.[58]

Although he did not advocate preventive circumcision, Acton followed Lallemand in arguing that one of the main causes of spermatorrhea was a long prepuce and/or the accumulation of secretions beneath it.[59] The invention of spermatorrhea was thus not a sufficient cause of the rise of preventive circumcision, but it made an important contribution to the cause in that it focused attention on the genitals and proposed that penile irritability was a common cause of diseases in regions remote from that part of the body. Without the mania for spermatorrhea it is unlikely that entrepreneurs like Lewis Sayre would have sought the cause and cure for paralysis and other obscure muscular problems in the condition of boys' penises.

Medical opinion in the 1870s was "greatly divided" between skeptics, moderates, and believers on the question of involuntary emissions, and the moderates tended to cite F. B. Courtenay's *On Spermatorrhoea*, a text first published in 1858. Courtenay did not doubt that there was such a thing as spermatorrhea, but he distinguished between "false spermatorrhea" and the real McCoy, the first showing no sperm in a urine sample, the latter coming up positive. He was critical of the cauterization treatment and quoted many examples of postprocedural complications, including bleeding, cramps, and persistent pain. He was fairly relaxed about occasional nocturnal emissions but expressed the usual views on masturbation. The main burden of the book was an attack on quackery and a critique of the medical profession proper for allowing them to prosper by refusing to take spermatorrhea seriously, thus driving men into their clutches.[60] Reviewing the book in 1871, the *Medical Press and Circular* praised it as "the soundest treatise on the subject of involuntary seminal emissions we have had to peruse for some time," though it regretted that the author had little to say about impotence.[61]

A stronger skeptic was Dr. Thomas Chambers, who in 1861 reported the death of a young man following cauterization by Richard Dawson, author of several books on spermatorrhea but not a licensed practitioner. The young man (J.S.) had first approached Dawson with a request for "an operation . . . for congenital phimosis" and afterward told him that he thought he was also suffering from spermatorrhea—as he would have learned to expect from the condition of his prepuce. Dawson, he wrote in a deathbed deposition, "asked me no questions about my symptoms" but immediately "passed into the urethra an instrument like a catheter, with a central piece and with lateral holes . . . which he filled with an ointment . . . [and] injected . . . by means of an apparatus at the end." Dawson repeated this procedure on several occasions, and after a couple of weeks J.S. was experiencing pains in the prostate, difficulty urinating, and a discharge of pus from the penis. Within another week he was dead. From his own deposition and the commentary of Chambers, it appears that J.S. first sought Dawson's help after reading one of his books, a copy of which was found in his room. The solution injected was not silver nitrate but a blend of zinc chloride and iodine, an equally caustic mixture (according to Chambers) that fatally damaged the previously healthy bladder and urethra. Chambers concluded his indignant account of this sad iatrogenic misadventure by affirming that spermatorrhea was "a purely imaginary disease," that semen may be "secreted in large quantities, and may be found frequently in the urine without . . . injuring the health," and that treatments like Dawson's were "useless, pernicious to health and dangerous to life."[62] Chambers further reported that J.S.'s father had also died after treatment by Dawson, but it does not appear that the latter was ever prosecuted or otherwise called to account for these incidents.

Among the skeptics, one of the more committed was Dr. George Gascoyen, who roundly attacked nearly all Lallemand's propositions in a lecture to the Harveian Society in December 1871. Gascoyen named Lallemand as the "father of spermatorrhoea" and observed that the disease was "a complaint scarcely known here until the issue of his book." Having read *Les pertes seminales* himself, he expected to find living proof of the disorder, but careful questioning of patients who complained of "debility" or the effects of masturbation revealed that most of them "were suffering from an unnatural excitation of the genital system, produced . . . by mental causes rather than . . . any real physical incompetency." Gascoyen criticized Lallemand for imagining that "he had discovered the cause of all the obscure symptoms met with in practice"; his book was "a striking example of how an able man can mislead himself when he has a theory to prove, and how he can unconsciously wrest facts and symptoms from their plain, simple meaning to interpret his own preconceived idea"—a comment equally applicable to many other toilers in the field of male sexuality. Gascoyen believed that spermatorrhea "as a disease has not been satisfactorily proved" and deplored the harm done by Lallemand's treatise, which had become the textbook of the "herd of charlatans who fatten upon the vices and fears of men" and an inexhaustible mine of information for those writing their own books on the subject. As a result of the wide circulation of these, the male public had come to dread spermatorrhea as much as gonorrhea or tuberculosis, and "their existence is embittered": some become "confirmed monomaniacs, and ruin themselves in their endeavours to be cured of an imaginary complaint." Gascoyen did not name Acton, but it is hard to see how he could have escaped such a dragnet condemnation.[63]

Such a robust attitude seems very reasonable to us, but it did not mean that Gascoyen doubted the injurious effects of "repeated masturbation or excessive sexual indulgence," or even of "nocturnal emissions and the irritable condition of the genito-urinary organs induced by these practices." On the contrary, lunatic asylums provided abundant evidence of the "mental derangement" induced by such indulgence, but it was "not the actual loss of semen which occasions the mental degradation, but the extreme nervous exhaustion which follows on the sexual act when too often repeated." Although this was no more than what Lallemand and Acton had themselves suggested, Gascoyen rejected spermatorrhea because he was a full convert to the nerve force theory of disease: emissions without orgasm were by definition harmless, since no nervous spasm was involved, and he actually doubted whether emission of semen that included a significant quantity of sperm could occur without sensation. Gascoyen conceded that many men experienced discharges of prostatic and other fluid in many circumstances but assured his listeners that such effusions were perfectly normal and not an indication of any morbid condition. He even went so far as to assert that the presence of sperm in such secretions was a sign of health rather than disease and evidence that "the testicular function is not impaired." Such good sense comes as a breath of reality in the hothouse of Victorian discussions of sexuality, but Gascoyen could not escape the wisdom of his time. Accepting that masturbation and excessive intercourse were harmful on account of the nervous strain involved, he was half in agreement with Acton and many of the quacks, and fully in agreement with them that sexual debility was a real condition that demanded medical treatment. Where he differed from them was in the emphasis he placed on the influence of the brain and nerves, which he thought could produce the symptoms of organic disease even when no physical cause was present, bringing about "a morbid excitability of the genital organs and of the brain until a state of complete nervous exhaustion is produced." The emissions of patients who reported sexual debility were really due "to an unnatural sensibility of the genital nerves . . . resulting from sexual abuse, masturbation, or some other cause." This stress on nerves was bad news for the nerve-laden foreskin.

Turning to treatment, Gascoyen pronounced himself strongly opposed to the *porte-caustique* as both ineffective (seminal loss being the result of a nervous condition, not "morbid conditions of the ejaculatory ducts") and dangerous: he knew of two persons who had died from the treatment and others who had suffered serious injury. In its place he favored the occasional insertion of a catheter to reduce congestion of the urethra; application of various ointments and drugs; and modifications to patients' behavior, particularly keeping themselves regular and not allowing their bladder to become full—"one of the most certain provocations of erection and emission." Hard physical exercise was also beneficial, since "the brain and the body are [then] too tired to run riot in libidinous dreams and practices." But Gascoyen's favored treatment was circumcision: if emissions arose from masturbation or venery, he was emphatic that "these practices must be discontinued; if from improper thoughts or conversations, all such subjects . . . must be avoided, as well as everything tending to venereal excitement. If the prepuce be long, so that the secretions accumulate beneath it and occasion erection from the itching and irritation, circumcision should be performed." After all that huffing and puffing, Gascoyen seems to have done a complete circle and come right back to the position of Lallemand on circumcision and of Acton on the desirability of continence.

Gascoyen's lecture is significant as the first sure sign that Lallemand's star was fading and as an indication of the growing reliance on and orthodoxy of nerve force theory in explaining male sexual disorders. He was no liberator: like Acton he regarded male sexuality as a minefield to be negotiated with trepidation and desire as a beast to be trampled with chemical and surgical means. His rejection of spermatorrhea was a consequence of his full acceptance of nerve force theory and the greater importance of mind over body; he did not doubt that masturbation and excessive intercourse were harmful but believed that the damage was caused by nervous stimulation, and especially the shock of orgasm, not the loss of semen. The focus of surgeons thus shifted from that problem to the danger of sexual excitement itself, particularly the nervous sensations experienced during acts of sex. Questioning spermatorrhea did not mean that sex became any less problematic for men; on the contrary, the emerging paradigm held that the greater the enjoyment and the more intense or prolonged the final orgasm, the greater the damage to the brain and nervous system. Measures to reduce sensation and make orgasm briefer and less intense must thus be beneficial to health, and the focus of therapy moved from minimizing emissions to reducing the nervous strain experienced in their procurement; Gascoyen was quick to recognize circumcision as the most efficient means of achieving this objective. His position suggests the somewhat surprising conclusion that it was the skeptics on spermatorrhea who were more likely to favor circumcision than its proponents; apart from Lallemand himself, they generally did not include it as a regular feature of their therapeutic arsenal. It was the younger members of the mainstream medical profession, embracing nerve force theory, who eagerly took up circumcision after the 1860s, while the older practitioners and the quacks continued to preach the dangers of seminal loss. Like Acton, they could not abandon belief in the latter, since their whole practice and livelihood were based on the premise that involuntary emissions (that is, without sensation) were harmful in themselves and represented a pathological condition that needed to be treated. Although some of them (like Dawson himself) still performed minor surgical procedures, unaccredited practitioners lost the right to provide medical treatment as the profession became more tightly regulated after the Medical Act of 1858, and they could not legally have done circumcisions: that weapon was now available only from the duly licensed. But there was also a theoretical basis to their reluctance. To put it crudely, the old guard saw the loss of semen as harmful and tried to preserve health by minimizing ejaculations: the fewer the emissions the better. The nerve force theorists held that it was the nervous strain of sexual excitement and the spasm of orgasm that were damaging and sought to promote health by reducing the intensity of the sensation: how many emissions you had did not matter so much, so long as the intensity and duration of the feeling were minimized. In this context, circumcision was the obvious therapy.

As belief in the harm caused by seminal loss declined, spermatorrhea did not disappear from the medical texts but was reclassified as a nervous rather than an organic disease. Here James Paget perhaps led the way. Although he was critical of some aspects of Acton's theory and practice,[64] he conceded that there was a disease that could be called spermatorrhea but averred that it was not an organic disease of the genitals; it was a disorder of the nervous system. In men with "over-sensitive nervous systems" or in whom the part of the spinal marrow near the genitals was "over-irritable,"

> emission of semen is apt to take place with much less than the normal amount of excitement. Hence it may take place . . . without erection and almost without sensation; sometimes from the mere friction of the dress in riding or walking. . . . This might be called spermatorrhoea; but even this is not a disease of the genital organs, it is a disease . . . of the nervous system . . . [most likely caused] by an irritable condition of the spinal marrow.[65]

The symptoms of Paget's version of the condition were an aching of the back and lower limbs, fatigue, incapacity for mental exercise, and "defects of will"; these were not the outcome of excessive seminal loss but "signs of a central nervous disorder" in which "the patients are full of apprehension, unable to divert their minds from their sexual functions," thus increasing the secretion of seminal fluid. Although spermatorrhea was thus really a mental disease, local treatment might help, for "if the unnatural sensibility of the sexual organs can be diminished the mind can be less distressed by emissions." Recommended therapies included cold enemas, galvanism, and catheterization "with or without caustic for the prostatic part of the urethra"—nothing less than Lallemand's cauterization. Paget commented that he had observed many cases in which the results of this technique had been "mischievous" but did not doubt that it was "sometimes useful."[66]

Following the discovery in 1879 of the microorganism that caused gonorrhea (*Neisseria gonorrhoeae*),[67] belief in spermatorrhea began to wane, but only slowly. By then its separate identity seems to have been well established, and its endorsement by someone with Paget's authority must have silenced many doubters. Its tenacious survival may be connected with the delayed impact of Neisser's work on the understanding and treatment of gonorrhea itself. Michael Worboys has recently shown that it took about a generation for Neisser's explanation for gonorrhea to be widely accepted and that his arguments were heavily contested in Britain; in the meantime old explanations and the old uncertainties of diagnosis persisted.[68] In his *Practical Treatise on Urinary and Renal Disorders* (1885), Robert Maguire took a cool look at spermatorrhea but concluded that it was a real disease. He acknowledged that occasional wet dreams were not harmful but agreed with Acton that if they occurred more than twice a week (a generous allowance) they were proof of a disorder that required medical attention. He deplored the exaggerations of the quacks but warned of the consequent danger that legitimate practitioners might regard such complaints too lightly and thus drive patients into their hands. Maguire reported several cases that indicate how seriously men took the warnings against seminal loss and how frightened they were, but he had little to add in the way of treatment for cases in which the condition was real. He cited Lallemand's conviction that a long prepuce was usually a local cause, especially in "uncleanly persons," and agreed that "its immediate removal" was the first step toward a cure.[69]

As late as 1894, the third edition of Quain's *Dictionary of Medicine* included an entry on spermatorrhea (by James Cantlie) in which the condition was defined as "a real or apparent discharge of seminal fluid . . . without voluntary sexual excitement." Like Courtenay, Cantlie distinguished between "true" spermatorrhea, where the discharge included sperm, and "false" spermatorrhea, where it did not. The cause of the disease was "local irritation," most commonly caused by masturbation but sometimes by a "disordered condition of the genital organs." He particularly cited balanitis, phimosis, and a long prepuce among several exciting conditions and pointed out that many of these could also be caused by masturbation. Going rather further than Acton, Cantlie considered nocturnal emissions as the first sign of spermatorrhea, leading to a condition of "extreme mental depression" in which "the sight of anything lewd, the act of defecation, or a chance irritation of the penis . . . is often sufficient to cause an abortive or . . . complete emission." The progress of the disease rendered the patient "physically and mentally a wreck, sleepless, listless, nervous, anaemic, and with an old and insipidly anxious look upon his muddy or pimpled face." Turning to treatment, Cantlie's first thought was circumcision: because local irritations must be removed, "a long prepuce should be cut off," balanitis cured, and rectal irritations be relieved. After that, masturbation must be stopped by painting the penis with iodine and caustics, which "by the pain they cause, prevent the patient meddling with the organ." Cantlie also recommended "counter-irritation" by the application of silver nitrate through a silver syringe-catheter, flexible tube, or urethrescope—essentially Lallemand's cauterization but with more modern instruments. Apart from such innovations, Cantlie listed a few old remedies: tonics such as strychnine, depressants such as belladonna, galvanism, cold hip baths, and enemas; he had no objection to "mechanical contrivances" to prevent masturbation but felt that attention to moral health was potentially more useful.[70] Such old-fashioned prescriptions indicate what little progress there had been in the understanding of male sexual health over the previous century. In the preface to the 1894 edition of Quain's *Dictionary*, the editors remarked that "never in the history of medicine" had progress been so rapid as during the twelve years since the first edition in 1882: "Not only has our knowledge of old and familiar facts been improved, but an entirely new development of our science has occurred, more especially with reference to the causation of disease [that is, the discovery of germs] and . . . the preservation of health," leading to the necessity for a "complete revision of the work."[71] But at least four entries were not revised in light of the new knowledge about the role of microorganisms in the genesis of disease: masturbation; spermatorrhea; penis, diseases of; and reflex disorders—all of which continued to embody old understandings of disease. Not modern bacterial explanations but such old-fashioned concepts as nerve force theory, the danger of seminal loss, and the teachings of Lallemand continued to provide justification for circumcision. Such conservatism offers strong evidence that the widespread adoption of circumcision was at least partly based on theories of disease causation that were already outdated at the time it was being popularized.

9 · The Besetting Trial of Our Boys

Finding a Cure for Masturbation

Fifty years ago . . . that sin was unknown at most of our public schools. Now, alas, it is the besetting trial of our boys; it is sapping the constitutions and injuring in many the fineness of intellect.

REV. E.B. PUSEY, 1866

Flee, therefore, this youthful lust. In the name of religion, in the name of soul and body, I ask you to avoid it. . . . Relinquished it is to be . . . though the effort be as painful as the cutting off a right hand, or the plucking out a right eye. The greatest teacher has spoken these stern words: "If thy right hand offend thee, cut it off, or if thy right eye offend thee, pluck it out; it is better to enter into life halt or maimed, than having two hands or two eyes to be cast into hell fire."

DR. WILLIAM PRATT, *A Physician's Sermon to Young Men,* 1872

While obstetricians were denouncing Baker Brown for exaggerating the prevalence of masturbation among women, the medical journals that printed their indignant letters about mutilation and lack of consent were demanding more vigorous action against evil habits in boys. At the same time as the medical profession determined that their duty to women's health obliged them to protect their genitals from surgical interference, they declared that the health and morals of boys were to be secured by the sort of operation that had been banned on girls. Concern about masturbation was nothing new, but what turned it into alarm was news that the practice was even more widespread than anyone had feared; the bearer of these grim tidings was, of all people, the Rev. E. B. Pusey, former Tractarian and leader of the High Church Anglicans, who had learned the fact from undergraduates at Oxford, in the course of the confessions he took as part of his revival of traditional rituals.

Pusey raised the topic in a series of letters to the *Times* defending the legitimacy of the sacrament of confession in the Church of England liturgy. He claimed that without the confessions he had taken he would never have discovered the extent to which boys were sinning against the seventh commandment and that the boys would never have had the opportunity to learn they were doing wrong. He thus advocated confession not merely because of its apostolic sanction but as a practical means of reducing the prevalence of masturbation: it provided the opportunity to tell the ignorant boys that it was a sin that would blight their life. In reply to a critic who wrote that such evils were best ignored lest they instruct the innocent in vice, Pusey replied that the ignoring plan had been tried but the upshot had been an explosion of the problem. He claimed that boys fell into the habit only because they were unaware of its physical and spiritual consequences and that confession was an effective means of finding out what they were doing and warning them against it.[1] The correspondence brings home just how seriously masturbation was condemned in the mid-nineteenth century: that a figure of Pusey's stature and calling should not only write to the *Times* about it but seek to use it as a lever for winning greater acceptance for the traditional Christian rituals he was intent on reviving offers a startling insight into the relationship between religion and medicine at that period.

The controversy aroused by Dr. Pusey's letters was comparable to the moral panics of our own time over computer games, Internet chat, and smoking among teenagers. Not all agreed that the problem was as acute as it was painted. Dr. Lionel Beale believed that Pusey had exaggerated and felt that the problem was magnified by too much supervision of schoolboys by clergymen ignorant of physiology and hygiene, who thus emphasized spiritual admonition at the expense of trusted remedies such as distracting hobbies and healthy outdoor sports that left "little room for sin." Beale revealed the doctors' aspiration to the traditional role of priest in his assertion that "the family Doctor" was "the right person to receive the confession" and would "give far sounder advice than the priest." He did not doubt that masturbation among schoolboys must be stamped out, but he thought that Pusey had done society a disservice by raising the issue in a nonmedical forum and was causing the same sort of harm as the quacks by drawing the attention of innocent people to a subject not properly discussed outside the surgery.[2] Dr. Pusey was supported by Alfred Meadows, MD, whose professional experience had convinced him that "the evil" was more common than many thought. He suggested that it was not the ignorance of the clergy that aggravated the problem but the apathy of the medical profession: distractions like hobbies and sport were all very well, but Dr. Beale did not seem to be aware "of the very early age at which this habit often begins." He knew of cases in which the perpetrator was as young as two years, and a colleague had told him of one in which it began at twenty months. In suggesting that "something more" than Dr. Beale's diversions was required, Meadows fell ominously into the language of Baker Brown: the cause of masturbation was not mental or moral frailty but a bodily infirmity or abnormality that could be fixed by the right medical treatment. "In the great majority of these cases," he wrote, "the habit originates in some local irritation." But like Beale, he concluded that boys needed a physician of the body, not of the soul.[3]

Dr. Pusey reentered the debate with a plea for cooperation. Scenting a takeover bid for a field formerly dominated by his enterprise, he hoped that a friendly merger could be arranged instead: "surely our professions ought not to be at variance; they might materially help one another. You have primarily to minister to the body, we to the soul; but since the body acts upon the soul and the soul upon the body, we need oftentimes your help, and sometimes . . . we may help you. . . . It is unphilosophical to set one preventive against another, when they are not only compatible, but ought to be united." Pusey denied that his estimates of boyhood and adolescent masturbation were exaggerated and insisted that the practice did not develop spontaneously (by some physiological process) but was nearly always taught by other boys (and occasionally by "unprincipled nurses"). He thus rejected the argument that "local irritation" was the most common cause and suggested that most boys succumbed to the temptation of their schoolmates because they had not been warned against the moral and physical consequences: "Elder boys teach it to the younger, mostly at the small private school at a very early age—commonly about eight, or from eight to twelve—and they, in their turn, to those younger than themselves. If the younger generation are warned in time, before they have contracted the habit, the plague, by God's mercy, might die out. But there should be some systematic effort among schoolmasters; for the infection spreads rapidly." Writing to a medical journal, Pusey emphasized the physical effects of masturbation, particularly madness: the medical head of one lunatic asylum had informed a friend of his that ten recent inmates admitted for "mental delusion" had all come from the same large school.[4]

This exchange revealed the positions of the "doves and hawks" in the antimasturbation drive, roughly corresponding to advocates of moral versus physical responses[5]—the former offering spiritual admonition and advice, the latter surgical and other medical interventions. The evidence from editorials in medical journals following the controversy is that doctors heeded Pusey's call for cooperation: spiritual and physical approaches were indeed seen as complementary rather than alternatives. The *Medical Times and Gazette* recommended a combination of fresh air, exercise, and cold bathing; warnings from parents not to listen to "nasty and prurient suggestions"; and appeals to self-respect and the need to avoid unchaste thoughts. Although the journal did not ignore physical remedies—"in a rickety child of two" masturbation was cured by circumcision—it was an Acton-esque regime, deploying religious instruction and moral feeling against "selfish sensualities."[6] Dr. William Pratt was also dovish. Despite his advice that masturbation would ruin mind and body, and his sinister reference to cutting it off (see the second epigraph to this chapter), he was a wimp when it came to treatment. All he proposed were cold baths, abundant work, plain food, careful reading material, religious faith, and prescriptions from trustworthy physicians like himself. Pratt denounced rascally quacks as vehemently as masturbation itself, but if all he had to offer were these outdated palliatives he was not making a good case for the superior firepower of the medical profession proper.[7]

A few years later the *Lancet* went for something stronger and stressed the efficacy of the surgical approach, as recommended by the main authorities quoted—Lallemand and Copland. In defining masturbation the editorial referred to the symptoms of spermatorrhea described by Lallemand: "nervous exhaustion and physical drain," which erects a barrier to "perfect bodily evolution," "diminishes mental energy and . . . leads to tubercular deposits in vital organs." Masturbation was always harmful to health, though its impact varied from one individual to another, and it was difficult to find cases in which it had definitely caused phthisis, epilepsy, and insanity. The editorial cited Copland in explaining how the foreskin incited boys to masturbation and why "the salutary oriental practice of circumcision" was therefore an effective cure: "The sebaceous secretions at the base of the glans soon become highly irritating, and when retained by an elongated prepuce, occasion irritation which suggests friction for its relief, and which also serves to direct attention to the penis. Hence the occurrence of erections, of pleasurable sensations increased by manipulation, and finally of ejaculation." Three possible treatments were proposed. First, the external cause of the irritation should be removed, and in cases of phimosis it was always salutary to circumcise; even when the prepuce could be retracted, the operation was beneficial. Second, if circumcision was not performed, an elaborate hygienic ritual was required to deaden the penis: "The prepuce should be fully drawn back at least twice daily and the exposed parts well washed with soap and water, then dried with a soft towel, and moistened with a lotion containing about four grains of sulphate of zinc to an ounce of equal parts of glycerine and distilled water. In this way slight sensations serving to call attention to the parts may be avoided." Note that the procedure was intended to promote chastity, not physical hygiene. Third, it was necessary to guard the penis against improper manipulation, best achieved by "keeping up a slight soreness . . . either by blistering liquids or tissue, tartar-emetic ointment, nitrate of silver. . . . The soreness should be sufficient to render erection painful."[8] With doctors demanding complicated routines like this, it is easy to see the origins of the myth that the uncircumcised penis was difficult to look after. Another hawk was Dr. Alexander Davidson, who regarded masturbation as a physical problem that could be overcome by surgery: "if we remove purely physical causes we might reasonably hope to greatly diminish this practice, and the only method which [is] . . . simple and complete is circumcision."[9]

Why circumcision remained an overwhelmingly upper-class phenomenon in Britain is largely explained by the intensity of the campaign against masturbation in the public schools. "Most educated people asked to have their sons circumcised," reported a Dr. Solomons in 1920, and he thought it "an excellent thing to do"[10] — for social if not for medical reasons. By the 1880s the penalties for a boy caught masturbating, either solo or in company, could be public humiliation, flogging, and expulsion, with consequent scandal and embarrassment to parents, who were accordingly willing to do almost anything to avoid disgrace and keep their boy in the educational stream that led, through Oxford or Cambridge, to a position in the British establishment appropriate to his family status. If circumcision was going to help, the destruction of his foreskin was a small price to pay. In the first half of the century, as we have seen, masturbation and other sex play among the boys was a pretty normal feature of public school life: the first words addressed to the young William Thackeray when he arrived at Charterhouse in the 1820s were "Come and frig me."[11] But as the century advanced, public schools cleaned up their act, and under the reforming zeal of Dr. Arnold they gradually became training camps for the inculcation of gentlemanly conduct and sexual restraint. What Edward Bristow has described as a "war on schoolboy masturbation" was declared in the 1880s by several headmasters who had been alarmed by the revelations of Dr. Pusey and the subsequent controversy of the late 1860s, as well as by medical testimony and their own experience as teachers. The leaders of the campaign were Edward Thring, headmaster at Uppingham, and the Rev. Edward Lyttelton, a senior master at Eton, then headmaster at Haileybury and at his old school from 1905.[12] Thring was well aware that in bringing many boys together, "a great public school . . . concentrates evil and creates the chance for evil to be infectious"; according to his biographer, he was a particularly zealous hound of the onanists. During the early years of his rule, Uppingham was free from "serious moral evil," and when it appeared later he grappled with it "with a strong hand, in some case of proven guilt punishing with unrelenting severity." Thring faced the issue of school morals "more fully and fearlessly than in any other of the great public schools," and his method was to "arm boys for the inevitable struggle with their own lower nature or against the influence of evil associates" by means of "frank and open treatment." As he wrote to a parent in 1880, "I plainly put before them the devil work of impurity, and warn them that I will pitilessly turn out any one who after such warning is found guilty"; after one such inquisition he expelled four boys.[13] A glimpse of how it might have seemed to the boys is suggested by George Orwell's recollection of an incident at his school in which a number of boys were flogged and expelled for group masturbation: "There were summonses, interrogations, confessions, floggings, repentances, solemn lectures of which one understood nothing except that some irredeemable sin known as 'swinishness' or 'beastliness' had been committed. One of the ringleaders . . . was flogged . . . for a quarter of an hour continuously before being expelled."[14] One of Ellis's case histories reported that he was asked to leave after his housemaster discovered that he masturbated, because he was "not a safe boy to be in the school."[15]

The boarding school dormitory, as Alan Hunt has observed, "readily lent itself readily to the imagery of contagion and corruption that were such established themes in medical, religious and social purity discourses." The headmaster at Wellington (E. W. Benson) went so far as to lay barbed wire on the partitions between the beds, while his counterpart at Gresham was so anxious about what boys might do by themselves that they were all required to have their trouser pockets sewn up.[16] The Church of England Purity Society established a committee of schoolmasters on the subject of masturbation,[17] and their spirit soon trickled down to the state education system. The high master at Manchester Grammar told the Royal Commission on Venereal Disease in 1914 that mothers must train boys as toddlers: "inhibitions must be imposed, and the child must be taught that there are certain parts of its own body it must not touch."[18] In line with more of Acton's recommendations, public schools introduced sport and games in the 1860s, and they became steadily more central to school life as the century passed. One aim (especially in team games) was to impose discipline and order, but the other (relying on prevailing theories that the body had a finite reserve of nervous energy) was to discourage boys from solo and group masturbation by wearing them out on the playing field.[19] Thring described games as "the weapon with which we anticipate sensual evils, and ward off their attacks," and in the 1890s Hutchinson Almond hailed football as "a moral agent": despite its toll of twenty-three deaths each year, "it is an incalculable blessing to this country that such a sport is so enthusiastically followed by all that part of our boyhood whom Nature has endowed with strong passions and overflowing energies. Its mere existence and the practical lessons which it teaches are with all the books that have been written on youthful purity."[20] That was a less than grateful reference to the efforts of people like Lyttelton, who wrote several detailed guides on the maintenance of moral standards for teachers, clergymen, and parents. The sort of emotional toughness and self-abnegation promoted by Dr. Arnold and his followers might well have encouraged boys to think of circumcision, like war, as a tribal ordeal that proved their manhood rather than a surgical operation that diminished it. Supporting a motion that "warfare was essential to the welfare of the human race," schoolboy debaters at Shrewsbury in 1910 argued that "war was no more cruel than the surgeon's knife and, in addition, made men of us."[21]

Edward Lyttelton wrote at length on purity policy in his privately circulated pamphlet, *The Causes and Prevention of Immorality in Schools* (1887). In his view the "gravest social question" of the day was "What is to be done to brighten the purity of the morals of the nation?" It was no use driving prostitutes off the street if men were not reformed, and the only way to do that was to stop them from masturbating when young: "Purify your schools, and the life of the upper classes will be purified, and with that the life of the whole nation."[22] Lyttelton's major theses were a development of Pusey's. First, masturbation was learned, not instinctive: boys were innocent until instructed in "foul practices" by other boys, who thus spread corruption throughout a school; second, the early arousal of sexual interest lead boys to prostitutes in adolescence. He warned that solitary vice was "prevalent to the most dangerous and deplorable degree" and the principal cause of immorality in schools, where "most boys" were addicted to the practice (12, 8–9). He was equally concerned with group masturbation, but believed that "if solitary vice could be stamped out, dual vice would be almost unknown" (29)—an opinion somewhat at odds with his conviction that boys taught it to each other. Following Acton, whom he quotes at length, Lyttelton reminded his readers that "the least defilement in boyhood enormously increases the difficulty of continence in manhood" and that vicious habits have a weak hold (which can be broken) at an early age, but that in a few years they would be "overwhelmingly strong" (15, 29). Also like Acton he was not drawn to surgical remedies but to moral persuasion and healthy, outdoor living: he suggested to teachers that they should include "the physical side of the question" in their talks but that there was no need to be too explicit "or in the least medical"; only in cases in which "every appeal to conscience is rejected would I dwell . . . on this aspect of the temptation" (26). Although Lyttelton did not mention circumcision in his booklet, his aim was much the same as those who urged the operation as an aid to chastity: to put the penis to sleep until marriage. He was thus one of the leaders of the moral force school, and probably the authority who the more hawkish Lawson Tait had had in mind when he criticized this approach to what he was sure was a physiological problem: "I have been consulted concerning epidemics of this kind . . . and have always found the chief difficulty to be that of persuading those having charge of the schools that the practice was to be regarded as a physical delinquency rather than as a moral evil; and that the best remedy was not to tell the poor children that they were damning their souls, but to tell them that they might seriously hurt their bodies."[23] If masturbation was a physical rather than a moral delinquency, then physical treatments were the appropriate response.

A number of physical interventions were tried before the medical profession settled on circumcision as the most efficient, including chastity devices, infibulation, blistering, castration, and cutting the main penile nerve. Each had its strengths and weaknesses as a preventive, but the general aim was to make erections painful or the penis too inaccessible, too immobile, too sore, too limp, or too unresponsive to permit rewarding manipulation. As the *Lancet* editorial suggests, blistering was one of the most commonly performed treatments before circumcision became widespread. John Milton advised bichloride of mercury mixed with potassium iodide and several other caustics, applied only once a week, "to keep the parts gently sore"; more frequent application was apt to alarm the patient "by the severe blistering and pain which [it] occasions." Milton insisted that it was "useless to reason with the patient"; the only way to break him of the habit was "to make the penis so sore that he is at once awakened by the smarting as soon as he commences any attempts at friction."[24] In the early 1860s John Hilton, professor of surgery at the Royal College of Surgeons, knew of "no way to prevent onanism except by freely blistering the penis, in order to make it raw and so sore that it cannot be touched without pain." He reported his "miracle" cure of a fifteen-year-old suffering from vague muscular and spinal pains—symptoms Hilton was sure were induced by masturbation. His suspicions were confirmed by the boy's guilty look when he examined his genitals, and he applied a strong iodine solution to his penis and left instructions that a fresh dose be applied each night for the next three weeks. At the end of that time the boy had been restored to health.[25] Other physicians preferred hot metal rods: applied to the skin they produced a gratifying burn and a blister that could last for weeks.

Various chastity devices were tried, ranging from such mild measures as mittens or tying the hands to the bedrail overnight to more extreme contraptions such as straitjackets and cages over the genitals, but some of these savor more of an entrepreneur trying to cash in on a potential market than a serious and professionally sanctioned tactic. These have been described and illustrated elsewhere,[26] but their general objective is suggested by the description of a cage for the genitals, kept in place by straps and secured by small locks, advertised in 1889. This was recommended for boys during periods when they were not under surveillance: "In the case of children the parent keeps the key, and if needful unfastens the apparatus for micturition late at night. . . . It is equally useful for older youths or men who find themselves unwillingly overpowered at night. Such a person must, at bedtime, place the key in a drawer or other place away from the beside; then, before it can be used, the temptation will have passed."[27] The problems with such devices are obvious. Apart from the expense, they were cumbersome, required constant adjustment, and relied on the good will and cooperation of the patient: how many men were seriously going to put the key out of reach? Even lockable cages for children were a nuisance: what parent or nurse wanted to be woken up in the middle of the night to unlock it so that the boy could have a leak? Hands could be worked free from mittens and restraints.[28] What was needed was a cheap, no-fuss, permanent fix that could be imposed not merely without the patient's cooperation but in the teeth of his opposition.

Surgical interventions meeting some of these requirements included infibulation, castration, and severing the dorsal nerve of the penis. Dr. Spratling recommended the latter, and in 1899 a Dr. A. Campbell Clark arranged the procedure for an inmate of a mental institution in Scotland. Clark had found mechanical restraints useless because "the fury of the patient" tore them to pieces, but he got the idea that "division of the afferent nerve" of the penis would eliminate both erection and sensation. A colleague performed the operation on a forty-nine-year-old man, and it proved successful: although he was "very much depressed for some time afterwards," he gave up masturbation and reported no sensation in his penis at all, except a faint one when urinating, and was "much improved mentally." Although Dr. Clark acknowledged that such a drastic step was not for everyone—it was a question for the family doctor and the friends of the patient to decide—"the mental result in this case justified the operation."[29] In Australia a Dr. Hamilton treated a female patient for "nymphomania" by cutting the nerves leading to the vagina, commenting at the end of his communication that he was persuaded to try the operation after learning that a Sydney surgeon "had performed a somewhat similar one for masturbation in a male, with satisfactory results."[30] Castration was occasionally used to treat spermatorrhea, and it was recognized as a possible resort in desperate cases: one anxious dribbler wrote to Acton in 1854, reporting that he had been cauterized twice without benefit and asking whether he should try castration.[31] Jonathan Hutchinson suggested that in the case of inveterate masturbators (such as those confined in mental hospitals) castration would "be a true kindness,"[32] but the idea did not catch on, and I have not encountered any British cases in which castration (either voluntary or enforced) was actually used in the war against masturbation. It was a different story in the United States, where the operation was not uncommon in orphanages and institutions for feebleminded children.[33] The reason is obvious. Severe treatments for masturbation were generally imposed by adults on children, not by adults on themselves, but castration would prevent the boy from continuing the family line and would thus be sought only by the most desperate parents. Men who desired treatment for their own masturbation or spermatorrhea were not likely to agree to anything so extreme. What was needed was something that would reduce the attractiveness of sexual activity while leaving the reproductive function unimpaired, like "Dr. Scoffern's" operation on the tongue.

A candidate in the form of infibulation certainly had its champions. The possibility of inserting a wire or ring through the foreskin to stop it from sliding back—creating an artificial phimosis, in fact—and thus preventing masturbation had been recognized by the author of *Onania*, who wrote that "to secure youth from wasting their strength by self-pollution or venery till that age [marriage], they are so careful in some countries, that they ring the men when they are young."[34] Robert James similarly observed: "It was a custom among the Romans to infibulate their Singing-boys, in order to preserve their voices; for this operation, which prevented their retracting the prepuce over the glans, and is the very reverse to circumcision, kept them from injuring their voices by premature . . . venery."[35] He was a bad prophet in predicting that infibulation was "not likely to be revived," and its leading promoter in the nineteenth century was Dr. D. Yellowlees, medical superintendent at the Glasgow Royal Asylum. He reported in 1876 that he had tried infibulation on eleven men under his care, with the most gratifying success, though his first case had been "a lad who was so extremely addicted to masturbation that his mother begged him to do what he could to prevent it." The results were "excellent," and the boy soon found work as a carpenter. Unlike later advocates of circumcision who asserted that the foreskin had no anatomical purpose and its removal made no difference to sexual function, Yellowlees appreciated that its importance in facilitating erection was precisely the reason why its immobilization could inhibit masturbation. Infibulation worked because "the prepuce was anatomically necessary for the erection of the penis. Its anatomical use was to give a cover for the increased size of the organ, if you prevented the prepuce going to that use you would make erections so painful that it would be practically impossible and emission therefore extremely unlikely." Yellowlees pierced the prepuce "at the root of the glans" with a needle, drew a length of silver wire through, and tied the ends together. He reported that his patients were thus "absolutely debarred from the habit" and that he was struck by the "conscience-stricken way in which they submitted to the operation. . . . The moral effect . . . was excellent, and one man was seen weeping over his [penis] in anticipation of its disablement." Those present at the quarterly meeting of the Glasgow Medico-Psychological Association at which he presented his report were impressed with his achievements, and Dr. Alex Robertson spoke for them all when he voiced the desire to be kept informed of progress with these cases: "Should they continue to prove beneficial in repressing this habit . . . we will all be glad to try it."[36] Robertson had himself reported favorably on the use of a silver ring to prevent erection in his account of a tour of American insane asylums in 1869.[37]

How widespread infibulation was outside mental institutions and orphanages is not clear. I have not seen other British reports, but there is evidence that it became more common in the United States, where Yellowlees' article was widely reprinted.[38] Even so, he was an indefatigable promoter of his fix, for he returned to the subject in his entry on masturbation for the authoritative *Dictionary of Psychological Medicine* (1892), edited by D. Hack Tuke (whose son Batty had been present at the 1876 meeting). Here he agreed with Dr. Pusey that treatment must be "at once moral and medical." On the moral side were warnings, exhortation to decency, and provision of other interests, while on the medical side lay "direct operative interference" of various kinds. Yellowlees dismissed blistering and cauterizing as only briefly effective and causing itchiness, which accentuated the evil. The best form of interference was "so to fix the prepuce that erection becomes painful and erotic impulses very unwelcome." After a grisly description of his method he concluded: "With the foreskin thus looped up, any attempt at erection causes a painful dragging on the pins, and masturbation is effectually prevented."[39] This solution remained rare, however, not because it was cruel but because it was cumbersome, unreliable, and impermanent. Inmates in mental hospitals were under constant surveillance, but what was to prevent older children from undoing the wires or pins when no one was looking? Even if they were inspected morning and night, there would still be opportunities to untwist, and few parents would be willing to monitor them with the necessary assiduity. Apart from the bother, the idea seems too kinky for the British middle class.

Another way to prevent the foreskin from fulfilling its anatomical roles of facilitating erection and providing sexual stimulation of all kinds by sliding back and forth was to remove the redundant tissue altogether. Before the practice of widespread circumcision had the effect of causing many people to forget that the penis was meant to include moving parts, it was assumed that boys masturbated by tickling, sliding, or otherwise manipulating the foreskin. In his eleventh-century guide for confessors, Burchard of Worms expressed the general assumption with a clarity rarely found in medical writings: "Did you make fornication with yourself alone . . . I mean that you yourself took your manly member in your hand, and so slide your foreskin (praeputium), and move [it] with your own hand so as by delight to eject seed from yourself?"[40] Few medical men have ever been as precise, but Dr. Spratling put the position plainly enough. The objective of the various methods proposed to discourage masturbation, he wrote, was to "prevent the mobility of the foreskin," but most of them were ineffective or caused too much resentment: chastity cages and infibulation were "unsatisfactory and unsuccessful"; castration was "not to be considered"; cutting the dorsal nerve was "a rational procedure, but rather too radical for constant routine practice." That left circumcision, in cases of masturbation "the physician's closest friend and ally":

> To obtain the best results one must cut away enough skin and mucous membrane to rather put it on a stretch when erections come later. There must be no play in the skin after the wound has thoroughly healed, but it must fit tightly over the penis, for should there be any play the patient will be found to readily resume his practice, not begrudging the time and extra energy required to produce the orgasm. The younger the patient operated on the more pronounced the benefit, though occasionally we find patients circumcised before puberty that require a resection of the skin, as it has grown loose and pliant after that epoch.[41]

Spratling recognized that it was not the irritation of the secretions that led to masturbation, nor the desensitizing of the glans achieved by circumcision that discouraged the practice, but the loose and mobile tissue of the foreskin itself, which both constituted the temptation and facilitated its gratification. Spratling's reasoning was not as widely enunciated as its plausibility warranted, but most of his colleagues arrived at the same conclusion, even if by a different route. A surgeon who had closely followed the debate over clitoridectomy and the subsequent trial of our boys informed readers of the *Medical Times and Gazette* that his extensive contact with Jewish people had convinced him that they were less beset by this trial than other communities; he "had long been inclined to attribute this circumstance to circumcision" and sought the views of his colleagues. The editor replied that he had been informed by "a Jewish surgeon" that the practice was "virtually unknown in Jewish schools" and commented that it was "well known that the removal of the foreskin diminishes the temptation and the facility. The skin of the glans becomes harder and less sensitive."[42] Responding to this exchange, William Soper (surgeon to the Jews' Hospital) showed how the outcome of the Baker Brown affair had cleared the way for circumcision as a cure for masturbation in boys, and how the Pusey controversy had highlighted the need for action:

> Now that clitoridectomy has so long occupied our attention . . . I must be pardoned for alluding to . . . "the Besetting Trial of our Boys." I gladly substantiate the remarks of one of your recent correspondents, and am assured . . . that the besetting trial does not exist amongst the Jewish boys. . . . the removal of a portion of the prepuce is for many years fatal to the practice, and the glans is well known to become greatly reduced in sensibility.

Were he to meet "a patient who practised the abuse I should have no hesitation in circumcising him."[43]

By the early 1870s, as Acton noticed, a significant number of doctors were calling for universal circumcision of infant males as the best means to guard against "sexual precocity,"[44] and they were able to cite an ever-increasing number of papers in medical journals which provided evidence that the foreskin was the major risk factor for masturbation. From then on the assertion that circumcision was an effective and acceptable prophylactic against the practice became steadily more confident. In 1873 Francis Cadell argued that "in boyhood . . . a long prepuce . . . might be an exciting cause of masturbation" and recommended "circumcision in boys between infancy and puberty whenever congenital phymosis caused the slightest inconvenience."[45] The following year a doctor sought advice on how to treat "excessive masturbation" in a seven-year-old and received two helpful replies. One reported that he had "never known a case to resist circumcision and bromide of potassium"; the other suggested that only treatment "of an heroic nature" would be effective. He was treating four children who engaged in the practice at every opportunity, and the result had been pallor, "loss of flesh and brain-power; the children are unable to compete with others at school, their minds having lost the power of retention." The treatment he adopted was "blistering the penis, or the application of a hot iron, so as to render the organ excessively sensitive to the touch." He had also tried the usual bromides, but what he really wanted to advocate was "the heroic treatment—I mean circumcision; and if you can gain the consent of the friends, the sooner it is performed the better. Removal of the prepuce will cause the glans to become hardened in texture and so limit sensibility, besides the moral effect of the operation, which is not readily forgotten. In a large Jewish institution with which I am connected, masturbation is unknown."[46] In 1876 Abraham Jacobi was emphatic that "masturbating children . . . must be controlled and frequently forced. Circumcision is essential."[47] In 1883 Mr. Fletcher Little listed "the dangers to health and morals attending the possession of an elongated prepuce" and urged "the circumcision of every male child a week or fortnight after birth"; he believed that the incidence of masturbation would then fall by 50 percent.[48] The case for circumcision received a powerful boost in 1890 when one of England's most prominent surgeons and medical teachers, Jonathan Hutchinson, published his "Plea for Circumcision," first in his own journal and then more authoritatively in the *British Medical Journal*. Discouraging masturbation and promoting continence were prominent among his reasons for urging widespread performance of the operation.[49] Prevention of masturbation was the most important advantage of circumcision discussed in M. Clifford's *Circumcision: Its Advantages and How to Perform It* (1893), and his explanation conformed to the general line that it reduced irritation from secretions, lessened the sensitivity of the glans, and turned boys' minds away from sex.[50]

Experts in the emerging field of pediatrics agreed. In his influential and much reprinted *Diseases of Infancy and Childhood*, L. Emmett Holt gave a list of the symptoms of masturbation as lurid as anything cooked up by the quacks and advised that "circumcision should be done if phimosis exists, and even when it is not, the moral effect of the operation is sometimes of very great benefit."[51] In his own textbook Edmund Owen advised that a boy who did not heed warnings against masturbation must be watched and "his hands tied behind him" if necessary. Since local irritation could have various origins, his bladder should be probed for calculus, and in such a way as to inflict pain and inspire fear: "The sounding should be undertaken without an anaesthetic . . . and the boy should understand that it may be repeated from time to time should occasion demand. It is well that some punishment be held *in terrorem*." Beyond that, since "a long prepuce . . . may direct unwholesome attention to the part and engender . . . a habit one would be glad to pass over in silence," any boy so constituted should be circumcised; masturbation was far less common among boys without a foreskin.[52] The medical consensus soon filtered down to popular manuals of child care and healthy living, such as Sylvanus Stall's *What a Young Husband Ought to Know*, which enjoined on parents "the duty of guarding their children against secret vice. . . . Where infants exhibit a tendency to handle their private parts . . . the family physician should be consulted to see whether circumcision is not necessary to remove local irritation and inflammation. This is found to be necessary in many instances."[53] In his influential text on adolescence (1904), Stanley Hall also affirmed that there was "much to be said in favour of circumcision" as a treatment for masturbation, since the foreskin was "a rudimentary organ with all the morbid tendencies these often exhibit," and removing it greatly lessened excitability. Hall's advocacy of circumcision is all the more interesting since he accepted that most of the old medical arguments for the harm of masturbation were exaggerated, cleanliness was less of a problem as civilization advanced, and phimosis was less common than previously believed. In their place, however, he felt that the "psycho-neural arguments for circumcision . . . have great force," particularly "its undoubted restraining influence on self-abuse, its tendency to withhold from sexual excess, and generally to stabilize . . . the vita sexualis."[54]

Attempting to found a new specialty in andrology in 1910, Edred M. Corner wrote extensively on the dangers of congenital phimosis and came up with the novel suggestion that masturbation was more harmful before puberty than after. Although he denied that the practice among adult men was responsible for "more than a tenth of the troubles attributed to it" and insisted that the excess, not the habit, was the problem, it was a different story before puberty, when "masturbation . . . is most harmful, not only to the mind and body, but to the development of the sexual glands themselves. . . . Precocious sexual stimulation does lead to imperfect development of the testicles when puberty arrives, as well as the premature cessation of their activity." Where he got this idea from he does not say, but he cites a Dr. Wrench as asserting that "nature. . . . has ordained that our reproductive powers should be idle until the time and age of marriage," and he thus follows Acton's line when explaining that the practical implications were continence until then and measures to discourage premature sexual activity. Treatment must be both medical and moral, and the former included removing sources of local irritation, such as a long prepuce.[55] If masturbation did more harm in infancy and childhood than in adult life, the earlier the foreskin was removed the better. As late as 1935 a correspondent to the *British Medical Journal* suggested that "all male children should be circumcised" because the "glans of the circumcised penis rapidly assumes a leathery texture less sensitive than skin" and the boy "has his attention drawn to his penis much less often. I am convinced that masturbation is much less common in the circumcised."[56]

Consensus there might have been, but it was not unanimity. Although no doctor could be found disputing the harmfulness of masturbation until the 1930s, there was disagreement as to whether circumcision was effective as a cure or preventive. Even an ardent advocate like Hutchinson acknowledged that it was difficult to collect data because of "the distasteful nature of the inquiry" and that "general impressions are all that can be had." He was nonetheless confident that circumcised boys were less subject to the maladies associated with masturbation and agreed with Mr. Curling that circumcision was valuable both in breaking the habit and diminishing the subsequent temptation.[57] Despite lack of statistical evidence, Hutchinson was convinced that masturbation was "very injurious to the nerve tone" and thus that circumcision was still desirable, and "imperative" if the foreskin was "unusually long or contracted at its orifice."[58] He had originally endorsed circumcision as a treatment for the congenital phimosis deplored by Cooper Forster back in the 1850s, and in his "Plea for Circumcision" he reiterated his belief that the foreskin was "a constant source of irritation" that "conduces to masturbation and adds to the difficulties of sexual continence." At the turn of the century he insisted that circumcision was necessary because washing the uncut penis led to undesirable excitement and thus to masturbation.[59] Medicine was not evidence-based in those days, but doctors less fanatical than Hutchinson were also interested in determining whether circumcised boys really did masturbate less. In this quest they naturally turned to the only population they knew in which the boys were routinely circumcised soon after birth: the Jewish community. There was plenty of anecdotal evidence that Jewish boys did not masturbate (or not as much), but at a time when Jews were striving to break down the last barriers of discrimination and secure full acceptance in English society, they were hardly likely to admit that masturbation was a problem for them even if it had been. Such was the universality of the taboo that when the Viennese doctor Eugen Levit published a pamphlet deploring the persistence of circumcision and urging his community to drop the rite as part of their reform program, he made the improbable claim that circumcision, by exposing the glans, actually provoked masturbation. When this was reported in the *Lancet*, it elicited a sharp rejoinder from "a Jewish surgeon" in London, who countered: "That the deprivation of the prepuce induces premature sexual excitement and onanism is quite opposed to experience and fact. On the contrary, the removal of the prepuce reduces in an extraordinary degree the sensitiveness of the glans penis; and, apart from biblical reasons, which have necessarily no place in your journal, I believe that the intention of the rite was to . . . advance . . . the chastity of the race by blunting mechanically the sensibility of the organ of sexual appetite."[60] The medical profession was divided on the issue and initially ambivalent about the propriety of Jewish custom. In 1876 the *Lancet* described the circumcision rite as "repulsive" yet criticized a "provincial newspaper" for condemning all circumcision as an "act of cruelty" and "outrage upon the laws of nature"; it replied that the effect was "often beneficial" and "sometimes needed as a remedy for sensual practices."[61]

The view that circumcision had the effect of reducing sexual pleasure, and had even been instituted with this objective in mind, was both widely held in the nineteenth century and in accordance with traditional Jewish religious teaching. Both Philo and Maimonides had written forcefully to this effect,[62] and Herbert Snow quoted the contemporary Dr. Asher (in *The Jewish Rite of Circumcision*) as stating that chastity was the moral objective of the alteration.[63] John Davenport quoted a certain Virey,[64] who had asserted that circumcision had been introduced among the Semitic peoples to prevent "the detestable and fatal practice of masturbation . . . for he observes that . . . the Egyptians, Hebrew and Arab legislators were desirous of putting a restraint on self-abuse, and therefore introduced the rite as an obstacle to a vice so frequent and so fatal in those warm climates."[65] Remondino claimed that the prepuce was the most frequent cause of onanism and quoted the opinion of Dr. Vanier that

> if the prepuce is lax, its mobility produces an irritation to the . . . nervous system of the child by the titillation in its movements on the glans; if too tight . . . it compresses the glans and by its irritation it leads the child to seize the organ.

In either case he regarded the prepuce

> as the principal cause of masturbation. . . . In children who have not yet the suggestions of sexual desire imparted by the presence of the spermatic fluid, the presence of the prepuce seems to anticipate those promptings. Circumcised boys may . . . be found to practice onanism, but in general the practice can be asserted as being very rare among the children of circumcised races.[66]

Remondino agreed that the ancient origins of circumcision lay in the desire of ancient Judaic lawgivers to discourage the sort of debaucheries practiced among their idolatrous neighbors in the Middle East.[67] According to a Dr. Beugnies, the proposition that circumcision diminished the sexual appetite was confirmed by the example of the Jews but contradicted by the reputation of "Mohammedans" as driven by "very strong sexual passions."[68] Less was known about the world's most numerous circumcising culture, but Muslims made up a high proportion of British colonial subjects, and the leading authority on their sex lives, Richard Burton, also reported that among Arab youths "onanism [was] to a certain extent discouraged by circumcision."[69] Since Jewish circumcision is performed at eight days, when the human body is not fully formed, and Islamic circumcision not until much later (between eight and twelve years, when the organs are more developed and nerve pathways have been established), the physiological and behavioral effects in each case could indeed be very different.[70] The subject intrigued nineteenth-century doctors in much the same way as some contemporary medical researchers have become fascinated with differences in the rate of HIV infection among circumcising and noncircumcising African tribes, leading them to the obsession that universal male circumcision is the best strategy against AIDS.

Since no one in those days was trying to conduct controlled clinical trials, however, empirical evidence was hard to come by. In 1890 Dr. Peachey reported a case of masturbation in a six-year-old, who "was cured by circumcision"; he continued the habit for six months afterward "but has now entirely ceased." The physician explained this by reference to the keratinization and hardening of the glans, which evidently "took some time to accustom itself to the irritation of the dress."[71] It is equally likely that it took the boy six months to realize he was not going to get back the sensations he was able to experience before the operation. Dr. Beevor, on the other hand, reported the case of an eleven-month infant who had been in the habit of masturbating since the age of four months; on him circumcision and bromides had no effect at all.[72] Responding to an inquiry as to the "generally received opinion as to the efficacy . . . of circumcision in infancy as a preventive of masturbation" in 1901, the *British Medical Journal* replied that there was "considerable divergence of opinion" but that "there seems to be no doubt that whenever a long prepuce exists with a contracted orifice the operation is indicated to prevent the genital irritation which results from smegma and other secretions apt to accumulate under the prepuce. This may become the exciting cause of masturbation in very early life, and more especially at the period of puberty."[73]

A longer reply from a "Consultant to the Children's Hospital" is an instructive instance of an authority setting a series of seemingly stringent conditions for circumcision that in practice turn out to have little limiting force. He wrote that circumcision was effective only "when there are clear and definite indications," namely, "(1) if it is noticed . . . that the infant has acquired the habit of fingering himself; (2) if there is a congenitally tight and long prepuce which causes difficulty in uncovering the glans, or if after having retracted the prepuce there is difficulty in drawing it forward again." These "definite indications" would easily be met in the vast majority of young boys, nearly all of whom both have a long, tight, and adherent foreskin (its natural condition at that age) and enjoy fondling it. Despite this, the consultant went on to make some sensible observations about the absurdity of preemptive surgery, suggesting that the circumcision of "every boy when an infant to prevent his becoming a masturbator . . . is pure quackery," and mentioning the (by then) unthinkable comparison with women and the flaws of single-factor reasoning:

> Women sometimes unfortunately develop the habit; are we therefore to advise some preventive operation . . . [on] all female children? The argument that, owing to circumcision, onanism is comparatively rare among Jews (. . . not proven) is on a par with the statement, frequently made, that owing to the same cause, cancer of the uterus is comparatively rare amongst Jewish women. It is the fallacy, too common in our profession, of arguing from one instead of taking all the concomitant circumstances.

The writer suggested there was a better case for universal preventive removal of the appendix, since the consequences of appendicitis were so much more severe than those arising from masturbation. He observed that surgeons who had performed circumcision as a preventive of masturbation had not found the results satisfactory and went so far as to suggest that the practice, "in the absence of special local conditions," was a thing of the past. In this judgment he was mistaken, for even his own precise indications would demand circumcision in the majority of cases. But what reveals the consultant's position in the "divergence of opinion" is his comment that most cases of masturbation arise from "mental deficiency or lowered moral tone, stimulated . . . by puberty. One or two filthy boys will corrupt a whole school. The habit is to be prevented by the avoidance of low companions, by the fostering of a high moral tone at our public schools, by encouraging everything (open-air exercise, unstimulating food, literature) to keep up bodily vigour."[74] On the hawk-dove spectrum he was a dove. The irony is that with his all-inclusive medical indications, arising from the same misunderstanding of normal genital anatomy that had given rise to the myth of congenital phimosis, even doves (and Frederic Truby King in New Zealand is a striking instance)[75] found themselves recommending all but universal circumcision. They might not call it routine, but because their "definite" conditions were really very inclusive, the result was much the same.

This chapter would not be complete without some discussion of whether circumcision really did reduce the incidence or rewards of masturbation. For my purposes it hardly matters, since there is no doubt that most late nineteenth-century physicians believed that circumcision was effective, or at least were willing to act on the assumption that it was. By the early twentieth century, as some of the letters to Marie Stopes suggest, the idea that circumcision was a useful treatment for masturbation had become as much an article of folklore as the harm of masturbation itself. C.W. wrote from Belfast: "I shall be much obliged for your advice on a 'disease' which has troubled me for the last 10 years, that of self-abuse. I started it when a boy at school, and it seems impossible for me to shake off the vice now. . . . Would you advise me to be circumcised?" In 1939 a twenty-four-year-old wrote that he had been addicted to masturbation since the age of seventeen, that he stopped after he married, but that he had separated from his wife and the urge was returning: "Has long foreskin: should he be circumcised?" he asked. Some men wondered whether circumcision might cure premature ejaculation, while others thought that circumcision could be the cause of that problem. There was clearly much uncertainty as to why circumcision was commonly carried out. Another correspondent asked: "Is circumcision really of any moral value, or is it merely a custom delivered to us from the East?"[76] The answer to that question depends on whether you are considering masturbation before or after puberty and what you mean by masturbation. When arguing that the main reason for the introduction of circumcision was the desire to discourage masturbation, I have often been met with the knowing reply that this could not possibly be right because the remedy did not work: "It never stopped me," they say. Such touching faith do these credulous skeptics have in the medical profession that they believe it would never have promoted a therapy unless it had been proven to be fully effective and free from adverse side effects, presumably after exhaustive clinical trials! It is, of course, a characteristic of quackery that its claims are never verified and its cures don't work, but it was not for want of trying in this case, and Victorian doctors did have good evidence (very good by the standards of the time) that circumcision reduced the incidence of masturbation, especially before puberty. This is a subjective area, where individual experience differs widely, clinching data are difficult to obtain, and Hutchinson's "general impressions" are all that can readily be had, but let us see if we can gain any insights from modern sex research.

In his study of sexual behavior in the United States, Alfred Kinsey confirmed the worst nineteenth-century fears: boys, even as babies and toddlers, did have erections and even orgasms, they did masturbate, and they did engage in sex play with other children. Worse still, the incidence of such activity increased as they got older: Freud's reassuring "latency period" was a myth. Kinsey found that both boys and girls masturbated before puberty and that many experienced orgasms at early ages. Indeed, with his narrow definition of masturbation he found that preadolescent orgasms arising from friction, either inadvertent or deliberate, or emotional impacts were actually more common than instances of deliberate manual stimulation, which he found to be comparatively rare. Kinsey pointed out that orgasms in preadolescent males were not readily recognized because there was no ejaculation but noted that "erotic arousal and orgasm . . . among younger boys and females appears to involve the same sequence of physiologic events that has been described for the older, ejaculating males."[77] His description of this sequence—flow of blood to the genitals, increased heart rate, loss of perceptive capacity, a degree of bodily rigidity, and a sudden climax and release, often involving a spasm or mild convulsion—corresponds closely to the symptoms of epilepsy so frequently noticed in young children by nineteenth-century physicians on the lookout for masturbation. Kinsey was not able to estimate the proportion of boys who experienced orgasm before puberty, but in his fairly small sample he found that 32 percent had achieved it by age one, 57 percent between the ages of two and five, 63 percent among six- to ten-year-olds, and 80 percent among eleven- to thirteen-year-olds.[78] Although Kinsey provides tabulations for social variables such as education level and religion, he unfortunately offers no breakdown on the basis of circumcision status: whether the presence or absence of the foreskin affected the incidence of these manifestations is thus not a question his tables can answer.

Striking evidence is provided by a recent study of differences in sexual behavior observed among Dutch and American boys aged from two to six years (table 9.1).[79] The authors attribute the differences to methodology or culture rather than anatomy—variations in sampling techniques or the effect of more positive attitudes toward sex and greater permissiveness in the Netherlands than in the United States. These could well be important factors, especially the latter, but it seems rather naïve not to mention the obvious fact that most of the American boys but very few (if any) of the Dutch boys would have been circumcised—routine circumcision being unknown in Holland. The differences in frequency of masturbation with object (0.8 versus 11.8 percent) and with hand (22.6 versus 57.4 percent) are so great that there is likely to be something more going on than just socialization. This suspicion is strengthened by the fact that there is a far smaller difference when it comes to showing sex parts to adults and talking flirtatiously; if socialization were the only fac-

TABLE 9.1 Frequency of activity observed (%), boys aged 2–6

	Dutch	American
Masturbates with object	11.8	0.8
Masturbates with hand	57.4	22.6
Shows sex parts to children	23.6	15.7
Shows sex parts to adults	26.6	25.6
Touches own sex parts at home	96.6	63.3
Touches sex parts of other children	28.7	8.9
Talks flirtatiously	8.4	8.5

tor, one would expect American boys to be just as inhibited in these areas. As it is, talk about sex seems to be the only field in which the American boys can keep up with the Dutch; when it comes to action, they are so far behind that one suspects they must have been physically disabled in some way.[80]

Circumcision may be less significant after puberty. It would have come as a surprise to Alex Portnoy to learn that Jewish boys did not masturbate: from the moment of puberty he seems to have done little else, as he "doubled over [his] flying fist" and "moved [his] raw and swollen penis" through a world of "matted handkerchiefs, crumpled tissues and stained pajamas." The clues here are *puberty, fist,* and *raw and swollen.* There is no evidence that Alex masturbated, or even played with his penis, before sexual maturity; it was a lifeless appendage then, belittled by his mother as "his little thing . . . that I used to tickle to make him go wee-wee."[81] When Victorian doctors complained that little boys masturbated, they were noticing two natural phenomena. First, infants and young boys naturally fondle and tug at their penis, and since their penis at that age is made up mainly of its foreskin, their fingers automatically find that first; by definition, they are then fondling and tugging at their foreskin. Many Renaissance paintings and engravings show baby boys doing exactly this.[82] Boys are probably genetically programmed to fondle their penis (as Hunter suggested) or prompted to it by slight itchiness, and the effect of such manipulations is to assist the gradual process by which the foreskin separates from the glans and achieves retractability, thus preventing phimosis. It is also probable that the fondling stimulates the development of neuronal pathways in the brain, thus enhancing erotic responsiveness and sexual functioning in later life. Two contemporary neurologists, noting that the foreskin is highly responsive sensory tissue (like the retina of the eye), have speculated that excision of the foreskin in infancy (before neural pathways have been established) causes sensory deprivation in the brain; that this deprivation produces neural re-organization that reduces sexual responsiveness and excitability; and that, this being a good thing, routine circumcision of infants should be universally performed.[83] This argument is very like that of the Victorians, who were the first to call the natural fondling engaged in by infants and boys "masturbation"—medical and other observers before the rise of the phobia having simply accepted it as part of normal juvenile behavior. Lallemand and Acton reported many cases of masturbation and orgasm in infants and children, but there was no unanimity on the issue. Yellowlees caught the borderline status of the phenomenon when he wrote that "masturbation, *so called,* is sometimes practised by very young children."[84] Obsessed with the danger of masturbation and believing that children should be sexless, Victorian doctors categorized this behavior as a pathological response to irritation caused by the "secretions" trapped under the prepuce, but their deeper worry was that boys enjoyed their work: that was enough for them to brand the activity as masturbation, irrespective of whether emission or orgasm followed.

Suggestive evidence from the nineteenth century is provided by some of Havelock Ellis's case histories. Of 55 males who provided brief sexual biographies for his studies in the psychology of sex, 30 mentioned that they had masturbated in childhood before puberty and 7 that they had masturbated in infancy. The only two who reported that they had definitely not masturbated before puberty had been circumcised. This is a small and perhaps unrepresentative sample, but the figures gain in significance because Ellis had not asked specific questions: respondents were simply telling the story of their own sex lives in answer to an open-ended invitation.[85] Circumcision status was not always given, but considering the ages of the respondents (late twenties to sixties) and the time when the histories were written (1890s), it is reasonable to assume that they were not circumcised unless they stated otherwise. Many make clear that they had not been circumcised, while the only two to state that they had been were the only ones to report no interest in masturbation until after puberty. None of the noncircumcised reported that he did not masturbate in infancy or childhood, and several provided details of their activities at early ages. One recalled that he masturbated frequently as an infant and that "nothing was done to prevent . . . the pernicious habit into which I was falling. Circumcision was perhaps little thought of in those days as a preventive of juvenile masturbation; at any rate it was not resorted to in my case. . . . A nurse discovered that I was practising masturbation, and I think she made a few half-hearted attempts to stop it"—without success.[86] Another reported that he was punished for playing with himself as an infant but that he was still able to achieve pleasure, and even orgasm, by rubbing his penis against the carpet while his hands were tied behind his back:

> My earliest recollection is being punished for "playing with myself" when I could not have been more than 3 or 4 years of age. I distinctly remember my exultation on discovering that I could excite myself (while my hands were tied behind my back for punishment) by rubbing my small but erect penis against the carpet while lying on my stomach. . . . I did what my desires and my instincts at that time prompted me to do. However, punishments and lectures failed utterly to break up this habit, and though I always wished and tried faithfully to obey my parents, I soon grew to indulge quietly in bed when I was thought to be asleep.[87]

The same man reported that he usually achieved orgasm ("a single thrill of pleasure that extended all over my little body") from an early age but experienced no emission until after puberty. Looking back with the benefit of late nineteenth-century medical wisdom, the respondent felt "reasonably certain that this precocity was due to an adherent foreskin which covered the glans tightly almost to the point of the meatus, and so kept up a continual irritation." A third respondent reported that after he had been initiated into the pleasures of masturbation by one of the domestic servants at the age of twelve, it was a year before he experienced his first orgasm, and another before his first emission.[88] It was a different story among the circumcised cases. One of these reported that he had been circumcised at the age of five "on account of the prepuce being too long" and that he found masturbation "a dry and wearisome formula" until well after puberty. During childhood and early adolescence his mind was full of masochistic fantasies involving bondage, flagellation, and other boys urinating on him. At school one of his mates "invited me to watch him in the process of masturbation," but "the spectacle left me quite unmoved." The other case (very probably circumcised)[89] reported no sexual excitability at all until after puberty and, unlike most of the uncircumcised boys, no nocturnal emissions even then. He reported that a "handsome groom" had tried to fool around with him when he was about seven but could not arouse him; it was only after puberty that he learned about "mutual self-abuse."[90] Two cases out of fifty-five are perhaps not significant, but they offer food for thought.[91]

Turning to the other clues, it is a fact known to those of broad social experience that circumcised and intact men have different masturbatory techniques and that the latter have a wider repertoire at their disposal. One of Ellis's case histories reported three techniques he used as a boy. First, he placed his penis through the handle of a pair of scissors and "flapped" it until "a strange, sweet thrill went over me from top to toe and a drop of clear liquid oozed from my member." Second, he "pumped" his penis by "slipping the prepuce back and forth." Third, he "grasped the organ at its root and violently jerked it back and forth."[92] Another method is to insert a finger between foreskin and glans and slowly rotate it, relying on those secretions to provide lubrication. The most popular approach among the uncircumcised is probably to use no more than the thumb and two nearest fingers—the thumb on the upper side of the penis, the fingers on the lower (frenulum) side—and, applying only light pressure, slide the foreskin back and forth over the glans.[93] As Kristen O'Hara has found, however, circumcised men require a tighter grip, heavier pressure, and a more violent action to get enough sensation to produce orgasm.[94] They typically make a fist with their whole hand, grip the penis firmly, and run the fist up and down the shaft; the fist thus becomes a foreskin substitute, but without lubrication the friction always produces chaffing, often soreness if done frequently, and sometimes bleeding from abrasion. Chester Eagle refers to the "puffy skin" seen round the collars of the circumcised penises of his schoolmates at Melbourne Grammar in the 1940s.[95] As a submission to the review of policy on routine circumcision carried out by the Royal Australasian College of Physicians in 2001 asserted, "it is far easier to masturbate if you have a foreskin." As the author explained:

> It is easiest with a normal foreskin not only to masturbate yourself, but also to masturbate someone else. The next easiest is with a loose circumcision (i.e. only a bit of the foreskin has been removed and there is a enough left to allow plenty of to and fro movement) and hardest with a tight circumcision—where there is little or no movement possible. In the case of a tight cut it is almost impossible to stimulate the penis satisfactorily without lubrication. Masturbating a tightly cut penis is too abrasive and painful.[96]

The Victorians were wrong to believe that circumcision might reduce sexual desire—that is stimulated largely by hormones, not discovered until the 1930s; following Carpenter and Kobelt's physiology, they believed that sexual desire was generated by the nerves concentrated in the glans. But they were evidently right to think that circumcision made sexual activity, including masturbation, more difficult and less pleasurable, and that was the main reason they favored it. Despite Hutchinson's frustration at not being able to produce proof, his contemporaries were convinced that circumcised boys of all ages, but especially before puberty, did masturbate less than the normal. Whether or not they believed the assurances of surgeons connected with Jewish schools that their boys did not masturbate at all, they certainly wanted to believe it, and they were prepared to act on the assumption that it was true. The vital consideration in their thinking was not so much the loss of the preputial nerves and the lessened sensitivity of the glans as a result of circumcision as it was the mechanical action of the foreskin and the enhanced functionality of the penis when foreskin, glans, and shaft worked together as a dynamic ensemble. Victorian doctors could thus argue that circumcision discouraged masturbation by removing the mobile sleeve that facilitated it, but that it did not significantly reduce the pleasure of legitimate sexual activity (marital intercourse) because that derived from the friction of the vagina on the glans. Some authorities (such as Hutchinson and Freeland) admitted that even this pleasure might be reduced by circumcision, but since they considered the only purpose of sex to be reproduction, and both masturbation and syphilis to be such serious diseases that sacrifices were justified, they did not consider this to be a deprivation to which boys and men had any right to object.

10 · This Unyielding Tube of Flesh

The Rise and Fall of Congenital Phimosis

In this unyielding tube the glans is imprisoned and compressed, often suffering the tortures that the "maiden" of the . . . Inquisition inflicted on the unhappy heretics. It becomes elongated, cyanosed and hyperaesthetic: the meatus of the urethra is congested . . . the glans [acquires] the long-nosed, conical appearance of the head of a field-mouse.

P. C. REMONDINO, *History of Circumcision*, 1891

No child should be allowed to grow up with a glans which harbours "smegma and other sexual secretions." There is no more revolting asset in an adult male than a foreskin which is not permanently retracted.

ERNEST SAWDAY, FRCS, *British Medical Journal*, 1944

The anatomists have never studied the form and evolution of the preputial orifice. They do not understand that Nature does not intend it to be stretched and retracted in the Temples of the Welfare Centres or ritually removed in the precincts of operating theatres. Retract the prepuce and you see a pin point opening, but draw it forward and you see a channel wide enough for all the purposes for which the infant needs the organ at that early age. What looks like a pin point opening at 7 months will become a wide channel of communication at 17. Nature is a possessive mistress, and whatever mistakes she makes about the structure of the less essential organs, such as the brain and stomach, you can be sure that she knows best about the genital organs.

SIR JAMES SPENCE, *Lancet*, 1950

In no area was the Victorians' loss of knowledge in sexual anatomy more cruelly expressed than in the theory of congenital phimosis—the proposition that the naturally nonretractable and adherent condition of the juvenile foreskin was a malformation, and one responsible for a host of diseases and disapproved behaviors. That such an error was held all but universally by the British medical profession for nearly a century (from the 1840s to the 1930s) is a tribute to the pervasive power of the masturbation phobia over this period and the refusal of doctors to subject hypotheses in sexual matters to empirical testing or verification. To maintain the infallibility of the authority figures on whose opinions they relied, doctors interpreted observed reality in the light of received theory. Even those who had reservations about circumcision as the best treatment had no doubt that phimosis in infancy was a disease requiring immediate attention, and this misconception is not dead in ex-circumcising cultures today.[1] For a century phimosis was the principal indication for cutting the foreskin from male infants and boys. The justifications offered were three: that the phimotic condition was abnormal and somehow wrong because it did not conform to an ideal image of what the doctor thought the penis ought to look like; that, by providing only a "pinhole" opening, it restricted the expulsion of urine and led to nervous conditions such as hernia and paralysis; or that, by trapping "secretions" and making it impossible to wash the penis properly, it would result in "uncleanliness" and give rise to a variable constellation of diseases, from cancer and syphilis to bed-wetting, masturbation, and fretfulness. The rise and fall of routine circumcision in Britain is closely correlated with the rise and fall of the myth of congenital phimosis.

Although the word *phimosis* is derived from the Greek (meaning "muzzled"), neither the term nor the concept appears in the texts of ancient medical writers. According to Frederick Hodges, the first recorded use of the word was by Roman medical writers, who employed it to denote a stricture or muzzling of any body part or organ, though not the foreskin. The first author to use *phimosis* with reference to the foreskin was Celsus, and by the term he meant an unusual hardening of the foreskin in adults—a rare condition now usually identified as balanitis xerotica obliterans and thought to be most commonly caused by a fungal infection.[2] Celsus also described a condition in adults in which the foreskin became nonretractable because of swelling or inflammation (most likely a venereal chancre), but he did not use the term *phimosis* to designate this. In the second century CE the Greek physician Antyllus used *phimosis* to indicate a condition in which the foreskin could not be retracted as a result of inelastic scar tissue or a "fleshy growth." He separately described another condition in which a previously retractable foreskin adhered to the glans because of ulcers or scabs, and he recommended treating the problem by syringing warm water beneath it.[3] So remote were these ideas from those of nineteenth-century physicians, and so anxious were the Greeks and Romans to preserve the foreskin and ensure a cosmetically attractive (that is, properly sheathed) penis, that the Greek physician Soranus (ca. 98–138 CE), in his famous midwifery manual, considered that lack of length, coverage, and tightness in the foreskin of a newborn baby was a defect known as *lipodermos*, which had to be corrected by gentle traction: "If the male neonate appears to be lipodermic, she [the wet nurse] should gently draw the foreskin [*akroposthion*] forward or even hold it together with a strand of wool to fasten it. If gradually stretched and continuously drawn forward, it easily stretches and assumes its normal length, covers the glans penis and becomes accustomed to keep the natural good shape."[4] Similar advice was given by Falloppio in the sixteenth century, and in the seventeenth by William Harvey, who nonetheless betrayed a certain loss of understanding as to the purpose of the maneuver by suggesting that the rationale was to make the penis bigger.[5] The folklore that penises could be enlarged by stroking and fondling at an early age was probably derived from the classical advice that inadequate foreskins needed to be gently stretched, but it survived in the animadversions of Acton et al. on nurses who tickled infants' genitals to soothe them and his concern that early retraction of the prepuce led to undesirable enlargement of the penis.

It was only in the eighteenth century that a recognizably modern understanding of phimosis emerged, but even then it was a condition described only in adult men, never in infants or boys. John Marten makes no mention of phimosis in his description of the "defects, diseases and infirmities" of the genitals, and describes only his treatment for a short frenum (frenulum breve), easily fixed by a snip to the offending filaments, in much the same way as recommended by Venette and later practiced by Ricord and Acton.[6] There is no mention of phimosis at all in Jane Sharp's *Midwives' Book* (1671), nor in any of the three eighteenth-century child-care manuals reprinted by Garland in 1985.[7] The conceptualization of phimosis as pathological defect in immature boys had to wait until the identification of masturbation as a disease agent had spread from the denunciatory texts into mainstream medical works, and from there the demonization of the foreskin followed. The increasing concern with phimosis in *adult* men was probably a response to the syphilis epidemic, which drove many to present themselves at doctors' surgeries with suddenly nonretractable foreskins as a result of swelling, ulceration, and other nasty side effects of sexual promiscuity. Such venereal infections often did produce sores that fused the foreskin to the glans as they healed and otherwise caused the foreskin to become less elastic and tighten. We have already seen the descriptions of these conditions by Pierre Dionis and John Hunter, both of whom stated that phimosis (nonretractability) in childhood was normal, and it is worth recalling Hunter's streetwise observation that boys commonly loosened tight foreskins by their ineradicable urge to play with their penis. This, indeed, was the advice given by Robert James for treating paraphimosis: cold water to make the erection subside; lubrication of the penis with olive oil or butter; and manual manipulation if that failed.[8] Such conservative therapies (especially the last) obviously became impossible once the masturbation taboo took hold. Thus the conjunction of the venereal disease epidemic and the masturbation phobia gave rise to the twin delusions that an adherent prepuce in boys was pathological and that preemptive amputation of the foreskin was an effective defense against syphilis and chancre.

In the late eighteenth and early nineteenth centuries the distinction between venereal chancre and phimosis was so blurred that the terms seemed almost interchangeable. William Buchan barely mentioned phimosis in his *Domestic Medicine* (1772), leaving the subject to be covered in his *Observations concerning the Prevention and Cure of Venereal Disease* (1796), in which he reported that phimosis was an occasional problem in adult men, usually associated with venereal disease, and that the best treatment was conservative: hot and cold poultices, fomentations, and bathing. Small incisions were sometimes necessary in severe cases. Buchan accepted the variability of foreskin length as a biological fact and did not try to impose his own standards of what was allowable:

> These parts are so differently formed in different men that some may be said to have a natural phimosis; while others have the reverse. I have seen the foreskin so long that above three inches of it were amputated [i.e., would need to be],[9] in order to discover the glans. In others the glans is never covered but remains exposed during life. Neither of these is attended with any considerable degree of inconvenience, unless in a diseased state.[10]

Buchan also warned that phimosis, and more often paraphimosis, was often caused by ill-advised interference:

> I have known some young men bring on a violent paraphymosis by acting on a wrong principle. One who had pulled back the skin and kept it there until it could not be returned without making incisions on both sides, said he did it on purpose to keep the glans cool. In this case, though the stricture was removed . . . the foreskin remained thickened.[11]

Most cases of phimosis caused by venereal infection could be cured by conservative treatment, and it was only in rare and obstinate instances that surgery was needed. Only after "all endeavours" to draw the foreskin back, using fomentations and so forth, had failed was it necessary to slit it open. Buchan was aware that this was a desperate step, since "many people" considered incision to imply "mutilation," and he was at pains to point out that such mutilation was necessary only when the problem had been neglected. Early treatment would ensure that no more than a small incision was required. He described any cutting of the penis as "mangling and maiming" and assumed that nobody would allow it to be done except to save his life, and that he would still regret it.[12] A similar classification of phimosis as a venereal disease was made in the 1820s by Sir Astley Cooper, who stated that phimosis arose from "slight inflammation of the cellular tissue, and effusion of serous matter into it." The cure was mercury, purges, and fomentations.[13] Although it was the consequence, not the cause, phimosis induced by venereal chancre or other infection was a serious condition, and treatment was certainly needed (not that the nineteenth century could offer any effective treatments). But the idea that phimosis (meaning nonretractability) was pathological in men neither infected with venereal disease nor suffering from other injury, and whose foreskins varied enormously in length and tightness, developed as a result of the confounding of these two quite separate categories. The outcome was the extension of phimosis as a disease condition to men who were perfectly healthy, and from there to infants whose tightly covered penises were perfectly normal.

The process by which the myth of congenital phimosis became consolidated as medical orthodoxy is obscure, but the idea gained ground in the 1850s. In 1846 the *Lancet* reported the case of an ailing and comatose eight-week-old infant whose prepuce was found to be elongated and with "an aperture only of the size of a pinhole" from which urine was dribbling. The examining doctor concluded that the problem was that the boy had never been able to empty his bladder, whereupon he slit the prepuce and reported that the symptoms vanished.[14] The interesting features of the case are that it is one of the earliest claims that a "pinhole" opening of the prepuce could lead to retention of urine; that no one used the term *congenital phimosis;* and that the physician reporting the case described such a problem as only "occasionally occurring in practice" and never previously described in print. Within thirty years such cases were popping up everywhere, and similar symptoms were being alleged in 60 percent of boys under four years of age.[15] Either the anatomy of the penis or the perceptions of doctors changed dramatically between the 1840s and the 1870s, and today the condition is nearly as unheard of as spermatorrhea.

Charles West's lectures on diseases of children in the late 1840s may have been an important factor in this transformation: as we have seen, he was one of the first to use the term *congenital phimosis*, to suggest that a narrow foreskin might make it difficult for a baby to urinate, and to urge circumcision if the preputial opening was "too small." He also asserted that the operation should not be delayed, since "adhesions are very likely to form between the glans and the foreskin, which render the necessary surgical proceeding more severe."[16] Since the most common cause of acquired adhesions in childhood are attempts to retract the foreskin,[17] it is likely that any rising incidence of this condition was the result of doctors, nurses, and parents following bad medical advice: that the problem was iatrogenic rather than congenital. As reported in chapter 6, Cooper Forster claimed to be the first English writer to identify the problem ("urinary irritation arising from long pressure, or congenital phymosis"), and he was probably the first to call it a "malformation" and to direct nurses to treat the condition by early retraction of the foreskin. "Every nurse should be directed to carefully wash away the secretion . . . which may easily be done by withdrawing the prepuce from the glans," he wrote, apparently unaware that this advice contradicted his observation that in young boys "any attempt to withdraw [the prepuce] over the glans is attended with much pain."[18] Hutchinson gave the term and concept currency in his article supporting Forster's paper, and probably in his many lectures to medical students, but the original source seems to have been Lallemand, who had identified phimosis (and particularly the "secretions" it trapped) as an important cause of early sexual excitement, penile irritation, and masturbation. Reflecting the conflicting influences of Ricord and Lallemand, Acton was uncertain and contradictory on the subject. It is possible that West and Forster had been influenced by the remarks of the American Edward Dixon, who had written in a text first published in 1845 that "natural phimosis" was a "deformity" of boys with "naturally too long a foreskin." He further commented that "the humane and enlightened rite of circumcision, if practised on all male children," would make the nervous affections arising from the phimotic condition "very infrequent," since they were "generally caused by a preternatural elongation of the prepuce."[19]

It might seem strange that a theory that emerged in the primeval 1840s was still influential in the 1930s, and is still held by some with scientific pretensions today,[20] but the long life of the concept was the result of its compatibility with both the nerve force and the germ theories of disease, or at least with early versions stressing filth and suppuration. According to nerve force theory, it was perfectly possible for the irritation caused by the trapped secretions, or even by no more than the friction of the foreskin over the glans, to provoke nervous imbalances that could lead to many diseases, from gonorrhea to epilepsy. Lewis Sayre relied on this notion to explain how an adherent prepuce could cause forms of paralysis.[21] Under zymotic and later germ theory, the accumulating secretions became "filth," which in the early phases "putrefied" and thus gave rise to disease poisons, and in the later stages either bred or nurtured the microorganisms that caused specific diseases. The concept of irritation was retained to explain how a disease like penile cancer, thought not to be caused by bacteria, could be generated from the secretions (as claimed by Abraham Wolbarst and most famously by Abraham Ravich, in his valiant endeavors to demonstrate that smegma caused not only cancer of the penis and cervix, but of the testicles and prostate as well).[22] Behind these concerns about real diseases rumbled the persistent ground bass that the main problem with phimosis in infancy and childhood was that it led boys into masturbation.

The idea that a nonretractable or adhesive prepuce was a source of apparently unrelated diseases was boosted by the labors of the orthopedic surgeon Lewis Sayre. Having discovered around 1870 that a wide range of childhood illnesses was apparently caused by a tight foreskin, he circumcised a number of boys suffering from various forms of paralysis, all of whom he reported were restored to health. Explaining the physiological basis for this miracle, Sayre employed nerve force theory to hypothesize that "peripheral irritation" from the foreskin produced "an insanity of the muscles," which then acted on their own accord, without direction from the brain. As he wrote in a paper called "Partial Paralysis from Reflex Irritation Caused by Congenital Phimosis and Adherent Prepuce," "many of the cases of irritable children, with restless sleep, and bad digestion . . . [are] solely due to the irritation of the nervous system caused by an adherent or constricted prepuce. . . . Hernia and inflammation of the bladder can also be produced by the severe straining to pass water in some of these cases." Sayre eventually consolidated his convictions in a book titled *On the Deleterious Results of a Narrow Prepuce and Preputial Adhesions,* published in 1888. Other doctors in the United States were quick to take up Sayre's impressive findings and push them further. Soon adherent prepuces were being discovered all over the country and their removal alleviating the symptoms of numerous childhood complaints; one doctor reported a case of "brass poisoning completely cured." Another suggested that, although it had never been calculated, the incidence of adhesive foreskins was probably higher than people realized. Since "a long and contracted foreskin" was so often a source of "secondary complications," he proposed that it was "always good surgery to correct this deformity . . . as a precautionary measure, even though no symptoms have as yet presented themselves." Christians had much to learn from Jews in this respect: "if circumcision was more generally practised at the present day . . . we would hear far less of the pollutions and indiscretions of youth." As David Gollaher observes, this declaration represented an important transition in thought: circumcision became not just a treatment for an existing problem but an anticipation designed to prevent potential "complications" in the future.[23] It was little wonder that crusaders for routine and universal circumcision leaned heavily on Sayre: Remondino declared that Sayre's discoveries about the nervous action of the prepuce meant that he "was to medicine what Columbus was to geography."[24]

Sayre's work was well known in Britain, where it was particularly popularized by Abraham Jacobi, John Erichsen, J. Arthur Kempe, and Edmund Owen. In a lecture reported in 1876 Jacobi warned that the foreskin often continued to be adherent after birth, with the result that "copious collections of smegma may easily occur and get rancid, and urine collect and get acid, a local irritation of the glans will result, and give rise to repeated attempts on the part of the little sufferer to get rid of the irritation by pulling at the organ—and in this way the habit of masturbation may be contracted." Jacobi accepted Sayre's claim that irritation of children's genitals "exerts a very widespread reflex influence" but doubted that instances of paralysis had arisen "solely from an adherent prepuce"; he suggested that masturbation was needed as an additional exciting cause.[25] It was possibly Erichsen, in his widely read and much reprinted *Science and Art of Surgery*, who did most to confirm congenital phimosis as medical orthodoxy and promote circumcision as the preferred treatment. He defined the condition as one in which the prepuce was elongated beyond the glans and so tight "that it prevents the proper exposure of this portion of the organ." (Note the judgmental word *proper*.) The effects were serious: atrophy of the penis; failure of the glans to develop; incontinence, retention of urine, hematuria, and priapism (as shown by Mr. Bryant);[26] and reflex paralysis, spastic contraction of the legs, and various other "nervous disturbances of a paralytic or spastic character," as demonstrated by Sayre. But the worst thing about congenital phimosis was its stimulation of premature sexual arousal: although most cases caused merely "local inconvenience," in some children "the retention of the sebaceous secretion—the smegma preputii . . . becomes a source of local irritation and inflammation from uncleanliness. The irritation thus kept up leads to local excitement, and favours the development of the habit of masturbation." So great were the evils arising from both congenital phimosis and even "an abnormally long though not phimotic prepuce" that it was "only humane and right from a moral point of view to practice early circumcision in all such cases." Indeed, Erichsen seems to have regarded phimosis as the wedge to encourage circumcision as widely as possible, as much for moral as "health" reasons: "Every child who has a congenital phimosis ought to be circumcised; and even those who, without having phimosis, have an abnormally long and lax prepuce, would be improved greatly in health and morals by being subjected to the same operation. It would be well if the custom of eastern nations . . . were introduced amongst us."[27] After such a modification, even boys not exhibiting phimosis could be expected to behave better.

In 1878 J. Arthur Kempe referred to a chapter on "phimosis as a cause of talipes and other paralytic affections" in Sayre's textbook *Diseases of Joints* in his own article on phimosis as a cause of rupture. Indeed, most of Kempe's article was taken up with citations from other authorities on problems caused by a tight prepuce: Edmund Owen on eczema induced by dribbling urine; Mr. Bryant on irritability of the bladder and priapism; and M. Malgaigne,[28] who claimed that one in every twenty-one children had a rupture. Kempe wanted to argue that most such cases were caused by straining to urinate through a constricted prepuce, but he was forced to confess that he had been "unable to find any mention of difficulty in micturition as a cause of hernia in children" and concluded that "the co-existence of phimosis and rupture seems hitherto to have escaped notice." Undaunted by the lack of precedent, Kempe set out to find some evidence and came up with statistics that made Hutchinson's "proof" of less syphilis among the circumcised (see chap. 12) seem rigorous. He examined "50 cases of congenital phimosis" in boys aged six months to four and a half years and found that no fewer than thirty-one had a rupture, including five with a double inguinal hernia. Kempe omitted to explain how these cases came to be available for study, but one assumes that they were brought to the children's hospital because there was something wrong with them, most likely an obvious or suspected rupture. Since most of the boys were aged less than two and a half years, the congenital phimosis from which they were "suffering" was the normal condition of their penis at that age; to Kempe, however, it was obvious that if a tight prepuce and hernia were found together, the former must be the cause of the latter, and all these boys were circumcised on the spot. Postoperative case details were not, unfortunately, provided, but Kempe assured readers that all cases were "much benefited."[29] Edmund Owen concluded a lecture on Sayre's orthopedic techniques with a digression on the prepuce, which began by blaming it for hernia and ended with bed-wetting. In Owen's experience, "the commonest cause of hernia in childhood" was "a small preputial or urethral orifice," and after that "the smegma-hiding or adherent prepuce," all of which gave rise to "frequent itching at the end of the penis." There followed an elaborate explanation of the nervous mechanisms involved in producing urinary retention during the day (and thus hernia) and relaxation (and thus bed-wetting) at night, complete with a fascinating diagram with a remarkable resemblance to a Victorian railway junction.[30] As late as 1890 the *Medical Annual* reported Sayre's discovery that "obscure nervous disorders in children may be due to a long or adherent prepuce."[31]

By the 1880s it was believed that every boy whose foreskin was not re-tractable within a few days of birth needed surgical intervention; the argument was over whether the deformity should be corrected by dilation and separation, a laborious process sometimes taking weeks, or by amputation of the adhesive tissue, a comparatively simple matter and one held to be less painful for the child. Even so determined a critic of circumcision as Herbert Snow accepted that "a perfectly healthy condition of the male generative organs is compatible only with perfect mobility of the prepuce over the glans," and he further conceded that it was "universally agreed" that "the adhesions between the prepuce and the glans can nearly always be broken down . . . during the first few weeks after birth."[32] Dr. Alexander Davidson followed Sayre's line in attributing a range of childhood complaints, from hernia to rickets, to a tight foreskin and claimed to have cured many such conditions by circumcision. He had an additional theory that early fondling of the penis did not loosen the foreskin, as Hunter had taught, but made it tighter still. In this scenario, the pent-up secretions caused irritation, which provoked the boy to seek relief by tugging at his prepuce, thus lengthening it and causing the orifice to shrink. Continued irritation led to manipulations, which gave rise to "masturbation in its most odious sense."[33] A few of Davidson's cases will show the quality of his reasoning and style of medical care, and how much they have in common with the theory and purported cures of Lallemand and Sayre:

> Case I. Aged seven years. Been ailing for a year, and under medical treatment. Previously active, intelligent and healthy. Now he is apathetic and unable to stand or walk; "plays with himself," and suffers from nocturnal enuresis. Prepuce long, orifice contracted, with inflamed edges, and very excitable. Circumcised. Nocturnal enuresis at once ceased; in a few days he tried to walk, and within a month walked a mile without support. Former intelligence had then returned.
>
> Case III. Aged three years. Very rickety and enfeebled. Frequently wakes crying, and is found grasping his erect penis. Nocturnal enuresis. Circumcised. Nocturnal disturbances entirely ceased, and health rapidly improved.
>
> Case IV. Aged five years, Paraphimosis with superficial sphacelation.

Has often been flogged for "bad habits." Circumcised. Parents believe that he has ceased to manipulate, and his health has greatly improved.

Although consistent with both the nerve force and the germ theories of disease, congenital phimosis as a pathological problem owed more to the former and is good evidence that circumcision was associated with a passing phase of medical theory, not with the understandings of disease that developed as microorganisms were studied. Even in the 1890s many doctors relied on nerve force theory to explain why the foreskin was a menace and should be removed. In 1891 Arthur Jackson blamed it for hip joint disease, "affections of the spinal cord," hernia, and epilepsy, and the last of these was particularly associated with congenital phimosis.[34] This connection had originally been advanced in the 1840s and was still quite respectable half a century later. In 1883 a Mr. Teale related a series of "epileptiform seizures" apparently caused by masturbation and cured at once by circumcision, which he recommended "as a preventive measure," and in 1895 a mainstream textbook listed "premature sexual excitement and masturbation" and "convulsions, epilepsy and hip-joint disease" among the baleful consequences of phimosis.[35] As late as 1907 another practitioner agreed that the adherent prepuce was a frequent cause of epileptic attacks.[36] There was also debate over whether phimosis was the main cause of bed-wetting. The English were more skeptical than the Americans,[37] but in 1913 it was reported that the problem was generally regarded as a nervous disease and best cured either by removal of the adenoids (given the "well known connection between enuresis and the adenoids") or by circumcision. One doctor believed the cause to be a "long, adherent prepuce" and had circumcised in 187 cases, of which he claimed 130 cures.[38]

Once it was accepted that the natural phimosis of the infant penis was a pathological abnormality, the stage was set for close to universal circumcision, but some doctors were unwilling to amputate and devised various regimes to dilate tight foreskins and separate them from the glans. These were invariably so time-consuming, elaborate, and agonizing for the boy that it is little wonder that many parents and physicians preferred circumcision, which at least had the virtue of being over comparatively quickly, but medical journals were full of correspondence from practitioners eager to share their favorite method. In 1879 Robert Parker advertised a pair of specially invented "dilating forceps" to be used in cases in which parents opposed circumcision or there was a risk of bleeding or infection. The prepuce had first to be detached from the glans by means of a button-probe, after which the forceps were inserted and opened to stretch the tissue; after four dilations of half an hour each on four consecutive days, the foreskin should be loose and the glans fully exposed. Parker actually preferred circumcision and urged it strongly in all cases in which the foreskin was long as well as tight, but he consented to stretching when the parents could not be persuaded.[39] Another practitioner learned an even more cumbersome method in 1883, involving the use of a probe to "break down the adhesions," followed by an unstated period during which the nurse was obliged to "draw back the foreskin once or twice a day to prevent it adhering again." There is a hint that this procedure might not have been entirely to the liking of the beneficiary in the comment that "on several occasions, owing to not having a good nurse to hold the baby, I have had to complete the operation at a second sitting"—implying that his struggles made it impossible to continue.[40] Noticing this difficulty, a reader wrote in with the helpful suggestion that a better way to keep the child quiet was to give him a few whiffs of chloroform.[41] Herbert Snow devoted a book to his own alternative to circumcision, without doubting that congenital phimosis was a condition that threatened the health of the boy and must be treated.

At the turn of the century the state of pediatric opinion was probably represented by Edmund Owen, who followed Remondino in asserting that a prepuce that covered the glans tightly could "prevent its proper development, rendering it corrugated and misshapen." It was important to retract the foreskin soon after birth because adhesions could render a boy "irritable and unmanageable," while the "reflex disturbances arising from preputial irritation" could produce conditions similar to spinal and hip disease. The prepuce of every "fretful, whining and neurotic child ought to be examined," and if there seemed to be "any redundancy, adhesions or retention of smegma, circumcision should at once be done." Owen brought in something from germ theory in explaining why a long prepuce was "a constant source of danger": because the secretions could not be cleaned away, they might decompose and suppurate. If circumcision was not performed, the nurse must draw the prepuce back and wash beneath it every time the boy had a bath. With tight foreskins, "dilatation [sic] with the blades of the ring-dressing forceps may suffice," but circumcision was preferable since "the daily drawing to and fro of a prepuce which is swollen and tender, on account of the forcible dilatation to which it has been subjected is likely to distress the child and to be objected to by the mother and the nurse."[42] It hardly needs pointing out that these elaborate rituals were possible only in well-to-do households with a nurse on permanent duty and the resources for frequent trips back to the surgery for the inevitable complications and possible second attempt. Many parents would prefer the quick snip because they could not be bothered: one doctor reported that he had tried the stretching regime but gave it up in favor of circumcision because he "never yet found a mother or nurse who could be relied upon to continue the daily retraction until [the foreskin] would remain permanently back."[43] It is also worth noting the persistence of nerve force theory in the idea that preputial irritation could cause disease, and of a somewhat outdated concept of infection in the notion that the secretions might decompose and suppurate: that sounds more like zymotic theory in the 1860s than germ theory in 1900. It is also apparent that all these careful directives must have done a lot more harm than good: as pediatricians since Douglas Gairdner have appreciated, nothing was more likely to cause scarring, bleeding, infection, adhesion, and genuine phimosis than all this poking, tearing, and stretching. Aside from being extremely painful, they had the effect of destroying the elasticity of the preputial sphincter, "preventing its proper development," and causing permanent deformity. A clue to the damage being inflicted is provided by a comment in the *British Medical Journal* from 1894, that circumcision should be performed "before adhesions have taken place between the prepuce and the glans."[44] Such intensifying adhesions could only be the result of attempts to retract the foreskin. By the end of the nineteenth century the most common cause of phimosis as a genuine disease condition was the misguided interference of the medical profession itself.

The extraordinary thing is that Victorian doctors had abundant empirical evidence that phimosis was normal in infants and that a retractable prepuce at or soon after birth was very rare. As the foreskin became more sternly anathematized in the second half of the century, so the incidence of congenital phimosis increased. In 1852 Jonathan Hutchinson had referred to the condition as "not common," but forty years later it had become "exceedingly common," and Remondino went so far as to claim it affected 95 percent of the uncircumcised.[45] In the 1870s Robert Parker described phimosis as "a tolerably common disease," and Abraham Jacobi acknowledged that a phimotic condition might "remain for months, and sometimes for years"; in most circumcisions "the operator is obliged to tear a portion of the prepuce from the glans."[46] In the 1890s even Remondino acknowledged that phimosis in infancy and childhood was normal, and pathological in only a minority of cases: natural phimosis was "the common lot, as a rule, and with some it remains so throughout life. As babyhood advances into boyhood and boyhood into youth, the prepuce gradually becomes lax and distensible." But he did not accept the logical implications of these observations and expressed his awareness in terms of reporting the views of other (obviously naïve and mistaken) authorities. He responded that the condition was "physiological" in infancy but that we did not know why it often remained until puberty, and he went on to quote conflicting statistics on the incidence of phimosis at various ages.[47] Snow recognized that "congenital phimosis may be said in some slight degree to occur in every newborn male child,"[48] and by the 1890s it was recognized that foreskin and glans developed as one structure in the fetus, but it was assumed without evidence that the two entities were meant to have separated by birth. Edmund Owen wrote that "in foetal life the mucous layer of the prepuce is always blended with the glans" but that "with approaching birth the adhesion melts away. Adherence of the prepuce after birth is the result of arrested development."[49] If Owen had any evidence for his final assertion he did not disclose it. A similar set of assumptions is revealed by (Sir) John Bland-Sutton (1855–1936), a leading gynecological surgeon, in one of the longest and most deeply researched articles on the penis published in the *British Medical Journal* before Gairdner's study of 1949. As you might expect from one of England's most avid practitioners of hysterectomy, described by one critic as "a criminal mutilator of women,"[50] Bland-Sutton was no friend of the foreskin.

Bland-Sutton began with an ominous aside that "the prepuce is liable to a variety of malformations and morbid conditions," followed by the assertion that the most common abnormality was "redundancy." By this he denoted a condition in which "the tubular process [*sic*] of skin may stretch for an inch or more like a miniature proboscis in front of the penis"—a common sight indeed, since it is the normal condition of the infant penis. Bland-Sutton conceded that this was not necessarily a problem so long as the foreskin could easily be retracted to allow the parts to be cleaned, but where this could not be achieved phimosis was present and circumcision was necessary. Congenital phimosis was "very common" and was caused either by "an abnormally long foreskin with a narrow orifice" or by adhesions between the foreskin and the glans. Relying on some recent studies of the development of the genitals in the fetus, Bland-Sutton made a slight advance from Owen in acknowledging that such adhesion was normal at birth but asserted that it "usually spontaneously disappears." Unfortunately, he had no idea as to how long this spontaneous disappearance was meant to take, nor what numbers were represented by the vague term "usually," and he thus followed Owen in assuming that it was all meant to happen very quickly. Failure to do so was retardation: "The so-called adherent prepuce of the infant is due to an organic connection between the glans penis and the non-differentiated preputial tissues, and results from the ingrowing epithelium above described not desquamating at the usual time, and is really in the nature of an arrested development."[51] The inability to specify the "usual time" betrays his failure to investigate this crucial question: one wonders why

Bland-Sutton did not conduct the necessary research. He was happier expatiating on the problems caused by an "abnormally long" prepuce, chief among which was difficulty with urination; the resultant straining could cause hernia and prolapse of the rectum. Apart from that, the dribbling of urine through a narrow preputial orifice caused irritation, which made the child fretful and peevish, and "may lead to reflex disturbances," as previously shown by Sayre and Davidson. In his discussion of acquired phimosis in adult men—in the eighteenth century, it will be recalled, a condition arising only from injury or venereal infection—Bland-Sutton reveals how far the demonization of the foreskin had proceeded; by 1907 even a loose and fully mobile foreskin was an object of fear and suspicion:

> Many men with a slight degree of phimosis or with a long but retractile prepuce remain uncircumcised, and so long as they are taught to keep the parts clean . . . the condition, though inconvenient, may not give rise to serious trouble. . . . There is no question that such a condition is often a hindrance to coitus and leads often to paraphimosis and balanitis, besides rendering the individual more prone to abrasions and slight fissures which may be infected with syphilis; moreover, a long foreskin is certainly a trap for the gonorrhoeal virus. . . . Apart from these evils, the margins of the preputial orifice are apt to be excoriated and fissured in old men, whose urine dribbles away from prostatic trouble.[52]

Despite the grudging concessions, nobody hearing his lecture could doubt that, even if he had not made much of a case for "the advantages of circumcision" to which he referred at the close, Bland-Sutton had convincingly shown the foreskin to be a troublesome appendage. The determination of doctors like him to circumcise even without persuasive evidence of benefit is vividly demonstrated by his failure to specify the time by which the "spontaneous separation" of glans and foreskin was supposed to have occurred, and by the fondness of other experts for circumcising even when the phimotic condition had cured itself. As one authority on "male diseases" wrote in 1910, although "many cases of apparent phimosis in babies get well from the natural stretching of the prepuce by erections," he would "strongly urge this little operation . . . [in early infancy] on sanitary and moral grounds."[53] By moral grounds he meant bad habits like masturbation, and it comes as no surprise that the author of this advice was the same Edred Corner who also warned that masturbation was maximally harmful in boyhood and that circumcision should be performed as a deterrent.

Corner recognized that "phimosis of some degree is natural in the babe and in the immature," yet he recommended rapid circumcision of all babes "suffering from" phimosis even when there was no evidence that they were "suffering" at all. As for grown-ups, "no adult male should be allowed to have any degree of phimosis." Corner followed Bland-Sutton in asserting that "redundancy of the prepuce" was congenital but ventured the extraordinary suggestion that it started causing irritation even before birth, claiming that its nonretractability was "generally a character acquired, possibly in utero, as the result of the irritation caused by the secretions of the preputial glands." The influence of Remondino's storytelling is also evident in his assertion that phimosis caused the glans to remain "small and poorly developed," though he did not go so far as to claim that it was forced into the shape of a mouse's nose. Corner was not taken in by old beliefs that phimosis caused hernia, however, with the consequence that he realized that recommendations for circumcision would need to be based on other grounds—"principally that of cleanliness."[54] The foreskin's main offense was that it kept the glans constantly moist and that this moisture "quickly undergoes decomposition, becoming malodorous and irritating both the glans and the prepuce."[55] Circumcision in infants could be avoided by any of the complicated processes suggested for "breaking down the adhesions" and keeping the foreskin retracted until the two surfaces had healed, but Corner strongly preferred circumcision as "more complete, more cleanly and more sure." Adult men might be able to escape circumcision by developing the habit of wearing the foreskin retracted (like Buchan's foolish youth): "The sensitiveness of the glans and the inner side of the prepuce can be allayed by the use of some spirit lotion. In a few weeks the oedema [i.e., bruising] will get less until at last a cleanly habit is acquired. There is no doubt that either this habit or . . . circumcision would do much to increase the comfort and cleanliness of many."[56] Like all the others, these routines were so obviously clumsy and bothersome that they seem to be mentioned only in order to demonstrate the superiority of circumcision; as Corner pictured genital anatomy, it was apparent to any reader that the uncircumcised penis required "increased care in maintaining cleanliness."[57] Despite his vehemence, it is not entirely clear what Corner considered the precise object and main benefit of circumcision to be. He was not trying to remove as much mucous membrane as possible (à la Freeland) to guard against the entry of syphilis nor trying to stop masturbation by removing the mobile sheath that made it so easy to do. His main object seems frivolous in comparison with the grand schemes of Hutchinson, Remondino, et al. to conquer syphilis, tuberculosis, cancer, and the like, and amounts to no more than trying to make the body easier to keep clean. In eleven pages the words *irritating* or *irritation* appear four times; *cleanliness* four times; *cleanly* twice; followed by *uncleanly*, *sanitary*, *washed*, *cleansed*, and *malodorous* with one appearance each. They might be appropriate to a manual of sanitation, but they suggest a limited perspective from which to try to found a new medical specialty in andrology.

The deepest problem with congenital phimosis was the dilemma it created for those who wanted to argue that the penis must be washed thoroughly every day but feared that it should not be touched lest masturbation ensue. In the late Victorian period cleanliness became an essential component of respectability and an important means of distinguishing nice people from "the great unwashed." Bodily cleanliness thus assumed great importance, but the hygiene of the genitals posed a problem. Obviously they had to be kept clean, but herein lay the equally obvious danger that the manipulation involved could be found pleasurable and give rise to bad habits. This uncertainty had been apparent in Acton,[58] and it became more explicit at the turn of the century. Genital hygiene had not been a concern of doctors before the eighteenth century and came to be seen as a problem only after the rise of the masturbation phobia: boys were then forbidden to touch their genitals, but how could they keep them clean if they were not allowed to touch them? Circumcision offered a path out of the thicket, as Hutchinson explained:

> The first advantage of removal of the foreskin is cleanliness. In adults the habit of withdrawing the skin and washing the glans has usually been learned. . . . In children it is [rarely] attempted; most boys would regard the attempt as indecent, and in many paraphimosis would result. . . . the practice would be injurious to the morals of the child, yet the accumulation of smegma and its decomposition is a source of annoyance. . . . Any irritation of the . . . penis is liable to produce reflex excitement of an undesirable character.[59]

The linkup of phimosis, hygiene, and masturbation was also made clear by M. Clifford, who wondered whether it was desirable to instruct boys to withdraw their foreskin in order to wash the inner surfaces:

> As a matter of fact it is rarely done, and hence the secretion, perspiration, dirt and so forth remain. . . . But if this want of cleanliness does not produce [balanitis] . . . the irritation . . . is very liable to give rise to [lascivious] ideas. . . . As age advances the habit of masturbation is very frequently to be attributed to it. But after circumcision the glans penis is always dry. . . . It loses much of its acute sensitiveness, . . . the mind is not directed towards the sexual organs, and a decided check is put to one of the vices . . . [of] early manhood.[60]

Contrary to Acton, the New Zealand child-care expert Frederic Truby King believed that instructing parents to wash their children's genitals was bad advice; it was in fact "one of the best means of teaching the child self-abuse," and the "natural parental instinct to chide or slap a child for 'fingering the privates' is sounder and more wholesome."[61] The Australian Zoe Benjamin was also aware of this dilemma, and in one of her books on child rearing she considered the various causes of masturbation and advised: "When bathing children, great care should be taken in handling and drying those parts of the body. They should be touched firmly so that no tickling sensation is set up, but not so firmly that the child is hurt"[62]—a fine line to tread. The final solution to the difficulty lay in removing the root of the dilemma, as recommended by the American Dr. William Robinson:

> The prepuce is one of the great factors in causing masturbation in boys. Here is the dilemma we are in: If we do not teach the growing boy to pull the prepuce back and cleanse the glans there is danger of smegma collecting and of adhesions and ulcerations forming, which in their turn will cause irritation likely to lead to masturbation. If we do teach the boy to pull the prepuce back and cleanse his glans, that handling alone is sufficient gradually and almost without the boy's knowledge to initiate him in to the habit. . . . Therefore, off with the prepuce![63]

Sanitary and moral issues were indeed the heart of the matter. The impact of the new medical perceptions on the public is evident in the case of the man who reported (in the sexual history he wrote for Havelock Ellis) that his own foreskin was very tight and remained partially adhesive until puberty, when he decided to tear the adhesions loose with a button hook. He had been left alone to find his own solution to an unusual condition, but his sons were not so fortunate: they "were afflicted with adherent foreskins to such an extent as to render circumcision necessary a few days after birth, in order that the function of urination might become fully established," he wrote, parroting the new medical orthodoxy.[64] This was the man who reported how much he had enjoyed masturbation as an infant and young child, despite parental efforts at restraint (see chap. 9); did he consider himself more humane than his parents because he had circumcised his own boys instead of tying their hands behind their backs?

Even in the 1930s concern about masturbation lay behind debates about whether various dilative regimes were an acceptable alternative to circumcision in cases of phimosis. A fiery controversy on routine circumcision was ignited in 1935 by D. I. Connolly, who cited the high incidence of complications from circumcision—including hemorrhage, ulcers, sepsis, and death—and asked if there was not "any reliable efficient method of treating severe phimosis other than by a cutting operation." By "severe phimosis" he meant the normal condition of the penis at birth, since his alternative procedure was to be performed within a week of that happy event. Connolly proposed yet another method for separating foreskin from glans, in this case rolling it back and keeping it retracted for "the next few days" (presumably, though he does not say so, to give the raw and probably bleeding surfaces time to heal). He claimed that the initial procedure took no longer than five minutes, but left it to the mother to keep the foreskin rolled back and held in position by means of some special rubber shields he had designed.[65] Several readers wrote in to commend Conolly for his initiative and to offer their own nostrums, including Cecile Booysen, who described a method she had learned from Geoffrey Keynes, which involved a very slow process of separation and stretching by means of conventional probe and sinus forceps. The advantage of her method was that it was done so gradually and gently that pain to the infant was minimized; the disadvantage was that it required "daily visits for one or two weeks," and she did not reveal how many parents were willing to undertake this marathon. In the same issue of the *British Medical Journal* R. Ainsworth made the revolutionary suggestion that phimosis was an imaginary disease, but his was a lone voice.[66] In the next issue the advocates of circumcision mounted their counterattack with the usual reasons as to why the operation was the only possible approach to phimosis, including the risk of hernia, bedwetting, "fits," cancer, gonorrhea, and masturbation. C. E. Gautier-Smith reacted violently to Dr. Booysen's innocent remark that her method could be carried out "without pain or risks" with the crushing retort that this sort of molly-coddling could only lead to masturbation:

> I have no doubt that the child exhibits no sign of pain but rather of pleasure, for as every child's nurse knows, nothing quiets a child so much as gentle manipulation of his genitals. At the same time nothing is more apt to start the habit of masturbation. . . . We are . . . familiar with the melancholy sight of a child of 3 or 4 . . . masturbating, and most investigators . . . are satisfied that this practice in the very young is the result of unwise handling by parent or nurse, which has taught the child the possibility of pleasurable sensation from friction in those parts.

Smith ridiculed the time and bother required by the stretching regimes proposed by several correspondents, and asserted that if the glans could be kept clean "only by regular manipulation of the foreskin, then it had better be left dirty or its covering removed surgically." He teased readers with an ambiguous and unanswered reflection as to whether it was any more necessary to cleanse the male glans than to wash out the virgin vagina, but he was satisfied that the lessened liability to cancer and syphilis was sufficient justification for routine circumcision of boys.[67]

This debate in the correspondence columns of the *British Medical Journal* was a watershed in the history of routine circumcision in Britain, revealing that many doctors were not happy with the practice, and also that there was growing consciousness that premature retraction of the prepuce actually caused rather than prevented phimosis, and often inflicted injuries that required circumcision later. An anonymous letter reported that "my brother and I both required this attention at school age. . . . I was foolish myself to listen to the advice of one of our maternity and child welfare staff, who stretched the prepuce of my elder son, with the result that he required at school age the operation he should have had as an infant."[68] Only Dr. Ainsworth was provocative enough to suggest that the boy would have required no attention at all if his foreskin had been left alone,[69] but he was a herald of things to come. It was in the 1940s that Douglas Gairdner studied the development of the prepuce and showed the theory of congenital phimosis to be a myth, and in 1944 a correspondent to the *British Medical Journal* asked whether the foreskin should be retracted in the child, the adolescent, and the adult. The surprising reply was that "special cleansing" was not usually needed before puberty, but that after that time it should be withdrawn and the interior washed "whenever necessary"—as with any other part of the body.[70] What was shaping up as the new orthodoxy did not go unchallenged. Ernest Sawday described this advice as "deplorable" and insisted that "no child ought to be allowed" to harbor sexual secretions. His policy was to circumcise all infants except those with an easily retractable prepuce or whose parents did not consent. "Very seldom have parents objected" he added, "and . . . I have told them clearly . . . that they are denying their child one of the greatest benefits with which a baby boy can start out on the road to life."[71] As the practice of circumcision declined, the evangelism of the remaining true believers became more fervent.

The problem until Gairdner researched the issue was that doctors believed that if the foreskin had not freed itself within a few days of birth it would never do so, and surgical intervention of some sort was thus essential. This was a serious medical error responsible for pain, suffering, and mutilation on a monumental scale, and it could have been corrected had the doctors gone back to the ancient and eighteenth-century texts or studied preputial development in normal boys in an empirical spirit. Instead, millions of boys were subjected to prolonged agony as grim-faced doctors, bustling nurses, and distraught mothers poked, stretched, and lacerated the most sensitive part of the boys' bodies. Even when amputation was not performed, their gruesome ministrations must often have destroyed the elasticity of the foreskin and prevented its sphincter from operating as the valve it was meant to be, as well as causing a deformed appearance, scarring, and often the very adhesions (arising as the torn surfaces healed) they were supposed to cure. Many came to the reasonable conclusion that circumcision was a kinder option. To appreciate the scale of the error, consider its equivalent in women: it would be as if doctors had decided that the intact hymen in infant girls was a congenital defect known as "imperforate hymen" arising from "arrested development," and hence that it needed to be artificially broken in order to allow the interior of the vagina to be washed out regularly to ensure hygiene. One can imagine any opponents of the operation being met with the clinching reply, "But it's so much more hygienic and easier to clean without the hymen." The various procedures carried out to treat congenital phimosis in boys makes Baker Brown's dexterous clitoridectomies look humane by comparison.

II · Prevention Is Better Than Cure

Sanitizing the Modern Body

Ninety-five per cent of the human race suffer from chronic blood-poisoning, and die of it. It's as simple as A.B.C. Your nuciform sac is full of decaying matter— undigested food and waste products—rank ptomaine. Now you take my advice, Ridgeon. Let me cut it out for you. You'll be another man afterwards. . . . I tell you this: in an intelligently governed country people wouldn't be allowed to go about with nuciform sacs, making themselves centres of infection. The operation ought to be compulsory; it's ten times more important than vaccination.

GEORGE BERNARD SHAW, *The Doctor's Dilemma*, 1906

For millennia the male's preputial cavity has acted as a cesspool for infectious agents transmitting disease.

GERALD WEISS, "Prophylactic Neonatal Surgery and Infectious Diseases," 1997

It is one of the puzzles of nineteenth-century medical history that the demonization of the foreskin as a source of ill health was accompanied by the denigration of its significance in the bodily system. It was a difficult balancing act to argue not only for the unimportance of the foreskin but also for the immense advantages of being without it, to assert its irrelevance to sexual function yet also its malevolence if left in place. A further paradox indicates the ambiguous connection of circumcision with what would be generally be regarded as medical progress: while doctors stressed its scientific basis as a modern therapy, they also sought to justify it by reference to the ritual practices of prescientific tribes not noted for their medical knowledge. In their search for authoritative statements in favor of these arguments, doctors leaned heavily on a supposed quotation from Philippe Ricord, revered as the century's leading expert on sexual matters by virtue of his work on venereal disease, and especially for decisively distinguishing syphilis from gonorrhea and identifying its three stages. In 1900 E. Harding Freeland headed an article on the need for universal circumcision as a preventive of syphilis with an epigraph on which he relied to support his contention that amputation of the foreskin was no serious loss: "The prepuce is an appendix to the genital organs the object of which I could never divine; instead of being of use it leads to a great deal of inconvenience, and the Jews have acted kindly in circumcising their children, as it renders them free from one at least of the ills to which flesh is heir."[1] The quotation was attributed to "Watson" in the *Edinburgh Medical Journal*, 1873, and it turns out that a Dr. Watson did quote this passage during a discussion of a paper by Francis Cadell titled "The Advantages of Circumcision," given in 1872. Watson expressed himself "surprised that Dr Cadell did not quote the greatest of all authorities on such matters, viz., Dr Ricord," who had made the statement "in one of his published clinical lectures." Watson then quoted the passage in full, including an additional sentence: "The prepuce is, in fact, a superfluous piece of skin and mucous membrane which serves no other purpose than as a reservoir for the collection of filth, especially when individuals are inattentive to cleanliness." As Watson then remarked, "this was very strongly confirmatory of Dr Cadell's views."[2] This Dr. Watson was Patrick Heron Watson (1832–1907), an active member of the Edinburgh Medico-Chirurgical Society and an authority on venereal disease, with several major publications to his credit.[3]

Given Ricord's conservative policy on amputation, his positive attitude toward the foreskin, and the absence of this passage from any of his publications that Watson would be likely to have read (see chap. 6, n. 35), it is improbable that Watson saw this statement in a text published by Ricord. It is more likely that he was recalling (and slightly misquoting) the passage as given by Acton in *A Practical Treatise*, and one of the misremembered details is significant. Acton attributed the comment to one of Ricord's clinical lectures, suggesting that he might have heard it while a student in Paris; Watson added the word *published*, implying that he had read it somewhere—which he no doubt had, but not where he implied. Despite its dubious authenticity, the quotation gave a great boost to the circumcisers' crusade by virtue of its simultaneous dismissal of the foreskin as a valueless inconvenience yet a serious threat to health and its accepted coining by someone with Ricord's authority, and it was much quoted by the anti-foreskin lobby. In 1890 Jonathan Hutchinson referred to the foreskin as "a harbour for filth," an expression obviously suggested by Ricord's reservoir; the following year Remondino misquoted part of the statement—"a useless bit of flesh"—in his own diatribe, attributing it to Ricord but without identifying the source.[4] In 1914 Remondino's misquotation was itself cited by Abraham Wolbarst, who referred to Ricord as "the famous master" who had judged the prepuce to be "a useless bit of flesh"—an opinion congenial to Wolbarst's demand for "universal circumcision as a sanitary measure."[5] The source of the popularity of this demand were developments in late Victorian disease theory, especially the theories of filth disease, autointoxication, sanitary science, and preventive medicine, all of which evolved in the context of new trends in multicultural and urban politics.

The Victorian imagination was haunted by the specter of the "epidemic streets" and the "fever nests," those unwashed urban pockets where overcrowding and lack of sanitation caused disease to fester, and from which epidemics spread to other regions of the body politic. As Anne Hardy has argued, the image received its original shape from the fear of typhus at midcentury, particularly from the description of the "fever houses" in Dickens's *Bleak House*—the putrescent slum of Tom-All-Alone's, "a villainous street, undrained, unventilated, deep in black mud and corrupt water . . . and reeking with such smells" that the visitor can scarcely believe his senses.[6] From those teeming backrooms the victims of pestilence were carried "like sheep with the rot," and from them the winds spread contagion to the better classes: "There is not a drop of Tom's corrupted blood but propagates infection and contagion somewhere. It shall pollute, this very night, the choice stream . . . of a Norman house, and his Grace shall not be able to say Nay to the infamous alliance. There is not an atom of Tom's slime, not a cubic inch of any pestilential gas in which he lives . . . but shall work its retribution through every order of society, up to the proudest of the proud."[7] Dickens's perspective emphasizes the point that what the respectable classes feared was contagion from the great unwashed, not that the working masses were about to expropriate the expropriators. He was using the miasmatic model of disease transmission, but the concept of the fever nest was taken over by the new theory of filth or zymotic disease, under which all diseases were thought to be related to lack of cleanliness and were preventable by sanitary interventions such as removing the nuisances where dirt could accumulate.[8] As Christopher Hamlin has argued, a central image in Victorian pathology was the corruption of the pure by contact with impurity, and its transformation into another impure agent that could spread further corruption.[9]

Circumcision established itself in the surgical repertoire during a period in which the causes of most illnesses were not understood, theories of disease were confused, no effective cures were available, and few preventives known. One of these was vaccination against smallpox, and the fact that it had been around since early in the century *and that it worked* goes far to explain why no one suggested that circumcision might reduce the risk of contracting that disease.[10] The crucial decades for the acceptance of circumcision as a valid preventive technique were the 1860s and 1870s, when germs were only a new and unproven theory, and many authorities denied their existence or agency. Apart from nerve force theory, there were four main alternatives to germs, all depending on either spontaneous generation or chemical processes, in the context of dirt, for their effects. Miasmatic theory held that diseases was caused by bad smells. Chemical theory held that filth decomposed and produced disease-causing poisons, and one of its strongest proponents, B. W. Richardson, argued that all bodily secretions were capable of generating poison: "a particle of any one of these poisons brought into contact with the blood," he wrote, could change that secretion "into a substance like itself." A seed-based scenario held that disease germs were particles of degraded bioplasm like seeds, which were thrown off by living beings and would be transmitted through the air and pass into the blood of others, where they would "sprout" and grow.[11] Probably the most influential theory was the zymotic, which held that disease was caused by rotting organic matter and that any organic matter could putrefy; if this got into the body it would cause the blood to decompose and ferment likewise. The biggest problem was sewage and household refuse, but any bodily product could putrefy and give rise to disease; even parts of the body could rot as a result of the accumulation of wastes.[12] Spontaneous generation (the idea that disease poisons were "constantly being generated de novo by the material conditions which surround us") was widely believed in the 1860s and 1870s, especially by medical practitioners and the "sanitary public," as William Budd, a believer in germs, complained;[13] the idea that disease factors could be generated by filthy matter trapped under the foreskin was all but required in this explanation. What all these theories had in common was dependence on dirt to produce or nurture whatever agency caused the disease, and it was not a new concept. Thomas Malthus had rejected the idea of disease as divine retribution and proposed instead that it was the result of having violated the laws of nature, particularly by permitting "dirt, squalid poverty and indolence" to accumulate. He referred to the London plague (1665) as evidence for this and commented that the subsequent "removal of nuisances, the construction of drains, the widening of the streets, and the giving more room and air to houses" eradicated this scourge and contributed greatly to the health and happiness of the population.[14] It was the sanitarian reform program a generation before Chadwick.

Zymotic theory arose by analogy with fermentation, recognized as a natural (and beneficial) process needed to turn dead organisms back into soil; but decomposition could also occur on or in the body, and specific forms of such putrefaction could give rise to different diseases.[15] This theory was most influential in the early years of Listerism, from the 1850s to the 1870s, and there is scarcely a disease that was not at some stage blamed on filth by somebody. In 1879 Andrew Fergus listed croup, diphtheria, dysentery, diarrhea, cholera, scarlatina, "fevers," measles, whooping cough, and smallpox—nearly all the Victorian killers—as zymotic diseases.[16] To preserve health, filth must be removed or, even better, prevented from accumulating in the first place; because it was difficult to tell when putrefaction became pathogenic, it was best to take a cautious approach and remove all organic matter before the rot set in.[17] There was much argument as to whether disease arose spontaneously from filth or whether it merely provided a favorable environment for disease-causing agents, and as germ theory developed in the 1870s it was the latter view that prevailed. Sir John Simon championed zymotic theory against the contagionists, since it seemed consistent with the germ theory and justified the sanitarians' war against dirt—the medium in which disease factors thrived. In a lecture given in 1870, the newly appointed professor of hygiene at University College, W. H. Corfield, admitted that "we know little or nothing of the causes" of diseases such as tuberculosis, cancer, and scrofula, but he was "certain that bad hygienic conditions favour the development of several of them, and may in many cases be the direct causes." He even thought that scurvy was caused as much by "bad hygienic conditions" and "damp, unwholesome dwellings" as lack of fresh vegetables.[18] Toward the end of that decade Charles Cameron dismissed spontaneous generation and accepted that disease was caused by a living organism, but he also maintained the traditional view that disease was related to filth and could be defeated by hygienic measures; as Michael Worboys sums him up, "all contagious diseases were filth diseases and could be subdued by the most rigid national and private cleanliness."[19]

The emergence of hygiene as a medical specialty was closely associated with the rising prestige of preventive medicine. In his *Manual of Hygiene* (1864) Edmund Parkes declared that hygiene meant clean urban environments, especially water supply and sewage disposal, and pure food—a bare minimum understood in a more comprehensive sense by Corfield to imply "the art of preserving health . . . during as long a period as is consistent with the laws of life; . . . it aims at rendering growth more perfect, decay less rapid, life more vigorous, death more remote." He explained that hygiene had become "one of the most important branches of medical science" because "its great object is to find out the causes of the maladies to which man is subject and . . . to make known the rational means of preventing or avoiding them."[20] He endorsed the old proverb "Prevention is better than cure" and affirmed that it was "prevention we shall study here, prevention of disease by removal of its causes." Andrew Fergus asserted that the greatest achievement of nineteenth-century medicine was to rediscover the importance of prevention—and it was a rediscovery because the preventative approach was not a new branch of medicine but one that reached back to "the most remote antiquity" when it was "better understood and more thoroughly carried out than any other branch of the healing art." He was even enthusiastic about the "strict and severe, we might almost say . . . brutal" measures employed to quarantine lepers as described in Leviticus and practiced in the Middle Ages, but insisted that "if we are ever to get rid of zymotic diseases, it will be by adopting the laws of Moses . . . [and] rigorously separating the sick from the healthy." He hoped that medical officers of health would soon have "the same stringent powers as they possessed in the times of Moses, who . . . acted directly under the Divine authority."[21] Sir John Simon's entry for "Contagion" in Quain's *Dictionary of Medicine* (1882) also stressed the importance of prevention, since there was little doctors could do once a disease-causing agent had entered the body. By the 1890s it was generally agreed that prevention was the great achievement of medicine in the Victorian era.[22] All of these partial accounts and metaphorical expressions were vague enough to be understood in many different ways, and it was easy to conceive of the human body as an urban landscape to which the usual sanitary measures could usefully be applied.

The value of hygiene as a preventive health measure was demonstrated both by the declining death rate from filth diseases and the example of an ethnic-religious minority whose numbers were steadily rising as a result of immigration and natural increase, and whose status was improving as secularism advanced and anti-Semitic prejudice declined. Between 1830 and 1871 all legal and civil discrimination against Jews was abolished, and they became eligible to sit in Parliament, hold civic offices, enter the legal, teaching, and medical professions, and take degrees at Cambridge and Oxford. The first Jewish MP (Lionel de Rothschild) took his seat in 1858, and by 1881 a further nine had been elected for the Liberals and two for the Conservatives; by 1874 England had a Jewish prime minister, a Tory charmer whom Queen Victoria far preferred to the earnest Mr. Gladstone.[23] In 1867 a Jewish doctor, in the person of Ernest Hart, became editor of the *British Medical Journal* and remained there for thirty years.[24] Most of the disabilities suffered by Jews had arisen not from racism or specifically anti-Jewish measures but from the fact that they were not members of the Church of England; the legal discrimination they had faced was little different from that affecting Catholics, dissenting Protestants, atheists, and any others unable to take the prescribed forms of official oaths. As the heroes of the Old Testament, Jews in England had been spared the sort of persecution they had suffered on the Continent by the egalitarian thrust and strong Bible consciousness of English Protestantism, and a recent historian, David Feldman, describes them as "fortunate," particularly in comparison with their co-religionists in France and Austria-Hungary, where anti-Semitism was on the rise as the nineteenth century drew to a close.[25] In Britain public opinion was more sympathetic to Dreyfus than to his accusers.[26] Most Anglicans were more familiar with the Ten Commandments than their Catechism, and every schoolchild knew how Moses outwitted the Egyptians, how David slew Goliath, how Joshua trashed the walls of Jericho, and how, in short, the ancient Hebrews had defeated all the bad guys and thus prepared the way for the Redeemer.

Since the main thing everyone knew about Jews was that they practiced male circumcision, it was inevitable that those with associative minds should wonder whether that custom played any role in their victories over the uncircumcised Philistines, though they remained tactfully silent about their later subjugation by the uncircumcised Greeks and Romans. Resilience in defeat and exile was then taken as further proof of the strength of either their culture or their racial heritage. In the 1850s Dr. Copland praised the Jews for maintaining their racial and cultural identity in the teeth of constant persecution,[27] and this idea became a recurrent motif of late nineteenth-century commentary. Corfield continued his lecture on preventive medicine by seeking hygienic directions in the works of Moses, which "teem with most excellent hygienic regulations, which the people were obliged to observe under pain of severe penalties." He singled out the rules for segregation of lepers and purification of persons and dwellings as doing credit to any set of sanitary provisions in his own day, and particularly praised circumcision as "one of the most salutary regulations that was ever imposed on a people, especially in an eastern country, where the . . . necessity of scrupulous personal cleanliness is so much increased. . . . What wisdom was shown by Moses, and by Mahomet in later times, in retaining this wholesome custom as a religious rite, and thereby securing its perpetuation." It was to the observance of such practices that many nineteenth-century writers on hygiene attributed "the singular immunity of the Jewish race in the midst of fearfully fatal epidemics."[28] Following this line of thought, in 1876 a Dr. Gibbon commented on "the immunity of the Hebrew race from syphilis and scrofula" although Edgar Sheppard, MD, thought the cause was not circumcision, as many seemed to think, but that the Jews were "more moral" than Christians and "carry their religion more into the details of their daily life," with the result that there was less drunkenness and fornication among them.[29]

Ernest Hart agreed wholeheartedly. A lecture he gave to the Sanitary Institute in 1877 was full of admiration for Moses the lawgiver and prophet, whose sanitary directions were so far ahead of his time that England was only just beginning to catch up with them. His sanitary code was "a system of laws which operate to prevent those fertile sources of zymotic disease which are to be found in the pollution of air, soil and water, and which prescribe effectual isolation of infectious diseases and rigorous methods of disinfection. . . . they include regulations admirably adapted to preserve personal cleanliness, dietetic care and sobriety." In explaining the better health and superior morality of Jewish people, Hart mixed up genetic and behavioral factors, but his strongest praise was for their well-ordered lifestyle and their care for children. As an effect of their religious adherence and consequent greater personal cleanliness, "Jews present a remarkable immunity from intermittent fevers, from cholera and other filth diseases; convulsions and tabes mesenterica of children, and from phlegmasia of the respiratory organs." He referred to a study by Dr. J. H. Stallard, *London Pauperism amongst Jews and Christians* (1864), which showed that Jewish children had "no hereditary syphilis and scarcely any scrofula" and argued that their "greater tenacity of life" was due to both "better maternal care" and "the inheritance of a better physical constitution than the Christian child." Hart believed that another factor was a more developed family feeling, "ensuring to their children and their aged and infirm parents a more active solicitude." He also acknowledged that there was less crime and illegitimacy among Jews, "chastity among Jewesses being more prevalent than with other nations."[30] Given Hart's evenhanded attitude toward the influence of heredity and environment, and his own Jewish origins, it is perhaps surprising that he did not mention circumcision in his lecture, but the silence was consistent with the tendency for modernizing Jews at this period to reject ancient rites and not to claim any health rationale for them.[31]

No such skepticism was shown by gentiles such as J. H. Kellogg and Alexander Davidson. Dr. Kellogg pointed out that the secretions from the "glands" of the inner foreskin often became "the cause of irritation and serious diseases," to prevent which and ensure cleanliness "Jewish law required the removal of the prepuce. . . . The same practice is followed by several modern nations dwelling in tropical climates; and it can scarcely be doubted that it is a very salutary one, and has contributed very materially to the maintenance of that proverbial national health for which the Jews are celebrated."[32] Dr. Davidson similarly suspected that "a nation like the Jews, whose ideas of sanitation were so far advanced as to include the 'dry earth' system of the nineteenth century, adopted the practice [circumcision] as much for its substantial benefits to health as out of regard to religious ceremonial."[33] The idea that Jews in poor urban areas were healthier than their neighbors was widely held in the late nineteenth century, and the reasons much debated. In 1884 the Rev. R. C. Billing, a rector in Spitalfields, commented that although they lived in "degraded conditions," their living standards were higher than their English neighbors, and "anything like contagious disease is not known among them, and that has been a great puzzle to the medical officers."[34] Many contemporaries noted the low incidence of tuberculosis among Jews, and Anne Hardy comments that their more stringent practices regarding the slaughter, preparation, and cooking of meat, a better and more varied diet, and cleaner homes probably contributed to this result, as well as to a lower incidence of typhus and cholera.[35] Their partial segregation must also have exercised a quarantine and thus had a protective effect.

At the turn of the century interest in Jewish child-rearing practices was rekindled when the Boer War revealed the poor physical condition of military recruits from working-class districts, intensified fears about imperial decline, and stimulated the search for measures to improve racial stamina. This was the second scare over physical deterioration. The first was in response to the Crimean War in the 1850s, leading to particular concern about venereal disease (and eventually to the enactment of the Contagious Diseases Act), calls for sanitary reform to raise the level of national fitness, and the rise of modern nursing as embodied in the efforts of Florence Nightingale. The second scare led to the establishment in 1903 of the Committee on Physical Deterioration, following alarmist articles in the *Contemporary Review* by General Sir Frederick Maurice, including one with the misleading title "Where to Get Men."[36] The committee was very impressed with what it learned of Jewish housekeeping, and particularly the care they took to prepare nourishing meals, keep their dwellings clean, and look after their children: "As regards poverty and the food for the children . . . we have had evidence from a great number of people that the Jewish mothers feed their children much better, and not only know what is best for them, but know how to cook it, and that they are more thrifty and more abstemious, and that it is the reverse with our Christian people."[37] Many witnesses backed up this view, but there was a strong tendency to place the issue within the maternal neglect paradigm, so powerful in the 1890s that it had generated ineffective legislation aimed at keeping nursing mothers at

home:[38] Jewish children were healthier because their mothers did not go
out to work. Charles Booth stated that they were "bigger and heavier" because mothers remain at home and look after the house (Q. 1165–74), and
this opinion was shared by Gen. Maurice (Q. 327), Dr. Smith (Q. 8524–27),
and several others. Dr. Eichholz, an inspector of schools, attributed the
poor condition of working-class children generally to poverty and ignorance, leading to malnutrition, exposure, lack of fresh air, overcrowding,
filth, and neglect by parents arising from overwork, smoking, and drunkenness (Q. 475). No one mentioned circumcision, and the overall impression a reader of the report receives is that the committee was out to
get working mothers, not the foreskin. As Maurice commented, the poor
physique of recruits was the result of poor nutrition in infancy, arising
from maternal ignorance; observers had found that "the health and long
life of the children of the Jews, whose women did not to out to work,
compared most favourably with that of the Christian population, the
women of which worked without adequate regard to their functions as
mothers. It does not follow that a stereotyped copying of the habits of
the Jews would be desirable, but . . . for the raising of a virile race . . . it
is essential that the attention of the mothers should be mainly devoted
to the three Ks—Kuche, Kirche, Kinder."[39] The committee's conclusion
was an endorsement of Hart's tribute of twenty-five years before: "Their
charity is unbounded; their morality is demonstrated by judiciary statistics; firmness and serenity of spirit are the most marked traits of their
character. . . . They rarely use alcoholic liquors to excess. Their religious
customs enforce cleanliness both personal and in their dwellings; and
two families are never found inhabiting the same apartment."[40] In their
sobriety, chastity, cleanliness, and family feeling, the Jews had become
model Victorians. Even if wholesale copying was out, maybe it was time
for the English to take a few tips.

Considering the prominence of the classics in English education, and
the prestige of ancient Rome in a comparably imperial culture, it is perhaps surprising that the sanitarians had so little praise for the aqueducts,
baths, and drains that were such a feature of Greek and Roman civilization, particularly as the construction of such facilities was such an important element of their own program. It would seem that the books of
the Old Testament were better known and more highly regarded than
classical treatises on the care of the body, and that the sudden mania for
the sanitary genius of a society of desert herders, with their earth closets
and stringent laws against lepers and foreskins, was related to their superior moral status as proto-Christians, far preferable to sensual pagans,
no matter how good their sanitary engineering. In his celebration of the
triumph of preventive medicine, George Newman took the story back to

the ancient Egyptians, whom he commended for inventing enemas, practicing circumcision, and prohibiting "sexual perversion or indulgence," self-abuse, contraception, and abortion. Their achievements were dwarfed by those of the Hebrews, whom he praised as "the founders of public hygiene," as embodied in eight great principles. These included the prevention of "defilement" from women who had just given birth or were having their period; circumcision to meet "the particular diseases then prevalent," namely, leprosy, venereal disease, ophthalmia, scurvy, and bone deformity; and "laws of sexual relationship and sexual health" to guard against "the abomination of sexual perversion." All these principles were equally important and together "accomplished an amazing service without parallel for the physical and moral redemption of man."[41] Although Bland-Sutton found that some parents resisted subjecting their boys to circumcision because they disliked the Judaic connotations, many doctors saw the association working in favor of the procedure. A striking instance was their praise for the large families commonly raised by Jewish parents. The high birthrate of Jews in London, especially recent immigrants, deeply impressed middle-class observers alarmed at the decline of the English birthrate,[42] and it was not long before circumcision was named as the responsible factor. Remondino cited promotion of fertility as one of the original rationales of the rite, and Bland-Sutton insisted that this was its main purpose: "it was to ensure fruitful coitus in order that the seed of Abraham should multiply according to the Covenant. A long foreskin is a recognised hindrance to convenient coitus."[43] As late as 1916 Henry Curtis referred to "the wonderful fertility of the Hebrew nation" as an argument for the routine circumcision of all males at birth.[44] The idea that circumcision promoted fecundity seems somewhat at odds with the proposition that it also reduced interest in sex, but it is consistent with the orthodox view that it only discouraged nonprocreative or recreational sex, thus allowing a husband to devote his energies to impregnation.

The germ theory of disease undermined the prevailing arguments for circumcision as a preventive of nervous illnesses by superseding the concept of nerve force and establishing that many diseases thought to be caused by imbalance in nerve force (induced in turn by an irritable foreskin or masturbation) were actually caused by bacterial infection. Many doctors seemed determined to circumcise anyway,[45] as shown by the increased incidence of the practice just as germ theory triumphed in the early years of the twentieth century, and their case was strengthened by their success in recruiting germ theory itself as a justification. The emphasis was no longer on the irritability of the foreskin but on its dirtiness: it was a "harbour for filth" and hence a reservoir of disease-causing germs. Hygiene, subtly changing its connotation from moral to physical, became the main argument for the procedure, and the old correlations between the low incidence of syphilis, tuberculosis, and penile cancer in Jewish men and their lack of a foreskin were brought out and polished up. The shift in the meaning of *hygiene* is very clear in the changing reasons given for strict penile cleanliness. Acton had insisted on daily washing of the foreskin and glans in order to guard against premature erotic arousal in young boys and masturbation in older ones. William Pratt similarly recommended a cold hip bath every night and morning because it was "invaluable for repressing all lewd affections of the body."[46] There was no mention of disease. With the triumph of germ theory the rationale changed, and by the 1930s Norman Haire wrote that either scrupulous cleanliness or circumcision was needed "for exclusively hygienic reasons, for the prepuce favours the accumulation of secretions and residues capable of creating a centre of infection." In the case of men with a "narrow prepuce," Haire painted as lurid a picture of the "process of infection" as anything penned by Remondino or Hutchinson: "The substances secreted under the prepuce decompose (specific odour); the product of this decomposition irritates the sensitive skin of the glans and causes till more copious secretion, which decomposes. The result of this vicious circle is acute inflammation, soreness of the glans and suppuration."[47] Haire's hostile attitude toward the foreskin is in sharp contrast to his reassurances that masturbation was harmless. Doctors before the nineteenth century had not been concerned with penile hygiene because masturbation had not been an issue and general standards of cleanliness were not high.[48] Acton's washing routine had nothing to do with preventing disease but was the equivalent of a cold shower. It was only after the rise of filth theory, and more intensively after the discovery of germs and the mechanisms of infection, that cleanliness was reinterpreted as a tactic for better physical health. The idea that circumcision was a wise decision because it discouraged masturbation certainly did not die (or not until the 1930s), but it was supplemented by an increasingly heavy emphasis on the role of the foreskin in raising a man's risk of contracting syphilis or cancer, and thus of encouraging circumcision as the closest thing doctors could devise to vaccination against these diseases.

Once it was agreed that the uncircumcised penis was by definition dirty, the proposition that it was a significant factor in the breeding or transmission of infection was axiomatic. Acceptance of the connection was facilitated by the influence of autointoxication theory in the late nineteenth century and by the peculiarly English way in which the theory of bacterial disease causation was received through the filter of Lister's antisepsis; Listerism and germ theory then modified each other to produce an understanding of disease and a surgical practice that stressed visible cleanliness and regarded tangible dirt (whether native or foreign to the body) as pathogenic. Listerism arose as a response to the high death rate in hospitals from surgical wounds as a result of infection, at that time identified as hospital gangrene, erysipelas, and pyemia. In the 1860s Lister began by using carbolic acid—as a spray during operations, as a bath on wounds, and as a film on dressings—because he believed the putrescent agents were airborne germs and that the objective must therefore be to exclude air. As time went by, and his method was criticized as cumbersome, he came round to endorse the cleanliness approach urged by his opponents (asepsis), and by 1887 he had abandoned carbolic spray and drenched dressings in favor of clean instruments and a sterile operating environment. Although the *Medical Times and Gazette* had denied that infection could be carried by medical men who "practised the cleanly habits of English gentlemen,"[49] the fact was that most germs came not from the air but from the hands and tools of the surgeon. This turnaround had the effect of making dirt seem more important than germs: even as correct theories of bacterial action reached Britain from Germany, obvious dirt was identified all the more vigorously as the pathogenic agent.[50] The immediate implication was that the obviously dirty appearance of a penis that had not been washed for a few days was of its nature disease ridden and disease provoking.

There is a certain irony in Lister's about-face, since in the 1870s he had been the one to argue that antiseptic cleanliness was not the same as aesthetic cleanliness, and thus that wounds that looked dirty were not necessarily at risk of putrefaction, against the more conventional idea advanced by the *Lancet* that cleanliness was a matter of appearance.[51] Lister also helped to pave the way for the circumcisers by suggesting that putrefaction was signaled by smell—"the odour of decomposition," and the idea that putrefaction was the decay of dead tissue or other organic matter in a typically zymotic process like fermentation.[52] Putrefaction was the model applied when it was argued that the secretions accumulating under the foreskin somehow started to decompose and became capable of generating disease. Sir John Simon's annual report for 1874 was particularly eloquent on the evils of filth, which he defined as the medium in which germs thrived and developed disease-causing properties; cleanliness was the best natural disinfectant.[53] Against this background and the complementary theory and practice of the sanitarians, the idea of making cities healthier by keeping them clean and removing dirt traps was easily transposed to the human body. As Michael Worboys has remarked, in the late nineteenth century the principles of sanitary science were increasingly extended from the streets and dwellings to the individual, and both Florence Nightingale and William Farr played a role in transferring "the prescriptions of the sanitary movement from the urban environment and the 'Great Unwashed' to hospitals and their patients."[54] This tendency was complemented by the vogue for prophylactic removal of organs liable to infection and disorder, which developed in the 1880s. Operations became more common and more ambitious as aseptic techniques improved and anesthetics became more widely available: "Bacterial aetiologies were also used to justify more radical excisions [such as] tubercular joints and infected wounds. The removal of tonsils, teeth and the appendix was understood to be either excising infected organs, or as a prophylactic, [that is] removing organs that were fertile soil for infection."[55] The most striking expression of this tendency was the vogue for removing appendixes, tonsils, teeth, and even the colon as the theory of autointoxication took hold.

Believers in autointoxication proposed that a neglected cause of disease arose from waste products lodging in susceptible parts of the body and putrefying to produce toxins that poisoned the system and gave rise to many symptoms of illness, from diarrhea and constipation to headaches and skin rashes. The idea was most spectacularly expressed in the proposition that food passing through the intestines could ferment and breed "ptomaines," leading Arbuthnot Lane to conclude that removal of part or all of the colon would restore sickly individuals to health. Other enthusiasts targeted the appendix, the tonsils, and the teeth, and practiced similar preventive or curative extractions. The theory was remarkably influential in exactly the period when the strongest claims were made for the advantages of circumcision, from the 1880s to the 1930s, and rested on an extension of germ theory and the application of hygienic principles of urban management to the human body. In the excitement of the discovery that many diseases were caused by specific microorganisms, it was not widely realized that most bacteria were harmless or benign, and hence assumed that all were bad and that the body and its organs were meant to be as sterile as Lister's operating table.[56] The various preparations offered to disinfect the digestive tract paralleled the elaborate rituals devised to keep the preputial cavity and penis squeaky clean. The concept was popular among the respectable classes because it spoke to the Victorians' anxiety about seething disorder down below; among doctors because it offered an explanation for obscure symptoms and thus maintained their claims to omniscience; and among surgeons because it gave them something to do.[57] Advocates of the theory had been heavily influenced by the sanitary movement, were fond of comparing bodies to drainage systems, and claimed to be practicing internally what the urban reformers practiced externally. "So widespread was the concern with sewers and cesspools," writes Hillel Schwartz, "that these images were turned back onto the human body."[58] Lane wrote that "any interference with the effluent of the main sewer of a town is followed by trouble in the drains of every house which discharges its sewage into it," and he referred to the colon as a "cesspool" and the digestive system in toto as a person's "drainage apparatus." If such dirt traps could not be kept clean, they had to be cleared away. Autointoxication theory was also related to discoveries about man's evolutionary development and particularly to speculations about the survival of "vestigial" organs from the distant past that might no longer be optimally functional. Lane described the "great bowel" as a "useless and dangerous structure" in the modern world, and another believer commented in 1901 that man had "adopted a vertical attitude, while his internal viscera are still arranged for a horizontal one," putting him at a disadvantage for defecation. In addition, modern civilization had so altered human food that people found themselves "with an internal mechanism which has to perform duties for which [it] is not properly adapted." The result was that "man is burdened with some feet of large intestine, a remnant which is probably not only . . . useless, but to which the origins of many of the ills to which flesh is subject can be traced."[59] It was by applying ideas like these that Remondino and Stanley Hall came up with their own ideas of the foreskin as a harmful evolutionary vestige, and Hutchinson gained credibility for his vision of the foreskin as a harbor for filth. You might indeed call Arbuthnot Lane the Remondino of the colon, and Remondino the Lane of the foreskin.

Other suspect body parts were the tonsils, the appendix, and the teeth. Appendectomies were never performed routinely, but they were frequently done when a doctor had no better explanation than appendicitis for diarrhea, constipation, headaches, nausea, or fatigue. The contrast with circumcision lay not only in the greater difficulty of the procedure, but also in the fact that appendectomies were usually performed on patients who had sought the operation and given consent, however ill informed.[60] Some authorities pointed the finger at the teeth. William Hunter believed that "oral sepsis" (infection in gums and teeth) was the real cause of many diseases, and he attacked conservative dentists for repairing rather than extracting teeth, thus allowing them to house cavities in which germs could thrive. He particularly targeted gold fillings and crowns, claiming that anemia, colitis, fevers, nervous disturbances, rheumatic problems, and kidney disease all "owe their origin to or are gravely complicated by the oral sepsis produced . . . by these gold traps of sepsis."[61] Peter Daniel went further to assert that oral sepsis was a factor in, if not the cause of, sigmoid, rectal, and anal cancer: he had found that all thirty-six such cases at one hospital were suffering from that sad condition. In obscure complaints, often ending in death, he claimed that the real cause would frequently be found in an overlooked infection in one of the small sinuses of "the mouth, nose, ear, etc" or "some cul de sac of the gastro-intestinal or urinary-genital tract"; one of the body's mucous surfaces was "invariably at the root of the evil"—including that of the foreskin. Daniel was sure that, like sepsis in the gums or teeth, "sepsis under a long or tight foreskin, with urethral infection, leads to desquamation of the epithelium of the foreskin and glans, to acute and chronic balano-posthitis, herpes, papillomatous warts, and soft sores. In every case of cancer of the penis I have seen, a chronic balano-posthitis has always existed."[62] There was thus a widespread movement in favor of the preventive or curative extraction of "vestigial" organs considered to be dirt traps and accordingly risk factors for disease, and it is likely that, had they been as accessible as the foreskin, many more colons and appendixes would have been routinely excised. The new demands of modern civilization demanded the sanitization of the body along with the cities. In some places, tonsillectomies did indeed become nearly as common as circumcision, though not done routinely on neonates.[63]

The image of the foreskin as a fever nest thus arose from the conjunction of zymotic disease and autointoxication theory with Judaic theology, all of which enjoyed privileged status in the late nineteenth century as an effect of the sanitary movement. The orthodox Judaic position on the foreskin was not scientific, but it was very clear. According to a Midrash text, the foreskin was "more unclean than any unclean thing . . . a blemish above all blemishes," and Rabbi Eliezer stated that eating with an uncircumcised man was like "eating flesh of abomination," and bathing with him was as though one had "bathed with carrion."[64] In this theological context *unclean* was meant in a spiritual sense, and the foreskin was only one of many natural phenomena declared unclean or otherwise taboo in the elaborate cosmology of ancient Judaism, but in the late nineteenth century the word acquired a distinctly physical application. Although William Acton had stated that the infant foreskin was normally free from smegma, Cooper Forster referred to the "masses of filthy secretion poured out by the glandulae Tysoni" in the 1850s,[65] and this accusation became a frequent refrain. Another doctor claimed that three-year-old boys often suffered from inflammation of the penis as a result of "smegma getting pent up," and as an army surgeon having to inspect soldiers for venereal disease he had been "much impressed by the length of their prepuces and the filth collected under them." In some cases he was obliged "to send them away to wash before anything could be seen."[66] By 1903 it was not generally thought that the filth itself was pathogenic, rather that it facilitated the absorption of viruses, particularly syphilis, but as late as the 1930s some doctors thought that smegma itself was a bacterium: "Has it occurred to anyone that a vaccine prepared from the smegma bacillus may possibly be of practical use—for example in connection with tuberculosis therapy?" asked D. I. Connolly.[67] Another army surgeon, writing under the pen name Musalman, managed to combine both zymotic and nerve force theory in a menacing disease syndrome orchestrated by the foreskin: "When one contrasts the clean, insensitive glans of the Musalman with the irritated, filthy, and malodorous condition almost invariably present in the Hindu and British soldier in India . . . there seems no room for doubt that the removal of the appendage is often a sanitary improvement. It is evident that the nervous irritation kept up by an irritable nervous membrane constantly covered with decomposing secretions . . . may produce very evil results."[68] Particularly lurid descriptions of the foreskin were penned by doctors who supplemented what they had learned at medical school with a class-conscious contempt for the poor. According to Abraham Wolbarst, "anyone who has worked in a male clinic must have observed that very few of the uncircumcised, at least among the poor and middle class, pay proper attention to the cleansing of the genitals. Times innumerable . . . the stench arising from the confined and retained balanic secretions has been almost unbearable, even in the absence of disease." He added that anyone who has "treated venereal disease in a large clinic patronised by uncircumcised men of the lower and poorer classes" knows the necessity for universal circumcision.[69] Although such a visceral recoil from the normal male genitals suggests a culturally conditioned and aesthetic attitude, more reminiscent of a certain Old Testament contempt for the uncircumcised foreigner than a scientific viewpoint, there was probably some truth in these complaints, if only because the "poorer classes" did not have access to well-appointed bathrooms. As for the better-off, Norman Haire reported that dirty genitals, in both sexes, were frequently encountered and that the cause was "ignorance and convention": "Women who spend hours every day over their toilet . . . often display to their gynaecologist sexual organs bathed with foul discharges. Men who pride themselves . . . on their 'morning tub' often think it quite superfluous to retract the foreskin and clean the glans, and are quite satisfied to go about with a sloppy, wet, evil-smelling penis."[70] As Hera Cook observes, the aesthetic revulsion here goes far beyond anything required by a medical appraisal; yet insofar as the complaint was fair, the condition was less likely to be the result of "ignorance" than all too meticulous adherence to the early advice of parents, doctors, nannies, and (moral) hygiene manuals, that you must never touch your private parts.

Apart from the mainly nervous complaints thought to be provoked by congenital phimosis, the most important specific diseases in which the foreskin was thought to be implicated were tuberculosis, cancer, and syphilis (see chap. 12). Remondino was a particularly ardent advocate of the tuberculosis link, and on this association he was able to cite French statistics from Algeria, showing that its incidence was highest among Europeans and lowest among Jews, with Arabs in between; he also cited letters from two physicians in Boston who both recorded their "impression" that tuberculosis was less prevalent among their Jewish patients than among the Christians, though they could offer no statistics. To fill this gap Remondino turned to figures collected by B. W. Richardson, which did indeed show that "the Hebrew race" seemed to suffer relatively little from this affliction. Of all tuberculosis patients at one hospital, 44 percent were "Saxon," 39 percent mixed race, 10 percent Celtic, and only 6 percent Jews.[71] These figures hardly seem telling to a modern reader, and it comes as no surprise to find that Remondino has not been entirely honest with them: as Richardson himself went on to explain, the statistics probably represented no more than "the relative proportions of the respective populations,"[72] or, as we might put it, the demographic profile of the hospital catchment. To Remondino, however, they were proof of "the immunity of the Jewish race from tubercular disease."[73] A true believer should not be afraid to offer bold hypotheses in support of his cause, and Remondino went on to assert that it was the uncircumcised condition of British sailors that brought tuberculosis to the South Pacific and that the disease could be spread by sexual intercourse: "Had it been the ancient mariners of old Phoenecia in the days of its circumcision, or the circumcised mariners of the ancient Atlantean fleets . . . instead of the uncircumcised sailors of modern England . . . it is safe to say that consumption would not now exist there." He commended the opinion of Dr. Bernheim, surgeon to the Israelitish Consistory of Paris, that sexual intercourse was a frequent means of tubercular infection because "the sensitive and absorbing covering of the uncircumcised glans" was "a ready medium for the transmission of the virus."[74]

Other believers in the theory that circumcision could prevent or even cure tuberculosis were the Americans S. G. A. Brown and Dr. Joseph Howe. Brown wrote that "the prepuce is an important factor in the production of phthisis," as proved "by the immunity of the Jewish race from tubercular affections."[75] Howe went into the subject in greater depth, but on the basis of an older theory of disease. Whereas Brown and Remondino framed the issue in terms of germ theory—the foreskin-softened glans was more vulnerable to penetration by the tubercular poison— Howe relied on nerve force theory—that the foreskin provoked irritation, which led to nervous imbalance and exhaustion, as well as masturbation, and thus greater susceptibility to tubercular attack. Masturbation led to "exhaustion of the nervous system," causing indigestion, lassitude, impoverishment of the blood, and susceptibility to "inflammation of the lungs"; consumption was thus the "effect of ignorant assaults on the genital organs, carried on through that part of the lifetime when the active forces should have been devoted to the protection and development of the rapidly growing tissues."[76] The foreskin itself could also cause organic diseases in a more direct manner, and Howe cited several cases of men afflicted by a variety of pathological conditions, all of which were cured, or at least alleviated, by removal of the offending tissue. Examining a forty-year-old man in an advanced stage of "pulmonary phthisis," Howe quickly discovered that he was suffering from congenital phimosis as well. He circumcised the patient on the spot, whereupon the latter is supposed to have said: "I know now that if that operation had been performed when I was boy . . . I would now be in good health, I would not now be dying from consumption." It was too late for a cure in this instance, but not in the case of a clergyman who complained of "a troublesome affection of the throat," which limited his voice and prevented him from preaching (perhaps another case of Acton's "clergyman's throat"). He also suffered from pains in his penis during intercourse, so Howe was quick to deduce that a tight foreskin must be the problem. He performed a circumcision, and the next time the man entered the pulpit he found that he had full command of his voice again. Howe describes several other cases in which circumcision relieved a variety of vaguely defined symptoms, such as lethargy, depression, and various forms of social incompetence.[77] Like the wonder drugs of the twentieth century, circumcision seemed to offer new hope to the victims of these mysterious and hitherto incurable conditions.

Although prevention of penile cancer was not often listed as a major reason for circumcision in the nineteenth century, this was the benefit promised in the earliest calls for the mass circumcision of infants and an association that later contributed to the radical extension of preventive medicine to include preemptive amputation. As early as 1852 the author of a report on cancer of the penis in a thirty-three-year-old man seized the opportunity to advance the new theory that congenital phimosis was both a malformation and a cause of other diseases and to urge the introduction of widespread circumcision. The report claimed that "congenital phimosis" was "notoriously favourable to the growth of cancer" because of its effect in causing "the retention of irritating secretions" and that this association had been noticed "by all who have recorded observations on the subject." One doctor reported that nine out of twelve cases of penile cancer showed congenital phimosis, while another asserted that Jewish men were "very rarely affected." Since there was no way of curing the disease once it had taken hold, prevention was the only hope:

> The connexion between the malformation and the disease is so palpable that, were cancer of the penis as common as small-pox, there is no doubt but that, before this, some public provision would have been made for the circumcision of every elongated prepuce. Does, then, its rarity constitute any good reason why this simple precaution should be neglected? The operation is totally devoid of danger and, if performed in infancy, is attended with but little inconvenience. If those engaged in the practice of obstetrics would undertake the matter, we feel sure that their trouble would meet a full reward, in the consciousness . . . of preserving a fellow man from a disease attended by a peculiar misery, and resulting in a very painful death.[78]

Such a radical proposal was remarkably prophetic, though far ahead of its time, particularly in its insinuations that uncircumcised men had a high risk of dying in agony from penile cancer and that circumcision was "a simple precaution" like vaccination, as well as in its helpful suggestion that strategically placed obstetricians could be enlisted to do the deed. Although anonymous, the article, as its fussy syntax suggests, is probably the work of none other than Jonathan Hutchinson. He was a sub-editor on the *Medical Times and Gazette* at the time, the case reported was under the care of his patron James Paget, and it embodied all his pet themes: the danger of phimosis, the freedom of Jewish men from disease, and the consequent desirability of mass circumcision of infants as a public health measure. Hutchinson returned to the topic thirty years later during a lecture in which he stressed the importance of early operations in all cases of suspected cancer. He believed that cancer had a "pre-cancerous stage" characterized by "chronic inflammation," which developed into full-blown cancer later: "Phimosis and the consequent balanitis lead to cancer of the penis; the soot-wart becomes cancer of the scrotum; the pipe-sore passes into cancer of the lip. . . . The frequency with which old syphilitic sores become cancerous is very remarkable." Hutchinson brought up an issue also raised in 1852—the difficulty of distinguishing syphilis from cancerous sores—and suggested that hundreds of lives would be saved if operations were performed at the "precancerous stage": "Instead of looking on whilst the fire smouldered, and waiting till it blazed up, we should stamp it out on the first suspicion.

What is a man the worse if you have cut away a warty sore upon his lip and, when you come to put sections under the microscope, you find no nested cells?"[79] It will be noted that Hutchinson's position here is more conservative than in 1852: he is not now advocating the preemptive amputation of healthy tissue, but only of tissue showing suspicious sores or growths, on the reasonable principle that if the doctor waits until cancer is proved, it is too late to do anything effective (though the man ends up losing his lip whether he had cancer or not).

Although Remondino devoted a whole chapter to the foreskin's complicity in the generation of penile cancer and quoted these remarks as evidence of the need for amputation before the appearance of any symptoms, he was not able to cite any authorities on the association. Most of his sources did no more than remark that cancer attacked the prepuce first and had nothing to say about the role of phimosis or "secretions" in this development, and he duly criticized them for failing to appreciate "the existence of the prepuce as an exciting cause."[80] The lack of evidence for the value of circumcision as a preventive of cancer is perhaps surprising, but it reflects the fact that cancer was not yet the frightening specter it became in the mid-twentieth century, and efforts had not yet been made to find an association. In the nineteenth century the bogeys were masturbation, insanity, syphilis, and tuberculosis, and as a prophylactic against those threats circumcision was urged with fervent conviction. The argument that early circumcision was necessary as a prophylactic against cancer of the penis and cervix developed only in the 1930s, mainly in the United States, just as the theory of masturbatory illness was collapsing.[81]

Such was the suspicion of the foreskin as a disease agent or risk factor that some doctors suggested that circumcision could prevent parasitic diseases of the urinary and digestive tracts. Between 1887 and 1909 James Allen, MD, consulting medical officer to the Natal Government Railways, claimed that one of these was a common African disease then called bilharziasis. His reports afford such an insight into medical logic, the ethics of the period, and the double standard regarding male/female genital inviolability that they are worth considering in some detail.[82] Bilharziasis, now known as schistosomiasis, is caused by a parasitic trematode worm (or fluke) that has a complicated life cycle involving freshwater snails and land mammals; humans commonly pick it up from rivers contaminated with animal urine and feces containing the eggs. A free-swimming form of the parasite penetrates the skin and lodges in the veins of the abdomen, causing anemia and a variety of chronic symptoms, and from which the females release eggs into the urine and feces, thus completing the cycle. The details of this saga, and particularly the parasite's mode of entry into the body, were not understood in Allen's day, but one school of thought held that the fluke or its eggs were swallowed with drinking water and thus got in via the stomach. Allen disputed this view, observing that the disease seemed to affect only those who bathed in rivers and contending (though with little confidence and no data) that boys were more often infected than girls or adults—a disparity for which he offered two contradictory explanations. "The real cause of the excessive number of boys affected," he wrote, was that they went swimming more often and did not dry themselves with towels, thus allowing the parasite to cling to the parts through which it invaded. This cause was thus behavioral and probabilist, arising from the boys' habits and their more frequent exposure to risk. The other cause worked differently and was related to Allen's conviction that the worm did not enter via the stomach but wriggled up the urethra: in this scenario the greater infection of boys was "mainly due to the ease with which the parasite can enter the urethra before the prepuce is retracted." One's immediate reaction here is that the reasoning seems back to front: on the face of it you would think that the valvelike structure of the foreskin, particularly in prepubescent boys, in whom it is normally quite tight, would be more likely to shut the parasite out or at least make its entry more difficult. But so completely had the foreskin been demonized, and so little did doctors remember about its anatomy and functions, that Allen blames this very feature for facilitating the penetration: "the prepuce plays a most important part in the entry of the parasite into the urethra. During . . . bathing the sack formed by the prepuce becomes filled with water and . . . the [fluke] would be guided almost directly to the mouth of the urethra by the prepuce and sustained until it effected an entry." Allen had no evidence that the prepuce did become a sac filled with water, nor that the parasite was guided thereby to the urethra, like a sheepdog urging wethers into a chute. Indeed, the proposition that it did was contrary to the understanding of congenital phimosis, which held that the problem with the foreskin of young boys was that it fitted so snugly over the glans that it could not even be retracted, let alone be loose enough to form a sac. Still, on a priori principles it was not illogical to argue that if the prepuce did form a sac, the worm might have more time to reach its target. All Allen was really doing was applying the medical slogan of the day: covered glans, bad; exposed glans, better; foreskin-free glans, best.

It was also Allen's experience that adults with a nonretracted prepuce were more liable to infection than those who kept it back or lacked one. He further suggested that in girls "the labia offer nearly as good sheltering places" for the parasite, and thus assist its entry to the same degree as the prepuce, but that their less frequent bathing and more vigorous use of towels to dry themselves made them less susceptible. The differing vulnerability of girls and boys dictated the difference in preventive steps. Ideally, and because of "protracted bathing and the impossibility of drying the glans penis on account of the prepuce," Allen asserted that "circumcision should be enforced in every country where bilharzia is prevalent"—though only on boys. Girls could protect themselves by wearing bathing drawers and drying themselves thoroughly afterward with a towel. But Allen seems to have been as much of two minds over the necessity for preventive circumcision as over "the real cause" of boys' greater risk. If circumcision could not be enforced, he felt that wearing tightly woven drawers and drying the penis carefully would probably work just as well.

Allen's report would not have been complete without a deferential nod toward ancient tribal wisdom. When he first advanced his theory that the prepuce was the major risk factor for bilharziasis (1887), he suggested that this was the real reason why the Jews and several African tribes had adopted circumcision as a religious rite: "It is very probable that in ancient Egypt the presence of this little fluke . . . in the waters of the Nile suggested the . . . operation and that the Jews . . . adopted the custom and carried it with them when they left Egypt, and that gradually the cause of its origin became forgotten, and it advanced from being a sanitary precaution to a religious rite." Circumcision was also performed by a number of African tribes where the fluke was prevalent, and it was "extremely likely" that circumcision originated "as a protection" against it and "will have to be practised again if the European or indeed any race is to maintain its normal vigour in the infested countries." This sort of teleological hypothesizing was typical of the period, but there are obvious difficulties with this theory, even ignoring the problem that modern archaeology has established that the Jews never were held captive in Egypt. If you accept the historicity of the Old Testament (as Allen did), it is hard to explain why it states that circumcision originated in Canaan as part of a territorial covenant with a divine overlord but says nothing about it as a health precaution adopted in Egypt; Moses' son is actually described as not being circumcised, suggesting that the Egyptian bondage led to the abrogation of the rite, not its adoption. Second, if the main victims of the parasite were prepubescent boys, it is hard to see why circumcision at or after puberty (as practiced by the African tribes Allen mentions)[83] would have any protective effect: according to Allen's own data, boys in the regions where the parasite was prevalent were not circumcised. But not to worry about mere logic and facts: confirming his speculations was the latest archaeological intelligence from the Nile valley, which offered "proof" that the ancient Egyptians were in the habit of circumcising prisoners of war and slaves. Allen naturally leapt to the conclusion that the practice might have become a religious rite later but that it originated as a sanitary precaution because its "protective influence" against bilharziasis was understood. The "fact" that the Egyptians circumcised their slaves, who could be expected to spend much of their time in the water, confirmed this, since their owners would not want their value reduced by illness or lassitude. Allen's medical ethics were as rough and ready as his scientific method. Seeking to learn more about the life cycle of the fluke and to establish that it did not develop inside the human body from eggs, he resolved "to experiment upon someone who . . . would be willing for a consideration to run the small risk of invasion. Such a man I found among the Indian attendants at Grey's Hospital in this town. On three occasions I injected into this man's bladder many eggs of the parasite containing vigorous embryos, and I satisfied myself that he retained those eggs for several hours, but the result was absolutely negative. The man did not become affected by the bilharzia." The Indian was luckier than many of the little boys who were the unwilling subject of doctors' experiments with the effects of circumcision.

12 · The Purity Movement and the Social Evil

Circumcision as a Preventive of Syphilis

The circumcised Jew is then very much less liable to contract syphilis than an un-circumcised person. This conclusion has, I believe, been long entertained by many surgeons of experience, but I am not aware that it has ever before been made the subject of demonstration.

JONATHAN HUTCHINSON, "On the Influence of Circumcision in Preventing Syphilis," 1855

Our great Mikado, virtuous man,
When he to rule our land began,
Resolved to try
A plan whereby
Young men might best be steadied.
So he decreed, in words succinct,
That all who flirted, leered or winked
(Unless connubially linked),
Should forthwith be beheaded.

The Mikado

By the dawn of the twentieth century the most important advantages of correcting congenital phimosis by early circumcision were understood to be deterrence of masturbation, syphilis, and cancer,[1] a trinity first proposed by Francis Cadell in 1873. In that paper he declared that the prepuce provoked "constitutional disturbances" in infancy, excited masturbation in boyhood, increased the risk of syphilis in adulthood, and was "an exciting cause" of cancer in old age.[2] Since protection against syphilis was such a clinching argument for circumcision, and probably the main reason for the rapid spread of the practice during the venereal disease scare of the early twentieth century, it deserves detailed consideration. That circumcision might be useful in treating or even conferring resistance to VD was not a new idea. As early as the mid-seventeenth century there are reports of amputations resembling circumcision in venereal cases, but only in adult men and as a last resort after conservative methods of treatment had failed. Joseph Binns treated a man with syphilitic ulcers on his foreskin by applying "a strong cataplasm" and scarifying the foreskin; when these measures failed he was forced to cut away the decaying flesh.[3] By the end of the century the practice was sufficiently widespread to come to the attention of Samuel Butler, who referred to it in his satire on the Puritan pedant Hudibras, whose knowledge of Hebrew he mocked as matched by another Jewish peculiarity:

> For Hebrew Roots, although th' are found
> To flourish most in barren ground,
> He had such plenty, as suffic'd
> To make some think him circumcis'd:
> And truly so he was perhaps
> Not as proselyte, but for Claps.
>
> *Hudibras* I.I.59–64

Despite the suggestion in the alternative last line ("'Tis many a Pious Christians case"), few men were keen to take a step that would ravage their penis even further. In the early eighteenth century a surgeon records having treated a man suffering from ulceration of the penis and resultant paraphimosis arising from venereal disease by the use of mercury and "a fourfold incision" to allow the foreskin to return to its proper position: "The glans incarn'd, and looks tolerably handsome; the extremity of the prepuce makes a sort of quadrangle . . . by reason of the cicatrix having a small knob which prevents it from playing freely over the glans; but from which it may at any time be freed by circumcision. As a martyr in the cause of Venus . . . [the patient] thinks he has shed blood enough already."[4] Even in the early nineteenth century, Ricord and Acton recognized that men were reluctant to submit to circumcision, and they were themselves loath to perform the operation except as a last resort in severely infected cases.

The proposition that circumcision conferred protection against venereal disease was first ventured as syphilis spread across Europe and doctors found themselves powerless to cure or even significantly alleviate its ravages.[5] The idea was sufficiently widespread in the late seventeenth century to attract the derision of Gideon Harvey, court physician to William and Mary, and in the mid-eighteenth century Robert James suggested a connection between the length of a man's foreskin and his vulnerability to venereal disease: "Those who have their foreskins naturally very long are very much more easily infected by impure embraces than others," he wrote in his *Medicinal Dictionary*.[6] These ideas had little immediate impact, but as we have seen they helped create a climate of medical opinion that eased the introduction of circumcision as a treatment for masturbation, spermatorrhea, and phimosis in the mid-nineteenth century. Venereal disease was rampant in the eighteenth century, but in the relatively relaxed moral climate of that period it was seen more as a recreational hazard than a serious public health problem.[7] In the more puritanical atmosphere of the Victorian age, however, it came to be viewed as "the monster social evil of the day," as William Acton put it, a "most destructive enemy" and a "foul and loathsome disease" implying "a breach of the moral laws."[8] Society was desperate to find an effective means of cure or prevention. It was in this context that Jonathan Hutchinson declared that circumcision provided such significant protection against syphilis that it should be widely performed on male infants.

While surgeon to the Metropolitan Free Hospital, Hutchinson recorded the incidence of venereal cases among his Jewish and non-Jewish patients during 1854 and came up with the following statistics:

TABLE 12.1

	Venereal cases	Gonorrhea	Syphilis
Non-Jews	272	107 (39.3%)	165 (60.6%)
Jews	58	47 (81%)	11 (19%)

On the basis of these figures he claimed that he had demonstrated a conclusion "long entertained by many surgeons of experience," namely, that "the circumcised Jew is . . . very much less liable to contract syphilis than an uncircumcised person," and the reason was obvious: circumcision rendered "the delicate mucous membrane of the glans hard and skin-like." Hutchinson did not explain why a penis modified in this way should provide such protection, nor what noninjurious alternatives might be adopted if it did, but doctors at that time were not expected to provide proof of inferences drawn from clinical experience, and Hutchinson offered more evidence for his claim than Tissot ever had for his. His explanation was also consistent with the medical knowledge of the period. James had referred to the greater vulnerability of long foreskins, and George Drysdale stated that circumcised men were "less subject to chancre, because the mucous membrane of the glans becomes hardened by exposure," with the result that it suffered fewer "excoriations" through which the poisonous matter could enter the body. Unlike Hutchinson, however, he did not assume that circumcision was the only answer, much less that it should be inflicted on everyone; instead, he suggested that "those who have much promiscuous sexual intercourse might imitate this, by drawing back the prepuce, and so keeping the glans habitually exposed." He also recommended condoms.[9] Such half-measures and incitements to fornication were not for Hutchinson: he thought it "probable that circumcision was by Divine command made obligatory upon the Jews, not solely as a religious ordinance, but also with a view to the protection of health. . . . One is led to ask, witnessing the frightful ravages of syphilis in the present day, whether it might not be worthwhile for Christians also to adopt the practice."[10] If Hutchinson was the author of the article on penile cancer published in 1852, he had already demonstrated his hostility to the foreskin, but such a small and unrepresentative statistical sample was a flimsy foundation on which to erect such an ambitious therapeutic edifice. All Hutchinson's observations showed that while gentile venereal cases had more syphilis than gonorrhea (60.6 versus 39.3 percent), Jewish cases had more gonorrhea than syphilis (81 versus 19 percent). Although Hutchinson insisted that the high level of gonorrhea among the Jews proved that less promiscuity could not have been the reason for the difference, the statistics revealed nothing about the relative susceptibility of cut and uncut men to venereal infection and could as well be cited to show that circumcision increased the likelihood of getting gonorrhea as to prove it offered protection against syphilis.[11]

Hutchinson's figures would hardly receive a second glance today, yet for half a century they were regarded as the "hard data" needed to prove that circumcision conferred significant resistance, if not immunity, to syphilis. That no one until the 1890s challenged them is an indication of how strongly the tide of medical opinion was running against the foreskin: any evidence would do. Hutchinson was not writing primarily as a venereologist seeking ways of reducing the incidence of syphilis but as an advocate of circumcision seeking arguments for its more frequent application to boys; it was his prior belief in the effectiveness of the operation against masturbation and congenital phimosis that led him to make his observations and communicate them to the medical press. He explains that he was "induced to communicate" his experience of venereal cases in support of a paper by "my friend, Mr Cooper Forster, recommending the more general practice of circumcision as a preventive of certain diseases of childhood"; he had "long held a similar opinion" that it was "the duty of the surgeon invariably to remove the prepuce of infants born with congenital phimosis."[12] It is thus evident that in trying to show that circumcised men were less vulnerable to syphilis, Hutchinson was really seeking evidence to support his colleague's policy of circumcising boys who exhibited signs of phimosis, and that the main problem with phimosis was that it provoked boys to handle their penis and thus fall into masturbation. Hutchinson's enthusiasm for circumcision was as much for its expected impact on behavior as for its physiological effects.

That (Sir) Jonathan Hutchinson (1828-1913) gained a reputation as Britain's leading authority on syphilis is a sobering comment on the backwardness of British venereology in the nineteenth century. He is chiefly remembered for "Hutchinson's triad," three signs by which congenital syphilis could be recognized in young children, but his contribution to the understanding and treatment of the disease was insignificant compared with that of Ricord and Alfred Fournier, to say nothing of the German researchers who identified the bacterium.[13] In personality Hutchinson was a reserved and gloomy Quaker whose watchword was self-denial and who rose early each morning to read the Bible and pray.[14] In 1890 *Vanity Fair* described him as "a great authority on defective and diseased eyes" and a "sensitive man who tends his patients with quite fatherly care," but a modern scholar comments that his attitude toward venereal patients was colored by "moral revulsion against sexual sin."[15] His youthful diary shows him rising before dawn to study his medical books and the Bible: his text for 28 December 1848 was Hebrews 11, to which he responded: "My supplications were poured forth at the footstool of almighty power for an increase of faith, lest, privileged to live under a great and glorious covenant of mercy, I might by any means fall short of the better things which God has provided for us." He was twenty.[16] Other favorite readings were the sufferings of Job and Saint Paul's Epistle to the Galatians—the one in which he reproaches them for continuing to practice circumcision, forgetful that Christ's sacrifice had made such fleshly signs of righteousness unnecessary. Hutchinson seems not to have approved of Paul, however, but to have agreed with "Dr Copland's renowned Dictionary of Medicine" that there would be much less masturbation among boys if the early Christians had not dropped the Judaic rite.[17] Hutchinson held deeply puritanical objections to nonprocreative sex and regarded methods of contraception with "disgust": such practices were "prejudicial to both moral and physical health."[18] Although he changed his mind on how best to control the spread of venereal disease through prostitution, he originally supported the Contagious Diseases Acts of the 1860s and even joined William Acton in urging their extension from garrison towns to the general population.[19] His own reasons for advocating routine circumcision owed more to moral sentiment than medical science, though he did his best to give them a statistical gloss.

The fact that in 1855 Hutchinson was more interested in phimosis and masturbation than in syphilis helps to explain why he took so long to make an effort to promote his idea for its surgical control. In the 1860s and 1870s the dominant strategy against syphilis was not a sanitary but a contagionist one, involving the inspection of prostitutes and the segregation of those infected under the Contagious Diseases Act. It was only with the repeal of this legislation and the development of new sanitarian and behavioral-moral strategies to prevent venereal disease, stressing cleanliness and control of the male sex drive (that is, physical and moral purity), that Hutchinson's ideas attracted widespread interest, and he returned to the subject with renewed zeal. There were some references to his original paper in the 1870s, but it was not until the 1890s that it made an impact. Before returning to the topic of Hutchinson's crusade for circumcision, I shall therefore survey the evolution of British policy on the control of prostitution and venereal disease.[20]

Although statistics were inadequate, by the 1860s it was feared that syphilis was running at epidemic levels, an impression derived from its high incidence in the armed forces. The feeble condition and poor performance of British troops in the Crimean War had shocked the nation, and much of the blame was placed on venereal disease. Statistics from 1864 suggested that syphilis accounted for 33 percent of army sick cases and affected 29 percent of troop strength, while in 1869 Sir John Simon estimated that 7 percent of the population as a whole was infected. In 1916 the Royal Commission on Venereal Diseases raised this to a minimum of 10 percent.[21] Although such figures hardly justified the declaration of an epidemic, there is no doubt about the emotional impact of syphilis, the threat of which terrified the late Victorian imagination in much the same way as AIDS does today. An article in the *British Medical Journal* described the victims as "wasted to skeletons by the frightful complications of these terrible maladies—the most wretched, miserable and loathsome objects that imagination can depict," while John Chapman wrote in 1869 that "thousands upon thousands . . . are the innocent and defenceless victims of a pestilence whose march is no secret, and whose attacks are so insidious that none can be certain of escape; many a trusting maiden . . . who gives herself in marriage speedily finds her joy turned to mourning, her health to disease, and . . . her beauty defaced by its loathsome poison; many a mother has to deplore the contamination, not only of her own constitution, but that of her child."[22] Such a critical situation clearly called for desperate remedies.

The first measures taken against syphilis were not desperate at all but involved a typically moderate British compromise in which prostitution, considered to be the most important means by which syphilis was spread, would be placed under limited supervision. The most significant single medical voice behind this policy was William Acton, whose study of prostitution (1857) mounted an argument for toleration and regulation in the interests of public health: prostitution was inevitable among a civilized population, and the only realistic option was to minimize its harm by supervision.[23] As Judith Walkowitz comments, he was "instrumental in generating an intellectual climate sympathetic to regulation," using the argument that something must be done to "stem the tide of venereal disease threatening to engulf the general population."[24] Acton's own research certainly did not confirm Hutchinson's claims about circumcised men being less susceptible to infection. His observations showed that venereal disease was rare in Brussels, and that among the Belgian troops the incidence of syphilis was only 1 in 56, compared with 1 in 4 among the London Foot Guards; he attributed the difference to a system of surveillance whereby the Belgian men were inspected each week and any found to be infected were required to reveal their sexual contacts, who were then examined in turn and sent to hospital for treatment if found to be diseased. He also felt that Belgian prostitutes were less aggressive than the English (they were kept in licensed brothels and not allowed to solicit in the street), leading to less patronage. Acton did not propose such an intrusive scheme for England, merely the provision of washing facilities for the soldiers, but the implication was there for others to draw.[25]

They were duly drawn in the Contagious Diseases Acts of 1864, 1866, and 1869, which provided that, in garrison towns, women deemed to be prostitutes could be apprehended, required to submit to a medical examination, and detained in hospital if found to be infected. Because the aim was to control VD in the armed forces, the acts applied only to named centers with large numbers of naval and military personnel. Although the acts were deplored by moralists, who saw them as condoning fornication, and by a smaller number of feminists who resented the way women had been singled out for blame and made liable for humiliating examinations, Acton believed that they had worked well and contributed to the decline of syphilis. In the second edition of *Prostitution* (1870) he wrote that they had "been attended with the happiest results, both as regards the health of our army and navy, and the sanitary and moral improvement wrought in the unhappy women who have come within the scope of its provisions."[26] So successful did Acton consider the acts that he made the fatal mistake of trying to get their scope extended from garrison towns to the whole population, an alarming suggestion that provoked a powerful moral backlash. Acton's policy was driven by the desire to curb venereal disease and the conviction that inspection of prostitutes was an effective strategy, and he realized that the opposition to the proposal was on religious rather than medical grounds, as well as concerns about "curtailing individual freedom," but he argued that such a degree of interference was minor and necessary both for the greater good of society and the health of the women themselves.[27] During the 1870s, however, the rise of both puritan morality and feminist sentiment began to affect the medical profession more strongly than before, and the alliance that had supported the legislation broke down.

As the *British Medical Journal* pronounced in 1870, control of syphilis was where "the territories of the physician and the moralist overlap," which is why it was "impossible for the sanitarian . . . to ignore morals. Syphilis is the product . . . of immorality. Increase immorality, and you increase syphilis."[28] A few practitioners regarded venereal disease as well-deserved retribution for sin. The most famous, Sir Samuel Solly, was reported to have said, during a discussion of Acton's paper on the control of prostitution, that "far from considering syphilis an evil, [he] regarded it . . . as a blessing, and believed that it was inflicted by the Almighty to act as a restraint on the indulgence of evil passions. Could the disease be exterminated, which he hoped it could not (*marks of disapprobation*) fornication would ride rampant through the land. He believed that . . . the best cure for the evil was the elevation of the moral character of society."[29] This attitude has sometimes been taken as representative of the medical profession as a whole,[30] but it was not a universally held opinion and certainly was not shared by the doctors at that gathering. Acton commented to general approval: "Statements similar to those made by Mr Solly he had heard from various persons . . . but he was not prepared to hear such language from a medical man (*hear, hear*)."[31] Acton particularly rejected the idea that, on account of ideological pressures, a cure should not be sought for the disease; such a fatalist attitude would stifle progress. The orthodox position was also expressed by the *British Medical Journal*: "Those who hold that venereal diseases have been ordained by the Deity for the chastisement of sexual sin are partisans . . . of a narrow-minded theology."[32]

The ink was scarcely dry on this editorial when its thrust was challenged by the campaign against the Contagious Diseases Acts, in the course of which Solly's position was revived with a vengeance and forced upon the public by an unlikely alliance of progressive feminists and extreme puritans in the social hygiene movement. Solly had been one of only three medical witnesses opposed to the regulation of prostitution to testify before a parliamentary committee, compared with twenty-nine who supported it,[33] but his views were held by the more extreme wing of the purity movement and soon came to be regarded sympathetically by many in the medical profession. With Ernest Hart as editor, the *British*

Medical Journal generally supported the Contagious Diseases Acts, and even their extension, on the ground that they represented the most effective way to contain the spread of VD. With his scientific and secular outlook, he called opponents of the acts "friends of contagion." Editorial policy changed briefly in 1869–70 under the editorship of Hutchinson, who was equivocal on the issue but coming around to the Solly-Josephine Butler position that making illicit intercourse safe merely encouraged immorality.[34] Although the policy did not survive Hutchinson's term, the *British Medical Journal*'s opposition to the extension of the acts in 1870 was a sign of the turning tide. In several powerful editorials Hutchinson argued that even the limited version was an admission that fornication by unmarried soldiers and sailors was unavoidable, thus sending a message to youth that a "deadly sin" was merely venial. Extending the act would worsen the situation by conferring legitimacy on prostitution and harming the cause of morality: "It will be increasingly difficult to convince the youth of the next generation that fornication is a sin, if they know that the police are openly employed in endeavouring to diminish its dangers. . . . The difficulties of parents and preachers in respect of this special sin will increase ten-fold." The editorial took a moral rather than medical line in asserting the importance of struggling with temptation, sought to exploit anti-European prejudice by a reference to France "laughing at our prudery," and criticized those who thought it was "no use in ignoring the facts of life." It chided the Sollys of the day for holding a "narrow-minded theology" but largely accepted their position: "syphilis and gonorrhoea do stand . . . as efficient scarecrows in he fields of forbidden pleasure," it wrote; if the government (by extending the act) spread the view that pleasure has been robbed of its sting, there will be "an increase in the number of those who err." Even more seriously, "if the promiscuous intercourse of the sexes should increase . . . whilst it is still only freed from physical risk, it is quite possible that there may be no gain as regards the reduction of . . . syphilitic misery. We may find that we have irretrievably lost in morality and gained not at all in health."[35] This was precisely the position Hutchinson argued in the 1890s when advocating widespread circumcision.

This line of argument was taken further by the social purity movement, whose target was not merely the Contagious Diseases Acts but sexual license in general. Back in 1851 Acton had asked, "If we are unable to curb the animal passions, should we not attempt to alleviate . . . the consequences which mankind suffers from their indulgence?"[36] The purity movement responded with a resounding "No: What we must do is curb men's animal passions," and ammunition for this project was not lacking in Acton's own work, much of which was itself devoted to the promotion of male continence. His views on prostitution, however, came under heavy fire from the opponents of the acts, who objected both to the inspection of prostitutes (as demeaning to women) and the implicit endorsement of fornication. As Frank Mort has observed, the campaign to repeal the acts represented the breakdown of the old medico-moral alliance and the rise of a new discourse in which medical science was to be subordinated to "moral law" and personal decency, which really meant abstention from sex: as the leader of the campaign, Josephine Butler, put it at a congress in 1877, the essential basis for individual and national health was "self-control in the relations between the sexes." The opponents of the Contagious Diseases Acts attacked male sexuality as the real origin of vice and disease: the Social Purity Alliance (established 1873) insisted that male desire was the origin of the immorality that led to prostitution and associated diseases, and that the "new and final solution" to these problems was to impose the obligation of restraint on them.[37] The campaign was waged by a coalition of diverse forces, but most of them did not aim at personal liberation; rather they hoped to equalize the double standard by imposing on men the same puritanical rules of sexual propriety that already limited women. The tendency of the movement was expressed in Christabel Pankhurst's later slogan, "Votes for women and chastity for men,"[38] and her allies wrote consistently of the need to enforce social purity and of venereal disease as "the God-ordained consequences of his sin" and "the bitter wages of sexual depravity."[39] In her pamphlet on how to end "the great scourge," Pankhurst relied heavily on medical opinion that sexual indulgence was not only unnecessary for men but damaging to their health. Promiscuous sex hurt innocent women and children by spreading venereal disease, and caused "bodily weakness" in men because "the sex act involves a very great expenditure of . . . energy," which ought to be put to better uses, she wrote, citing Acton and other medical authorities in her support. She did not specify circumcision but did suggest that, in the interests of self-control, medical assistance in the form of drugs to lower the sex drive could be provided to the weak willed: "Self control for men who can exert it! Medical aid for those who cannot!"[40]

In its emotional rejection of state regulation, the British approach to prostitution and VD was so different from those adopted in European countries that Peter Baldwin has called it a *Sonderweg*. He provides a subtle and comprehensive analysis of the social and political bases for the defeat of the Contagious Diseases Acts: the laissez-faire tradition, the nature of the parliamentary system, the operation of the lower courts, the organization of the army, and the power of the purity movement. For my purposes it is the last of these that is the most important. Baldwin shows that the opponents of regulation were less interested in control-ling VD than in stamping out vice—they wanted to eliminate prostitu-tion not so much because it spread disease but because sex outside mar-riage was immoral.[41] As a result of their pressure, brothels, homosexual acts, and nude bathing became illegal, pimps could be flogged, and pros-titutes could be arrested merely for being on the street, but there was no attempt to criminalize the transmission of VD, to make it reportable, to require that the infected be examined or reveal their contacts, or to stop them from marrying—all measures that were tried in Continental coun-tries. The focus was public morals rather than public health.[42] The aims of the purity movement were similar to those of the author of *Onania:* to resurrect and give force to the old Christian discourse of the flesh, though its methods and social basis were quite new—a combination of lower-middle-class respectability, a few puzzled civil libertarians, and an assertive feminism that sought to "enlist the state and its coercive powers on behalf of changing male behaviour through the repression of vice and public immorality."[43] Baldwin stresses how different this move-ment was from similar antiregulatory campaigns in Europe, which were more libertarian in spirit, more focused on disease, and more inclined to favor sexual freedom for both men and women rather than stronger re-pression. The British movement, he argues, was not an outgrowth of lib-eralism but was driven by a moralizing and conservative variety of fem-inism which held that women's "natural purity" should set the standard for society, and thus educate or otherwise assist men toward sexual re-straint. It is easy to see how measures such as circumcision would not meet much opposition in such circles.

With the repeal of the Contagious Diseases Act in 1883, the blame for syphilis thus shifted decisively from fallen women as the infectors of men to licentious men as the seducers and infectors of innocent women.[44] As the problem became redefined as male lust rather than female depravity, the focus of the control strategy moved from policing the bodies of pros-titutes to controlling the male sex drive, and in this context any means that curbed men's sexual exuberance was considered useful. In places today where the spread of AIDS has been contained through safe sex ed-ucation, it may seem strange that the first, and in some ways the princi-pal, target of the social purity movement was masturbation. The practice was viewed not as a safe substitute for intercourse but, in Acton's and Lyttelton's terms, as a premature awakening of the sex drive that would lead boys to prostitutes during adolescence.[45] As Joanne Townsend com-ments, the downward path showed the boy who masturbated and read salacious books "growing into the man who seduced women, consorted with prostitutes and married to infect his wife and children with the fruits of his profligacy."[46] Following the logic of Acton's theory that so long as the sexual tap was not turned on, desire would never be a problem, the nurse and hygiene expert Lavinia Dock declared that the very first thing to be done to control venereal disease was "prevention of all habits known as self-abuse or masturbation" from early childhood onward, and she hinted that circumcision might occasionally be necessary to assist this endeavor.[47]

Some purity campaigners were quite explicit that circumcision would as be as effective in protecting against syphilis as in discouraging secret vice. In a book on child management directed at mothers, Mrs. M. I. Henry advocated the mutilation of the genitals of both boys and girls in the interests of continence. "Satan has been quick to realize the fertility of childhood for his sowing," she wrote, and had "planted the seeds of moral leprosy in the delicate flesh of the smiling babe, and claims early youth for his sickle"; today "there can scarcely be found a child whose sexual organs are not abnormally sensitive." Even the "guileless flesh of childhood" carried "a spot of irritation and uncleanness which bred diseased imaginings," but luckily God had provided an antidote in the form of "physical correction by which the child should be restored to something like what he would have been if he had been conceived and born in sinlessness instead of sin." Society had woken up to "the hygienic importance of a certain operation, kindred to the old rite of circumcision, in which is found the physical remedy for an evil that kills the soul" and which was necessary in infants because they were incapable of "acting from principle or by faith." In fact, the operation was so "kindred" as to be indistinguishable: circumcision both discouraged impurity like masturbation and promoted an unselfish character:

> This harmless operation in the flesh of the little child removes the principle cause of that peculiar irritation that leads to secret vice, giving physical freedom from that downward-dragging self-consciousness which it engenders; and a chance to grow the wings of a noble self-forgetfulness.

Accepting the doctors' argument that circumcision was preventive medicine for the body, Mrs. Henry went further to suggest that it was good preventive medicine for the soul as well:

> Circumcision stands as a remedial agent with vaccination. It is a means of correction which must needs be applied before there is anything to diagnose in the case, if you would make sure of the most satisfactory results. Every child does not need it; but it will do no harm to any; and if you wait for such developments as would lead the family physician to so order, you risk leaving a taint on the child's memory which can never be removed.[48]

Circumcision would not only discourage children from masturbation, and thus lead them away from risk of disease indirectly, but protect them directly from syphilis:

> As a religious ordinance circumcision is still in existence among the Jews, and as some special forms of venereal disease became more and more manifest among other nations, while the Jews went almost entirely free, the discovery was made that the old rite ... had a value for both boys and girls as a cleansing and preventive process.

Circumcision was thus urged for its effectiveness in both modifying behavior and producing physical changes that made the body less susceptible to venereal infection.[49] A more prominent member of the purity movement who endorsed circumcision was Ellice Hopkins, described by Frank Mort as one of the "new breed" who wanted the law to "protect" women and children, educate men into self-control and chastity, and reform working-class morals, and who supported the use of the criminal law to enforce decent conduct. Motivated by Evangelical religion, she particularly targeted male sexuality as the problem and male lust as the main cause of prostitution.[50] In her widely read book *The Power of Womanhood*, Hopkins urged mothers always to be present at their sons' bath, because "often evil habits arise from imperfect washing and consequent irritation; and many a wise mother thinks it best on this account to revert to the old Jewish rite of initiation by which cleanliness was secured."[51]

The success of the purity movement in securing the repeal of the Contagious Diseases Acts was related to the reclassification of syphilis from a contagious to a filth disease. As we have seen, the major argument over disease control in the 1870s was between pro- and anti-contagionists: the former advocated measures to quarantine infected individuals from the healthy, while the latter (sanitary reformers) urged environmental modifications to eradicate the "fever nests" from which diseases spread. The contagionist approach was expressed in both the Contagious Diseases Acts (directed at prostitutes), and the Contagious Diseases (Animals) Act of 1869, passed to control an outbreak of cattle plague and other diseases of livestock, and which empowered the authorities to quarantine infected animals and ban imports. Both pieces of legislation were based on the same contagionist understanding of disease, as illustrated by a remark in W. R. Greg's discussion of prostitution in 1850: "The same rule of natural law which justifies the officer in shooting a plague-stricken sufferer who breaks through a cordon-sanitaire justifies him in arresting and confining the syphilitic prostitute who, if not arrested, would spread infection all around her."[52] The repeal of the Contagious Diseases Acts in 1883 reflects the general spread of sanitarian ideas and the rise of preventive approaches to health, with the result (as Michael Worboys comments) that "concern about people and their behaviour rather than the environment and its pollution became factors of growing importance."[53]

Syphilis was never formally classified as a zymotic disease, but the idea that it could be generated or at least spread by filth and prevented by cleanliness gained ground from the 1860s. The idea was implied in Acton's proposal to provide washing facilities for the London troops, and at the same meeting Holmes Coote suggested that syphilis was like a filth disease, to be controlled by the same sort of sanitary regulations that were improving the health of the cities: "The chief evil of which prostitutes had to complain was dirt, and the proper means of ablution. . . . There was nothing peculiar or specific in the disease . . . it was mainly caused by filth."[54] The intimate connection between syphilis and filth was pictured more vividly in a passage in Etienne Lancereaux's *Treatise on Syphilis* (English translation, 1868) from the medieval William of Saliceto, which not only used that very word but specifically blamed the foreskin for trapping it. Describing venereal sores on the penis he referred to "ulcers and pustules that arise because contact with women is followed by the retention of 'filth' or 'venomous material' between the glans and the prepuce."[55] Hutchinson certainly read Lancereaux's treatise, but I have not been able to establish whether he made particular note of this reference. It would probably have impressed him if he had noticed it, and the idea of all that festering matter beneath the foreskin became such a refrain among later writers on the connection between venereal disease and circumcision that one could easily assume it was in wide circulation. In 1871 the Royal Commission concluded that it was "not improbable that the venereal contagion" was "like other diseases which are partly engendered and always aggravated by neglect of cleanliness." The commissioners rather mixed up sanitarian and contagionist principles in suggesting that the disease was in decline as a result of "the various sanitary regulations which have been enforced," as well as "the increased activity of the police"—a reference to the Contagious Diseases Act.[56]

It was Jonathan Hutchinson, however, who led the push to reclassify syphilis as a filth disease, more appropriately controlled by sanitarian than segregationist measures. J. D. Oriel has described him as not much interested in bacteriology and his response to the discovery of *Treponema pallidum* in 1906 as "cool,"[57] yet he had predicted that the cause of syphilis would be found in a microorganism (or "cryptogamic germ," as he put it) and had shown quite an advanced understanding of how the disease was transmitted. In a lecture to the London Pathological Society in 1876 he stated that syphilis was "due to one virus which, having been introduced into the body by contagion, develops within it, with tolerable uniformity as regards stage and time"; the disease depended on "a living material which is capable of self-multiplication, which breeds in the blood and tissues, and which is destined to pass through various stages of development."[58] As Lindsey Granshaw has commented, Hutchinson accepted that specific germs caused specific diseases, but understood their mode of operation in a sense that emphasized the role of dirt: "[He] expressed his belief in the germ theory in a way that had strong similarities with an older, additive view of dirt—the dirtier the wards, the more likely it would be that wounds would putrefy—and its corollary of emphasis on cleanliness. . . . [He] allowed that germs caused sepsis, but . . . argued that they were carried by diseased patients, or on dirty instruments. . . . Strict cleanliness would thus result in a germ-free environment."[59] By the early twentieth century Lavinia Dock could refer to syphilis as a "filth disease" like any other, pointing out that "knowledge of the breeding place or native haunt of its germ is of the utmost importance for practical hygiene" and to prevent "filth diseases" attacking "cleanly living individuals." The breeding places for venereal disease were prostitution and sexual promiscuity, and the only way to control it was by attacking those evils.[60] Despite his insights into bacterial causation of syphilis, however, Hutchinson seems to have heeded the *Lancet*'s editorial advice to "spare us another debate on the germ-theory" and its hope that his "belief in the cryptogamic origin of syphilis will not lead to a search for such organisms at the exclusion of . . . far more important points."[61] It was thus left to the French and German bacteriologists to make the discoveries that led to the development of means to cure the disease, while Hutchinson himself turned from pursuing the cryptogamic germ to attacking the dirty parts of male bodies that he thought might harbor it. As he stated in 1895, "the space between the glans penis and the prepuce is very apt to harbour the virus, a fact forming one out of many reasons for . . . circumcision at an early age."[62]

Not that the transition in thought and practice was as sharp as this rather schematic analysis implies. In the control of venereal disease there were three contending (and partly overlapping) strategies: (1) regulation of prostitutes; (2) enforcement of greater cleanliness by provision of washing facilities and other means; and (3) behavior modification. Although the first was strictly a contagionist approach and the second a sanitarian one, both were recommended by sanitarians and often described as sanitarian measures; the third meant chastity to the purity campaigners and those under its influence, though it could equally imply condoms, had anyone but the radical George Drysdale been recommending them, or other forms of safe sex, had the concept been invented.[63] Circumcision was consistent with options two and three. Under the sanitarian paradigm, a foreskin-free penis that did not trap filth was by definition cleaner and thus less disease-prone than the natural variety; under the behavioral paradigm, a circumcised boy was considered less likely to get into the habit of sexual gratification through early masturbation, to be generally less interested in sex, and thus to be less likely to seek out prostitutes later on. It need hardly be said that there was a strong element of wish fulfillment in all these strategies, and that they all failed dismally.[64]

The new emphasis on prevention was related to the general rise of preventive medicine and more specifically to the realization that, once syphilis had got into the body, it could not be got out. Acton and the young Hutchinson had been reasonably confident that judicious use of mercury could cure a person of syphilis, or at least arrest the progress of the disease and save him or her from its final ravages, and the policy of confining prostitutes in hospitals until they were pronounced cured implied that a cure was possible. Hutchinson still seems to have believed this in 1876, when he compared syphilis to a yeast in the blood: "If mercury can kill or retard the development of the yeast plant of syphilis, it is very probable that it . . . may do the same for the yeast of typhus, typhoid or smallpox."[65] But during the following decade it was realized that no amount of mercury could kill the disease or permanently halt its progress, meaning that the only effective means of control was prevention. As John Bristowe put it in 1884, "it is now generally admitted that syphilis . . . is incapable of absolute cure, and that it will run a definite course in respect of duration, no matter what steps are taken to arrest its progress."[66] It was thus unfortunate that moral considerations prevented doctors from recommending condoms. Soft rubber became a feasible option after the invention of a vulcanization process in the 1850s, wearable condoms became available in the late 1870s, and it was well understood that they provided effective protection. In 1879 a humorous squib in the underground erotic magazine *The Pearl* pictured a horse race ("The whoring handicap") with various venereal phenomena as the horses and concluded: "The sporting prophets say that if French Letter had not been scratched she would have altered the result of the race."[67] Indeed, as Baldwin comments, it was the very effectiveness of condoms that made them so unthinkable.[68] How widely condoms were used is the subject of some debate. Norman Himes and Michael Mason suggest that they were quite cheap by the 1850s, and thus affordable, although disparaged by most birth control advocates as awkward or immoral.[69] But Angus McLaren argues that they were still too expensive for most people and unpopular because uncomfortable and inconvenient, and too closely associated with men who frequented prostitutes to be permitted in respectable households.[70] That they were unacceptable as a birth control measure, however, does not mean that they were not more widely used as a preventive against venereal disease; Drysdale did not recommend them for the former purpose but urged them strongly for the latter: "It is not impossible that to this instrument humanity may in part be indebted for the total eradication of the syphilitic disease."[71] But to adopt condoms was to legitimize both birth control and casual sex, and to most respectable people that was the sin of fornication. Szreter has shown that this was the main reason why condoms did not come into general use until the 1930s, following the Church of England's change of policy, the relaxation of opposition by the medical profession, and the development of latex (allowing the manufacture of a more sensuous product).[72] Until then, most doctors were vehemently opposed to condoms, partly because they deplored birth control and partly because many believed that removal of the penalties for fornication would only encourage it. The purity feminists rejected condoms for the same reasons: as a pamphlet of the 1880s explained, any use of contraception would only multiply promiscuity and strengthen the sexual appetite, thus "brutalising" the emotions and leading to animalism. In 1912 another tract warned that contraception facilitated "the indulgence of uncontrolled passions" both within and outside marriage.[73] The mood was ripe for harsher measures.

Hutchinson's enthusiasm for circumcision revived with these developments. In 1890 he issued "A Plea for Circumcision" in which he described the foreskin as a "harbour for filth, and a constant source of irritation. It conduces to masturbation and adds to the difficulties of sexual continence. It increase the risk of syphilis in early life, and of cancer in the aged."[74] Three years later he advised circumcision of baby boys as essential "whenever the prepuce is unusually long and contracted" but advantageous for all boys.[75] He returned to the topic at the turn of the century with a lecture, "The Advantages of Circumcision," delivered at the Polyclinic and widely reported in British and U.S. medical journals. He considered that the strongest argument in favor of "the general practice of circumcision" was that it "would reduce the prevalence of syphilis," in support of which opinion he pulled out his old statistics from 1854, "which proved" that although gonorrhea was as common among Jews as among Christians, syphilis was "much less frequent." This fact showed it was not superior morality that gave Jews their "comparative immunity" but some "adventitious advantage" that could only be "the absence of the prepuce"—and not surprisingly, for it would be "difficult to contrive an appendage more likely to facilitate the implantation of the syphilitic virus." Hutchinson assured readers that no measure for the prevention of syphilis was as efficient as circumcision, but he made no mention of condoms, a silence consistent with his opposition to contraception as morally unacceptable and physically harmful, and echoing the stance of his 1870 editorial: any measure that made "irregular sexual intercourse less dangerous" was "injurious to decency . . . and detrimental to the moral conscience of a community." Circumcision did not present this drawback: "Effected in early infancy, and with other avowed objects, it would silently become the means of preventing . . . a loathsome and misery-producing disease." The value of the operation would be enhanced by its effect in diminishing the sexual appetite: "The only function which the prepuce can be supposed to have is that of maintaining the penis in a condition susceptible of more acute sensation than would otherwise exist. It may be supposed to increase the pleasure of the act and the impulse to it. These are advantages, however, which in the present state of society can well be spared, and if in their loss some degree of increased sexual control should result, one should be thankful."[76] In other words, in controlling syphilis, circumcision was preferable to condoms or health checks because it would discourage premarital and extramarital sex.

With the advance of social purity, and despite their obvious flaws, Hutchinson's figures became hot property. In the new sanitary/preventive atmosphere, they came to be regarded with such reverence that they were still being cited as proof that circumcision reduced vulnerability to syphilis (and even gonorrhea, so little attention did later writers pay to his fine print) in the 1940s.[77] As enthusiasm for circumcision spread among the medical profession, Hutchinson's "oft-quoted statistics," as Herbert Snow referred to them in the 1890s,[78] were increasingly valued as the sort of hard evidence scientific men needed. Dr. Cadell claimed that circumcision would "diminish the secretion from the glans . . . and thus render the mucous surface less susceptible to the venereal poison." In the discussion of Cadell's paper, Dr. Watson supported this view by reference to Hutchinson's article, which showed that although "the proportion of Jews to Christians among the out-patients was as *one* to *three*," the proportion of syphilis cases "was only as *one* to *fifteen*." He repeated Hutchinson's comment that this "was not the result of any higher degree of morality on the part of the Jewish population" because "one half of the cases of gonorrhoea occurred in Jews"; it had to be the foreskin.[79] A couple of years later a book in favor of circumcision by an Egyptian writer cited Hutchinson's observations as proof of "the immunity of the circumcised from venereal diseases."[80] In 1883 a surgeon asserted that if every male child were circumcised soon after birth, "venereal infections would become much less common," and in 1893 M. Clifford claimed that if this simple operation were adopted, many common diseases (including syphilis and masturbation) would become extinct: "The prepuce tends to keep the surface of the glans penis moist and . . . little cracks . . . are liable to occur on and around it. These may easily be inoculated by any noxious or contagious matter. . . . Hence they are often the starting point of chancres or syphilis in young persons, and of cancer in the aged."[81] The wording was modeled on Hutchinson's. In 1900 another surgeon commented similarly.[82] On the basis of his experience as a military doctor in India, B. R. Foott thought that the "filth collected" under the foreskin "no doubt assists in the absorption of the syphilitic virus, and very likely the reason why a hard sore is generally on or near the corona glandis. If the glans is always uncovered it is not so sensitive, it is cleaner, and no smegma or other dirt can collect to cause irritation."[83] Remondino also cited Hutchinson's "proof" of "less syphilisation among circumcised men" as a powerful argument in his own case against the foreskin, and he followed his mentor's reasoning in accounting for the phenomenon: "the absence of the prepuce and the non-absorbing character of the skin of the glans penis made so by constant exposure."[84] But he departed from Hutchinson's original article by suggesting that it was not only via the glans that the disease entered the body but through the tissue of the foreskin itself, and he weakened his argument with the concession that circumcision was not the only reason for the Jews' immunity to syphilis: the "well known chastity of their females" was another factor[85]—a direct contradiction of Hutchinson's original point that morality had nothing to do with it.

Hutchinson's statistics surfaced again at the turn of the century in an important article by E. Harding Freeland that was probably as influential as the original communication. His thesis was nothing if not ambitious: "if it were possible to secure the efficient circumcision of every male in infancy not only would many of the disorders [of] . . . the genito-urinary organs . . . be prevented, but . . . the incidence of that scourge of humanity, syphilis . . . would be materially diminished."[86] Freeland acknowledged that he was advocating "the universal practice of an operation which has for its object the wholesale removal of a certain healthy structure as a preventive measure" and recognized that he therefore had to provide "good evidence" that (1) the operation was free from risk; (2) the removal of the foreskin would inflict no physical disability; and (3) the benefits of the amputation were substantial and commensurate with the sacrifice. On the first point Freeland contented himself with the assertion that the risk of the operation was "infinitesimal." On the second he conceded that circumcision "dull[ed] the sensibility" of the penis and thereby "diminish[ed] sexual appetite and the pleasurable effects of coitus," but countered that this was no bar to procreation and thus not a serious deprivation. On the third point he produced Hutchinson's statistics, which showed "not only that the incidence of syphilis is far less frequent among the Jews but that the incidence of gonorrhoea is far more frequent, thus clearly proving that their comparative immunity from syphilis is not due to their excessive morality, but rather, in the absence of any other reason, to circumcision." Freeland claimed that his own experience as a ship's surgeon treating circumcised Lascars and uncut Europeans and "Sedi boys" confirmed this picture,[87] though he was unable to produce figures. In their place he offered evidence from authorities on syphilis that the majority of primary lesions (73 percent) in uncut men were found on the prepuce or retro-preputial fold and that between 25 and 46 percent of them occurred on the prepuce proper. He therefore predicted that universal circumcision, by abolishing the site of most infections, would reduce the incidence of syphilis by 49 percent.

Despite Freeland's statistical precision and general tone of triumph, it is not immediately apparent that the site of the initial sore proved as much as he thought it did. As one of his cited authorities, John Hunter, had pointed out, one function of the prepuce is to provide the slack necessary to accommodate the penis when tumescent, unfolding as the erectile tissue expands;[88] when erect, the penis is entirely covered by what, in its flaccid state, is the foreskin. It follows that if syphilis enters the body through the part that has been inside an infected vagina, the initial lesion must be either on the glans or on the covering of the penis shaft, and if it is on the latter when erect, it will probably appear on the foreskin when the penis is flaccid. Although the suggestion that the foreskin itself was the point of entry for whatever caused the disease departed from Hutchinson's original explanation that it was the foreskin-softened glans that played the Trojan horse, Freeland downplayed this difference in trying to explain why circumcision should provide the prophylaxis it manifestly did. With the glans permanently exposed, the retro-preputial fold obliterated, and the frenum completely excised, the "pocket-like folds which . . . favoured the retention of secretion are smoothed out" and the risks of irritation, excoriation, and "implantation of disease germs" are minimized. The "thickened condition of the epithelium of the glans" was "an additional barrier to any local infection." These were ambitious claims but backed up with little more than impressions from clinical experience. Nor did Freeland have solid evidence for his assertion that the primary sore was usually found on the prepuce. In the days before its demonization, Buchan had written that chancres could be found anywhere: "Though chancres are not confined to any particular part of the body, yet they generally appear on the glans or prepuce, and frequently on the frenum. . . . Sometimes I have seen them on the back of the penis, and even on the scrotum and pubis," as well as fingers, lips, and other nongenital areas.[89] Drysdale had similarly pointed out that the chancre was not necessarily confined to mucous membranes and could be found anywhere on the body, "provided the contagious matter be introduced beneath the skin."[90] Like Remondino, Freeland made up in rhetoric what he lacked in data, and much of his paper was taken up with emotive descriptions of the ravages of syphilis and sheer vilification of the body part he considered guilty of abetting it: "Anyone who has taken the trouble to compare the dry, pink-parchment-like cleanly appearance of the glans of the circumcised with the sodden, swollen, uncleanly structure which is frequently presented to view when the prepuce of the uncircumcised is retracted cannot fail to have been struck by the contrast."[91] This sounds more like an aesthetic preference than a scientific judgment.

In the United States Abraham Wolbarst relied on Hutchinson's statistics to support his call for "universal circumcision as a sanitary measure" in 1914. Citing Remondino's summary rather than the original article, as well as the figures on the site of the primary chancre reported by Freeland, Wolbarst asserted that "these data show conclusively that there is far more syphilis among the uncircumcised than among those who have been circumcised."[92] He had collected statistics from his own patients that showed that although gonorrhea was more common than syphilis in both the circumcised and the normal, the difference was smaller among the latter (59 to 41 percent, compared with 78 to 22 percent for the circumcised). This was inconsistent with Hutchinson's finding that there was more gonorrhea among the circumcised, but the point Wolbarst wanted to emphasize was that while 41 percent of his uncut venereal patients sought treatment for syphilis, only 22 percent of the circumcised did so.[93] The suspicious feature of the samples is that they included an equal number of cut and uncut men (400 each) at a time when most adult men in the United States were not circumcised, suggesting that they were far from representative. There is thus no reason to think that Wolbarst's figures bore any relation to the actual number of cut and uncut venereal cases throughout the United States, and it seems likely he made his sample 400 each for ease of calculation. All he had demonstrated was the ratio of gonorrhea to syphilis among his patients, not the respective rates of venereal disease among the circumcised and intact populations; although this is the only statistic that would prove anything, it has always been difficult to achieve. Wolbarst himself acknowledged that figures could be "distorted to prove almost any contention,"[94] and he sought to buttress his claim with the results of an informal poll of his medical colleagues. He did not reveal how many letters he sent, but he quoted from fifteen replies. Not surprisingly, most of these (eleven) agreed that the uncircumcised were more vulnerable to syphilis (though many of these asserted that they also exhibited increased susceptibility to gonorrhea, herpes, masturbation, and other problems demanding circumcision); two were undecided; and two were firmly of the view that there was no difference at all. Given that only about 25 percent of U.S. males at this time were circumcised,[95] it would not be surprising if three-quarters of patients with venereal disease were uncut. In the twentieth century Wolbarst's article acquired something of the canonical authority that Hutchinson's had enjoyed in the nineteenth. It was summarized by the British *Medical Annual* in 1915, and in 1950 a critic indignantly quoted his figures in opposition to Gairdner's submission that there was no proof that circumcision conferred protection against syphilis and thus that it was not a valid reason for preventive circumcision.[96]

As the response to Wolbarst's survey indicates, there were always skeptics of the association between circumcision and reduced liability to syphilis. Gideon Harvey (ca. 1640–1700) rejected another authority's opinion that a denuded glans helped prevent contagion because "the virulency, otherwise being hidden under the prepuce" finds it easier to enter the body: "for which reason he asserts that the Jews, because they are circumcised, may venture with less danger: a gross mistake certainly; we grant them less pockified for want of occasion, it being a capital crime to miscolate themselves with Christians, notwithstanding at Venice I was told of two Armenians, who are likewise subject to the law of circumcision, that were abominably clapt. To the contrary the prepuce is rather a defence since those whose glans is well covered come off with less harm."[97] This remarkably astute judgment anticipated the conclusion of many nineteenth-century European observers that any reduced liability to common diseases observed among Jewish people was the result of personal habits and the quarantine effect of segregation.[98] With sympathy for circumcision running so strongly in nineteenth-century England, doubters were few, but one was the rationalist Charles Drysdale, who thought that Jews should speed their integration by dropping circumcision, not by encouraging everyone else to do it.[99] Another skeptic was Herbert Snow, who criticized Hutchinson's statistics: while the testimony of such an eminent figure "cannot but receive considerable weight," caution was needed because of his "evident bias in favour of radical measures." He mentioned the obvious but usually overlooked point that the figures showed that Jews were more prone to gonorrhea, but he concluded with the very fair comment that the data were simply not sufficient to prove anything.[100] An interesting example of the difference between received wisdom and actual observation is provided by Arthur Powell, surgeon to the police hospital in Bombay. Having practiced among a mixed Hindu and Muslim population, he had formed "a very definite impression" that syphilis was "much more common" among the uncircumcised Hindus and commented that his "belief in the protective value of circumcision is held by most surgeons. Mr Hutchinson . . . notes the immunity of Jews as compared with Christians." But when he checked the actual figures he found a different story. Out of an average strength of 1,570 Hindus there were 209 syphilis cases, compared with 105 cases among 523 Muslims, giving a rate of infection of 13.3 percent among the uncut and 20 percent among the circumcised. As Powell remarked with some surprise, "these figures are quite opposed to one's preconceived opinion."[101] Like that of the doctors in Wolbarst's poll, Powell's impression of more syphilis among the uncut was probably a consequence of there being fewer circumcised patients among his clientele.[102]

Although it remained a selling point heavily touted by advocates of routine circumcision, the belief that the foreskin seriously heightened vulnerability to syphilis faded from the medical mainstream as the twentieth century advanced. Following the First World War and the Royal Commission on Venereal Diseases, it became a fringe and rather quackish preoccupation, although not as cranky as Hutchinson's unshakable conviction that leprosy was caused by eating rotten fish.[103] In his influential and much reprinted textbook on syphilis, he himself discussed circumcision only as a vector of syphilis, not as a preventive at all;[104] and he was silent on the topic in his lengthy introduction to D'Arcy Power's *System of Syphilis*, published in 1914. The report of the Royal Commission (1916) made no mention of circumcision, condoms, or any other method of prophylaxis, but it did publish estimates of deaths from syphilis broken down by social class, suggesting that there was no correlation between circumcision status and resistance to infection.[105] In 1921 P. Fiaschi listed "circumcision of all male children" among eight prophylactic measures against venereal disease. He discussed sex education, better training of doctors, and use of condoms and Metchnikoff's ointment (both of which he disparaged as too complicated for the average "horny-handed individual"), but when it came to circumcision he made do with a bare assertion and an appeal to Old Testament precedent: "I do not think any medical man can raise any objection to this small surgical procedure, having in view the great assistance it gives to the personal hygiene; it tends to avoid venereal infection, chiefly syphilis. Moses discovered that the same conditions obtained with his hosts in Egypt as result of their sojourn there as we did and his order was centuries ahead of the times."[106] Fiaschi was not the first to bolster a weak medical case with appeals to religious precedent.

Discussion of the association then seems to have died down until the debate on routine circumcision of 1935, when those who supported the practice were quick to cite protection against syphilis as one of its most irrefutable advantages. "F.G." wrote that if "the removal of the prepuce lessen[s] the incidence of syphilis . . . then circumcision is surely a duty in all cases"; C. E. Gautier-Smith agreed: "the increased liability to syphilis and cancer in the uncircumcised is sufficient justification for removing the foreskin."[107] Against these views, H. M. Hanschell from the Seamen's Hospital VD clinic pointed out that there was "no convincing evidence yet presented of less incidence of syphilis in the circumcised," though he let slip that he personally found circumcised penises less disagreeable to handle.[108] More tellingly, V. E. Lloyd and N. L. Lloyd referred to a study they had conducted at Guy's Hospital in 1932 which showed that "there was no lessened risk of acquired syphilis in the circumcised."[109] Like most of the others, this was a fairly impressionistic survey of venereal patients at a hospital, along the same lines as Hutchinson's pioneering observations but involving a larger group (499 men) and a more rigorous analysis of the data. Unlike Hutchinson and Wolbarst they did not neglect to calculate the proportion of syphilis cases among their cut and uncut patients, separately grouped. The Lloyds cited Hutchinson's findings, then referred to other studies that seemed to confirm them, including the one by Wolbarst, whom they criticized for failing to distinguish syphilis from soft chancre and thus making it impossible to calculate the number and proportion of syphilis cases. Their own figures showed a slightly higher incidence of gonorrhea among the circumcised but no significant difference in the incidence of syphilis—20.2 percent among the circumcised and 21.9 percent among the not circumcised. The authors reasonably concluded that "it appears that the absence of the prepuce is not the important preventive factor in the acquisition of syphilis that is commonly believed."[110]

Although the development of Salvarsan and Metchnikoff's ointment, washing after intercourse, the establishment of venereal disease clinics following the First World War, and the later use of condoms helped to reduce its spread, syphilis remained incurable until the introduction of penicillin in the 1940s brought it quickly under control.[111] The claim that circumcision could protect men from syphilis has a long history, but it has more often been made in texts arguing the need for circumcision than in dedicated studies of venereal disease. Despite Hutchinson, few reputable books on syphilis even mention circumcision, let alone discuss it as a prophylactic, and in a recent survey of the medical literature, R. S. Van Howe concluded that "no solid epidemiological evidence has been found to support the theory that circumcision prevents STDs or to justify a policy of involuntary mass circumcision as a public health measure."[112] Exponents of the claim that universal circumcision would eliminate or "materially diminish" the incidence of syphilis have generally been inspired by other motivations: Hutchinson et al. by the desire to discourage masturbation and promote continence; Remondino by a personal crusade against the foreskin as a "moral outlaw"; and Freeland by an aesthetic preference for a dry and "pink-parchment-like" glans. Today we see this debate recapitulated, almost word for word, in the claim that circumcised men are significantly less vulnerable to HIV infection, and thus that universal circumcision of infants is the only way to defeat AIDS. It is a touch ironic that a recent claim to this effect, in trying to prove that the foreskin rather than a host of other epidemiological, social, and behavioral variables is the key factor in HIV transmission, has shown, like Hutchinson with gonorrhea, that circumcised men are more vulnerable to syphilis.[113] It would seem that incurable STDs still elicit the same premodern tendency to blame anatomy for the action of microorganisms.

13 · The Stigmata of a Gentleman

Circumcision and British Society

There is certainly much to be said in favour of the more general adoption of circumcision. Apart from the fact that it lessens the sensitiveness of the glans penis and minimises the risk of venereal infection in after life, circumcision dispenses with the necessity for methodical hygienic measures, failing which the secretions accumulate and decompose, giving rise to excoriation and irritation which . . . pave the way to the formation of disastrous habits in early life.

"The Advantages of Circumcision," *Medical Press,* 19 September 1900

Most educated people asked to have their sons circumcised; he thought it an excellent thing to do; it helped to prevent hernia due to straining, and later it helped in preventing masturbation. The ordinary schoolboy was not taught to keep himself clean, and if he were taught he thought too much about the matter. No anaesthetic was necessary when circumcising infants—in fact it was harmful.

British Medical Journal, 5 June 1920

He was in lots of pain for weeks after. He screamed whenever he did a wee and he screamed the first time I put him in the bath after the operation. After that he wouldn't go near the bath for two weeks. His penis got infected and he needed antibiotics to clear it up. He kept crying and saying "I wish I had my old willy back."

Mother's report, *Practical Parenting,* June 2002

By the outbreak of World War I the circumcised penis was the mark of the English elite, or at least of its younger members. Whatever their descendants might insist, late Victorian fathers seem not to have worried that their sons would look different from them and generally acquiesced in doctors' recommendations. Better health than they had enjoyed and a stricter morality than they had practiced were the promises, and no one could argue with that. A sign of the times was a new breed of quack, calling himself a "specialist operator," who sent circulars to families that had announced the birth of a son in which he sought "to show the importance of the youngster being circumcised without delay, and offers to do the operation within half a minute in an ordinary case," as the *British Medical Journal*'s sarcastic summary put it. Among the "moral and physical reasons for its performance" were sure protection from "obscure nervous disorders" and "exemption and immunity from disease." The *BMJ* ridiculed the advertiser's bad grammar, but he was merely taking advantage of the scare created by the medical profession, and his language echoed the warnings of the orthodox health experts.[1] The pamphlet, like the doctors who mocked it, did not suggest that the fathers ought to avail themselves of this new aid to health; as David Gollaher has observed, it was a service to be enjoyed only by a "group of patients who could not object."[2] The advantages of circumcision were considered so persuasive that in 1900 the *Medical Press* flagged the possibility of the operation being made as compulsory as vaccination,[3] and in the 1920s a fair indication of what parents were being told is provided by a popular medical guide, *Harmsworth's Home Doctor and Encyclopaedia of Good Health*. First they were given the impression that the normal foreskin made urination difficult if not impossible in infants, and second that paraphimosis was a common problem. Next they were informed that because "the advantages of circumcision are so great, and the operation so trivial," it was possible that "the rest of the human race might well follow the example of the Jews and Mahommedans and make it a compulsory rite." After that they were advised that circumcision was "an aid to moral and personal cleanliness. . . . When the glans is continuously covered by the foreskin it remains moist and very sensitive. A moist glans is very susceptible to infection, especially as a narrow foreskin prevents the daily cleansing. . . . A sensitive glans is a positive danger to growing lads, as it fosters early sexual excitement, and is provocative of self-abuse." The author of the entry appreciated that the objective of circumcision was to ensure that the glans was permanently exposed and acknowledged that other methods of securing this outcome, such as stretching, might also work in some cases, but circumcision was preferable because less troublesome: "Dilation of the end can sometimes be carried out, but the process is painful and tedious. Hence the operation should be performed."[4] It was advice that many parents of the middle, professional, and upper classes duly heeded.

In 1907 Bland-Sutton reported that circumcision was increasingly common in London hospitals and that the operation was performed on

894 boys at the Hospital for Young Children in 1906, but he acknowledged that parents often had to be pressured into agreeing to it: "Mothers often strongly object to have their baby boys circumcised, not only from dislike to subjecting them to a surgical operation . . . but also from a feeling of revulsion in subjecting them to a process which is regarded as a rite in other religious communities. My own experience in this matter has been that when the advantages of circumcision are explained to them, they yield."[5] In 1888 a practitioner had to use all his professional authority to persuade the parents to let him circumcise their "strong, healthy eleven-year old" for bed-wetting—a problem caused, he was sure, by the boy's elongated prepuce. It was only when he promised that the operation would prevent masturbation as well that they reluctantly gave their consent.[6] An indication of the brutality that could follow such persuasion is provided by the case of a man who sought psychiatric treatment for impotence some time in the 1920s. During the course of his analysis it emerged that he had been circumcised, as he thought in early infancy, but that it had not occurred to him to mention the fact because he had imbibed the prevailing wisdom that it was of no importance: "a natural hygienic operation etc." Further questioning and discussion with his mother, however, brought forth a different story:

> During his infancy his mother was from time to time advised on matters of child hygiene by a medical practitioner who was a close relative of her own. He seems to have had a mania for performing the operation of circumcision, and very few children who came within his ken escaped this fate. His own children were circumcised. In spite of the fact that our patient's prepuce and glans were normal in every respect, this surgeon never failed to impress on the patient's mother the inestimable advantages to be obtained from circumcision. . . . On the occasion of a particular holiday visit the mother's scruples were finally overcome, and she consented to have the circumcision performed on her child. The final step in gaining her consent took the form of visiting the nursery. The patient was awakened out of his sleep by having his bedclothes abruptly pulled away. He woke up to find the sinister figure of the doctor leaning over the bed. His penis was unceremoniously seized by the surgeon's left hand, with the right the motion of cutting was imitated and the mother, who stood on the opposite side of the bed, was asked to note how simple a matter it was to cut off the foreskin, or words to that effect. She was rather concerned at the whole performance, and observed that the son showed signs of panic, but she did not interfere with the demonstration. The technique must have been rather crude, because the process of healing was delayed. The wound had to be dressed daily, and each dressing

aroused agonized anticipations and was followed by wailing protestation. One protestation in particular took the form of a reproach directed at his mother. The day after the operation he is said to have cried out to his mother, "Why did you let him cut it off?" After a week's dressings the wound began to heal by granulation, and there is no exact record of its subsequent course. There was, however, no doubt in the mother's mind that the experience was an agonizing one for the child, and she regretted her decision for a long time afterwards.[7]

Not only she, one suspects.

Circumcision never became as common in Britain as it later did in Australia and the United States, where greater social equality and a more elaborate insurance system allowed all classes to benefit from medical advances, and where fewer skeptics were found doubting that the practice was an advance. At the height of its incidence circumcision affected only 30 to 40 percent of British boys, but this was not distributed evenly through the population: while two-thirds or more of public school boys were cut, the proportion in the working class or living in rural areas was much lower; as Erichsen's surgery complained in 1889, the operation was "still not practised often enough, especially among poorer patients."[8] Circumcision probably reached its peak around 1930 and was already in decline by 1935, when a long-running controversy in the correspondence columns of the *British Medical Journal* revealed that as many doctors were against the operation as in favor. Examination of army conscripts in 1953 (men born in the early 1930s) showed that 34 percent were circumcised.[9] A similar survey in 1956 of RAF recruits born between 1930 and 1936 found an overall circumcision rate of 34.4 percent, but with significant variations depending on education level and birthplace. The incidence of circumcision in Scotland and Wales was noticeably less than in England, and lower in rural than in urban areas generally. The incidence for Britain as a whole was 32.8 percent for those who got no further than elementary school, 36.6 percent for grammar school boys, and 41.9 percent for those from public schools. The highest incidence of circumcision was among English public school boys (47.5 percent) and the lowest (18.6 percent) at urban elementary schools in Scotland.[10] A survey of boys born in 1946 found that only 24 percent were circumcised, but the class differential was again striking: 39 percent among professional groups and only 22 percent among manual and unskilled workers.[11] In 1949 Gairdner reported a circumcision rate of 67 percent for thirteen-year-old boys at public schools, 50 percent for five- to fourteen-year-olds at rural state schools, and only 30 percent for five- to eleven-year-olds at primary schools in Cambridge.[12] In many working-class communities circumcision remained a Jewish peculiarity. Richard Hoggart (b. 1918) recalls that Jewish men were reported to have "a great, bare, foreskinless purple mushroom," which was rumored to make girls more excited than the variety of penis normally found in Leeds. The older boys countered that "the way the foreskin rolled back on entry" afforded "an even greater thrill."[13]

In explaining these differentials, MacCarthy and colleagues suggested that women from "the salaried and professional classes" were more likely to follow medical advice and attend ante-natal clinics and child welfare centers than were the poor. Their children were also "more likely to be vaccinated, immunized and have their tonsils out." Mothers were probably following the advice of their doctor when they authorized circumcision, particularly as it was common for obstetricians "to charge an inclusive fee for maternity care and to circumcise the child as part of the service."[14] By this time, just as the medical profession was abandoning faith in circumcision, it was evident that parents had thoroughly absorbed the propaganda of the previous century. In an informal survey of mothers in 1946–47, Alex Comfort found the following justifications (in descending frequency):

1. Advised by doctor, usually because of nonretractable foreskin at birth.
2. Advised by nurse or midwife.
3. Desired by (circumcised) father.
4. Family custom.
5. Jewish or Muslim religion.

The reasons for advising circumcision given by nurses were

1. Adherent prepuce at birth.
2. Cleanliness and ease of washing.
3. Prevention of masturbation.[15]

Another doctor reported in 1950 that "one mother was most anxious for the operation . . . because her own doctor had convinced her that when the boy grew up lack of cleanliness would lead to local irritation, thence to masturbation, and thereafter down the steep and slippery slope of total moral degradation."[16] Nineteenth-century attitudes were evidently still powerful.

Much of the social differential can be explained in MacCarthy's terms: unlike the poor, the richer classes could afford inessential medical care, and they were more likely to be exposed to the advisory literature. But there may be a further factor in the popularity of the operation among middle-class parents, related to the belief that masturbation caused mental deterioration and the promise that circumcision would lead to behavioral modifications desirable in those who wanted to get ahead. Nicola Beisel has argued that moral crusades like Anthony Comstock's Society for the Suppression of Vice (New York, 1870s-1890s) derived their strength from parental anxieties about whether their children would equal or surpass their own position in society. He exploited parental fears that carnal indulgence would render them unfit for desirable jobs and social positions—that they would not be hired or would be excluded from the right circles and networks because their habits, reputation, or appearance made them seem untrustworthy or unsuitable.[17] Such a perspective seems equally applicable to the English purity movements of the same period, targeted as they were at middle- and upper-class males,[18] and particularly to their anxiety over masturbation. Doctors hammered the point that it would damage boys' minds and bodies in ways that would unfit them for decent jobs, and many reported cases of schoolboys who lost the power to concentrate and failed their exams because of their addiction. As Sylvanus Stall warned, "the bright boy that stood at the head of the class is gradually losing his power to comprehend and retain his lessons. He memory fails him. His mind begins to lack grasp and grip. . . . Gradually he loses his place and drops back towards the foot of the class."[19] If a boy could not even get through school, what hope was there of reaching university and acquiring the degree and connections necessary for success? Comstock himself claimed that the worst effect of obscene literature was that it led to masturbation, and he quoted a "prominent citizen" who claimed that self-abuse was "a thousand times worse where it is occasioned by obscene plates," whose impact on the mind "remain[ed] throughout life." Comstock played deliberately on parental fears that their son might fail at school and introduced the idea that the most likely reason for failure was being "ruined" by vices taught by other boys: "What is more beautiful . . . than the youth of manly form . . . his face radiant with the bloom of a pure blood, a countenance bespeaking a conscious rectitude and unyielding integrity. . . . How proudly the father . . . places him in some select institution of learning, where he can be qualified for future positions of trust and honour!" Alas, their dreams of upward mobility are shattered and their sacrifices rendered vain when he comes under the influence of evil companions, "a black stain is fixed indelibly" on his imagination, and he becomes a wreck of his former self.[20] Beisel concludes that Comstock's rhetoric of moral corruption was really about "the social downfall of upper and middle class children."[21] She does not mention circumcision, but Comstock's argument was that children were not threatened by the sexuality of those who were likely to corrupt them (prostitutes, other boys, and so forth) but by *their own sexuality*—"their own unleashed desire." Means to curb and repress their sexual urges would thus make them less vulnerable to moral infection and would be an important way of protecting them from dealers in dirty pictures and suppliers of information about masturbation and contraception. Applying Sayre's reflex neurosis theory in an article arguing that evolution was trying to abolish the clitoris as well as the foreskin, Robert Morris suggested that a schoolboy with learning difficulties might really be suffering from eye problems caused by preputial adhesions. If he was circumcised so as to restore normal vision, "the expert baseball pitcher might become an Alexander von Humboldt."[22] What ambitious parent would not be tempted to give it a try?

Despite the popularity of the practice there was no unanimity among doctors as to the best time for circumcision, the appropriate technique, or the level of skill required. Although an increasing number of boys were cut in infancy and often soon after birth, the custom of allowing the mother's obstetrician to do it in much the same spirit as he tied the umbilical cord never developed as it did in the United States. Most boys were not circumcised as a routine (that is, automatically before they left hospital) but because they had an adherent prepuce or were later caught playing with their penis. Circumcision was also common in childhood, particularly just before a boy started school, as a precaution against picking up the habit of solo or group masturbation from his new mates. The decreasing age at which the operation was performed arose from the difficulty of giving children an anesthetic and the related problem of immobilizing them if one was not used. Edmund Owen commented in 1897 that "some surgeons advise that the operation be done under the influence of cocaine: for the adult this answers well, but for children it is far better to give chloroform. Children are frightened by the restraint, by the sight of the instruments, or of a little blood, and before the operation is well begun they may be struggling to be free."[23] Newborn babies were less trouble. Samuel Newman appreciated that infants "may be held down by two assistants and the operation done without any anaesthetic"; he bound his own patients "to a board after the Indian fashion of strapping the papoose," thus inventing the circumstraint.[24] Corner recommended that the operation be done "in early babyhood" because it gave "the minimum of discomfort" and no anesthesia was required: "Up to 6 months of age a healthy baby is very easily nursed, as it leads the life of a vegetable."[25]

The technique of circumcision was never standardized during the period it was common in Britain, and many different methods were in use. As Herbert Snow commented in 1890, "an immense variety of operative procedures . . . might be quoted," but "the contradictory . . . advantages claimed for each" suggested that none was found "entirely satisfactory."[26]

Most doctors used the freehand approach, with either scissors or scalpel, and many had his favorite protocol. In 1883 a Dr. Macleod proposed "an improved method of circumcision" for congenital phimosis, which he defined as a situation where the foreskin has a "more or less narrow orifice" and is adherent to the glans. An improved method was desirable because it was difficult "to separate the inner layer [of the foreskin] from the tiny glans, wet and slippery with blood" as it always was. The virtue of Macleod's reforms was that they made it easier for doctors to see what they were doing and thus limit damage to what they intended:

> The last case operated on, in a child of two years, scarcely admitted the point of a probe through the orifice of the prepuce, but by dilating this orifice forcibly with "sinus forceps," and the addition of a few tiny snips with scissors round the margin . . . the foreskin could be drawn back until the point of the glans showed itself. Further retraction was prevented by the adhesions . . . but these were easily broken down by means of a probe passed between the prepuce and the glans, and this done until the corona glandis was exposed[27]

—thus permitting the necessary scissoring and suturing. The development of task-specific instruments showed that, in the spirit of invention, the British lagged behind the more entrepreneurial Americans. In 1883 R. J. Lewis announced the production of an "instrument to facilitate the performance of circumcision in children," endowed with all the versatility of a Swiss army pocket knife. It was described by the *Edinburgh Medical Journal* as a complex arrangement consisting of blades, a thumbscrew, a device to give traction, and a bistoury to finish up with.[28] In 1889 W. W. Sinclair, resident surgeon at Selaugor, Malaya, urged the adoption of a clamp used by Muslims on eight-year-old boys. The article was accompanied by illustrations of the bamboo original and an improved steel model made in London. Sinclair had found operations with this device "so simple, rapid, clean and safe" that he recommended it to the profession. He also reported that the local Muslims initiated girls in a similar manner, by nipping off part of their clitoris, but that the clamp was not needed for this procedure, though he stopped short of commending this example of an "ancient operation" to his modern colleagues.[29] In 1936 a pair of "special circumcision forceps" was developed by surgeons at Guy's Hospital because they were concerned that "the operation . . . entails considerable needless haemorrhage and the results were to say the least inartistic."[30] It was considerations like these that lay behind British doctors' disenchantment with circumcision in the 1930s and A. P. Bertwhistle's "Plea for a Standardised Technique," in which he expressed surprise that every modern textbook described a different method. He was also concerned that the results were "by no means uniformly good" and commented that a repeat operation was often necessary "because of cicatrization of a foreskin left unduly long, and an objectionable lump [near] . . . the frenum." Bertwhistle's technique called for "two pairs of Spencer-Wells forceps, one pair of blunt-nosed scissors . . . one pair of dissecting forceps, a needle, and a simple, inexpensive instrument . . . resembling an army button-cleaning stick." He thus belonged to the school that believed most operators took too little foreskin, insisting that it was "important . . . to remove enough of the prepuce, otherwise scarring may call for a second operation." Such an elaborate procedure, culminating in the need for many stitches, was hardly likely to recommend itself to those seeking speed and simplicity, and it is little wonder that this method was forgotten when the Gomco clamp became available in the late 1930s.[31] Described by its modern champion as "a model of excellence in design and innovation," it promised all the ruthlessness demanded by Bertwhistle, with such ease of operation that even the least-skilled operator could wield it without incurring an unacceptable level of complications.[32]

There was also much disagreement among doctors as to how much tissue should be removed. Some (like Dr. Spratling) urged the maximum possible, others the minimum needed to expose the glans, yet others a middle course. Erichsen's *Surgery* warned doctors to be careful "that too much skin be not removed,"[33] but Freeland complained that most cut away too little. He insisted that the "the fraenum should always be removed" as well; in this way "the folds . . . on either side are obliterated, and the oedematous nodule which is liable to form at this point is prevented."[34] George Fullerton assured readers of his home medical guide that it was impossible to remove too much of the prepuce, since "to have it short is conducive to cleanliness," and both Sir W. Ferguson and Professor Humphrey thought it "best to amputate the structure as radically as possible."[35] Hutchinson also urged a tight job.[36] Circumcision was not classified as serious surgery (and thus reserved to specialist surgeons) in the carve-up of professional turf but was generally regarded as a minor procedure, like scratching off a wart, which any GP, intern, or medical student could accomplish. In 1950 even an advocate of universal circumcision admitted that it was usually performed by "house surgeons who are not properly taught and do not stay long enough to observe the results. The operation is the Cinderella of surgical instruction."[37] Fullerton commented that the operation was "perfectly safe and requires no anatomical knowledge on the part of the performer," but the messy results of many operations did not bear out such confidence: as even an advocate like Edmund Owen admitted, "circumcision is often badly done."[38] One of Havelock Ellis's case histories reported that when he was a boy he found circumcised organs "disagreeable," particularly the "much-ridged penis" of the son of the headmaster at his school.[39] There was no elaboration of what "much ridged" meant, but "heavily scarred" seems a reasonable translation.

It was indeed the consistently disappointing results that lay behind the constant search for new techniques. Commending his own method in 1894, one doctor stressed that it ensured "no inflammation, no discharge, no swelling, no pain, and no crying or screaming," suggesting that such sequelae were often encountered.[40] Hutchinson confessed that hemorrhage was a serious problem and that "many children have died after the operation in consequence of carelessness in this matter." Other risks were poisoning of the wound by unclean instruments and the introduction of syphilis by the dressings; he knew of at least seven cases in which a Jewish circumciser communicated syphilis by unclean lint and had been consulted in another in which a surgeon did the same by his instruments.[41] It is thus not surprising that Clifford began his account of the advantages of circumcision with an assurance that its divine sanction and long history were proof that it was really quite safe: "From this early period . . . the operation has been regularly practised, and amongst some peoples has been performed as a religious observance up to the present day. This fact alone is strong proof that distinct advantages must have been recognised to follow the operation. . . . Had there been reason to suppose it dangerous or even detrimental in the slightest degree, parents would never have allowed their children to be submitted to it." This reassurance was not exactly confirmed by Clifford's admission on the facing page that he had "met with so many instances where . . . circumcision has been performed in a bungling manner, where the wound has been a long time healing, and where afterwards the parts have been . . . deformed"; indeed, his main reason for writing the book was to reduce the incidence of "the various complications and troubles likely to be met with in conducting the operation."[42] The story as told to other doctors was evidently somewhat less comforting than the narrative supplied to parents. A contributor to a surgical textbook in 1895 explained that although the operation was "deemed insignificant," care and judgment were required to avoid complications; these included excessive skin removal, infection (leading to cellulitis or erysipelas), infection with syphilis or tuberculosis, and hemorrhage.[43] In 1907 Bland-Sutton admitted that syphilis and tuberculosis were sometimes communicated in ritual circumcision and that "infants have died from bleeding and sepsis when the operation has been performed by medical men," but he evidently felt that such casualties in the battle against disease were acceptable wastage: "These things only serve to show that an element of risk pervades all human actions."[44] Even in 1916 a supporter acknowledged that, as usually performed, circumcision often entailed "unnecessary loss of blood and the formation of troublesome haematoma," leading to "that small but regular percentage of deaths from haemorrhage which is reported annually."[45] In 1950 a surgeon listed eight complications of circumcision that he was regularly called upon to treat: bleeding; removal of too much skin; removal of too little mucosa; skin tags; urethral fistulas; amputation of part or all of the glans; amputation of the entire penis; and stitching of the skin edge to the glans.[46] Although common, these adverse outcomes must be seen in perspective: at the turn of the century all operations were risky. When doctors said that circumcision was safe they meant that the incidence of complications or death was less than the norm, perhaps only 10 percent, compared with the 20 or 30 percent death rate that was usual in other surgical procedures. How acceptable you considered that percentage would depend on how necessary you considered the procedure.

Little evidence has come down about whether the unwilling beneficiaries of circumcision were grateful to have been relieved of their preputial burden. Douglas Gairdner found that in discussions among men, "those still in possession of their foreskin have been forward in their insistence that any differences which may exist in such matters [aesthetic and erotic] operate emphatically to their own advantage."[47] This view is confirmed by one of Marie Stopes's correspondents, who mentioned his bitterness at "having been served by this inhuman operation,"[48] and there is other testimony that suggests there must have been many boys who wept along with Dr. Glover's patient and the boy who wanted his old willy back, as the sad case of the classical scholar and poet Alfred Housman (1859-1936) suggests. Alfred seems to have enjoyed a happy childhood, but in 1872 his mother died, and the following year his father Edward married his cousin Lucy, an evangelically minded woman from London. Around the same time Edward gave his son, then aged fourteen, the man-to-man talk that was becoming the standard Victorian father's warning against masturbation, but he did not leave it at mere advice: he decided to have Alfred and his four younger brothers circumcised as well. Housman's most recent biographer has no explanation for the decision, though it could have been the influence of his purity-minded new wife, or a response to emerging medical wisdom: as we have seen, the 1870s were the decade in which the idea of circumcision as a precaution against masturbation really took hold. Whatever the reasons for it, the operation provoked considerable resentment among the boys, as one of their sisters recalled later: "It was severe treatment, mentally and physically, for well-grown boys, and a great mystery at the time to the younger ones who made open complaint, with a mixture of importance and resentment, of the ill-treatment which had befallen them."[49] Alfred made no surviving reference to what was done to him, but there are signs in his subsequent life and career that it left a mental as well as a physical scar. Shortly after the operation he visited London and was deeply affected by the Greek and Roman antiquities in the British Museum, especially the nude male statues—which would all have shown either an intact prepuce or no penis at all as a result of breakage. Taking part in a family competition for a poem about the ruins of Rome in 1874 or 1875, he penned the following melancholy lines:

> The city is silent and solemn
> That once was alive and divine;
> And here stands the shaft of a column,
> And there lies the wreck of a shrine.[50]

Ancient ruins are a conventional theme for elegiac verse, but it would be understandable if ruined shafts and broken columns had a particular poignancy for him at this time. It is also interesting that, as a scholar, Housman went on to specialize in the branch of classical studies concerned with the recovery and restoration of incomplete and mutilated texts, and also that he does not seem ever to have established a sexual relationship with anyone. He experienced the misery of unreciprocated crushes on university athletes while an undergraduate, but the only sexual activity in which he is thought to have engaged is with male prostitutes in Paris (though he might have had a Venetian gondolier as a lover for a time). Graves suggests that the misbehavior of a governess and his father's warnings against the perils of sexual desire made him think of "sex between men and women as something rather dirty,"[51] but it is equally possible that his penis was so badly injured by the surgery that he was not physically capable of normal sexual activity with anyone.

Housman is better known today as a poet—author of *A Shropshire Lad*—than as a classical scholar, and it is in his poetry that one finds the strongest evidence for his sadness at the mutilation of his penis. The wistful tone of most of the poems, their reverence for the teenage male body, their sense of its vulnerability and transience, the scarcely concealed erotic interest in the lads yet the sense that nothing could be hoped from them, all point to a sensibility charged with regret and conscious of loss. Apart from the elegiac mood of *A Shropshire Lad* overall—a powerful factor in the collection's popularity during the slaughter of young men in the First World War—several of them make specific reference to past wrongs and injuries. In "The Welsh Marches" (poem 28) we read:

When shall I be dead and rid
Of the wrong my father did?
How long, how long, till spade and hearse
Put to sleep my mother's curse?[52]

Housman has insisted that the poems are not autobiographical, but such a direct statement makes you wonder. In the ironic poem 45 there is an even more direct reference to the concept of injuring the body in order to save the soul—exactly the view of the doctors, purity campaigners, and others who urged circumcision to prevent masturbation:

If it chance your eye offend you
Pluck it out, lad, and be sound:
'Twill hurt, but here are salves to friend you,
And many a balsam grows on ground
And if your hand or foot offend you,
Cut it off, lad, and be whole;
But play the man, stand up and end you,
When your sickness is your soul.[53]

One can imagine this as Housman's sarcastic parody of what his father or the doctor might have said to him about the long-term health benefits of his operation. Indeed, it is eerily reminiscent of Dr. Pratt's advice in his *Sermon to Young Men:* had Alfred seen the pamphlet, or had his father read it and taken its advice literally?

W. H. Auden once referred unkindly to Housman's sexual obsessions as "something to do with violence and the poor," but since he too resented having been circumcised, it is surprising he did not show more empathy.[54] Scholars have drawn attention to the prominence of violence and humiliation in Housman's verse and connected it with his teenage ordeal. As Dick Davis writes, "his father's decision to have the boy . . . circumcised must have had a dramatic effect on someone who was . . . worried by his sexuality for other reasons. As his poems everywhere attest, violence perpetrated by or against young men held a fascination for him which was almost certainly erotic in origin, and the maimed male body seems to have been a source of deep physical attraction."[55] *Attraction* may not be the right word, but the fascination, whether excited, curious, or horrified, was certainly there. Housman himself reflected on comments such as these in cryptic but suggestive terms:

They say my verse is sad: no wonder.
Its narrow measured spans
Rue for eternity, and sorrow
Not mine, but man's.[56]

If this seems to shift the explanation for his melancholy from his personal situation to the human condition, a statement in a letter toward the end of his life brings it right back home again: "I did not begin to write poetry until the really emotional part of my life was over; and my poetry . . . sprang chiefly from physical conditions, such as a relaxed sore throat during my most prolific period, the first five months of 1895."[57] Can one really believe that a passing sore throat exerted a greater influence than his permanently scarred dick?

A pair of famous brothers who resented their circumcision were John Maynard and Geoffrey Keynes, both of whom were circumcised in childhood to stop them from masturbating.[58] When interviewed in 1979, Geoffrey (b. 1887) recalled being taken to the doctor at the age of three; he could not remember when Maynard (b. 1883) was done, but if it was at the same time he would have been seven. Their father's anxiety about masturbation may be judged from an entry in his diary from 1894 that "Maynard was very sad this morning because the pockets of his overcoat were sewn up." Sewing up pockets was commonly recommended to make it harder for boys to interfere with their genitals, but it is not clear whether this precaution (when Maynard was eleven) was taken before or after his operation. It seems more likely that he was circumcised earlier but still kept up or had resumed his bad habits. The subsequent lives of the boys suggest that the experience left them scarred in subtle but detectable ways. Although Geoffrey does not mention the incident in his reticent memoirs, he told Robert Skidelsky that he had "never forgiven his parents" for what they did to him,[59] and there is plenty of evidence that the memory remained to haunt him. In one revealing passage he describes how "deeply affected" he was by an episode at primary school, when a boy who had been caught encouraging two others to have a competition about who could piss the furthest was flogged in front of an assembly. He reports this incident as his most vivid memory from his early years and comments that the triviality of the offense deserved no more than "reprimand and a smile," suggesting that he felt a deep affinity with other boys punished for playing with their private parts. Years later, he tells us, he found a "charming wood engraving" from about 1790 by Thomas Bewick, showing two boys having a similar contest at the edge of a pond. He reproduced this in his memoirs, commenting: "What Bewick had regarded as a harmless joke, the Victorian schoolmaster magnified into a major offence demanding brutal punishment."[60] To the Victorians, of course, nothing relating to the genitals was harmless or funny, but the headmaster's victim was perhaps luckier than Keynes himself and boys in the United States, where those caught holding pissing competitions were sometimes punished with the loss of their foreskins.[61]

And there are other signs. Without explanation he prints an engraving by William Blake, "The Circumcision" (of Jesus), in which a tiny baby is dwarfed by a stand of threatening adults. From an early age Keynes liked Housman's poetry and used to go for long walks with his future wife, reading aloud from *A Shropshire Lad* as they went. In 1934 they had dinner with Housman, and he recalled that they had an interesting "psychological discussion" in which the poet agreed that "we did not forget the horrid things that had happened to us, as psychologists said we do."[62] Being English gentlemen they probably said no more than that, but each knew the bitter truth behind the observation.

The fact that circumcision in Britain was far more common among urban and professional groups than among the workers and rural laborers casts a revealing light on the proverbial preference of upper-class English homosexuals for working-class lads, ploughboys, and Italian sailors. It has usually been assumed that they were attracted to their superior physiques, greater virility, and less sophisticated manners, but it seems probable that their foreskins were another factor. As Davenport-Hines comments in his biography of Auden, middle-class Englishmen's "frantic hunting for rough trade" was "related to their pleasure in foreskins, and their identification of them with real men, rather than the effete and circumcised of their own class," whom they regarded as partially emasculated.[63] Encountering a Norwegian sailor on a beat during World War II, the English MP Tom Driberg (b. 1905) was ecstatic over his "long, uncircumcised, and tapering, but rock-hard erection," a response suggesting that Driberg did not encounter such a feature as often as he could have wished and perhaps regretted that his own organ did not sport it.[64] Alan Turing, the computer pioneer and principal inventor of the Enigma machine, which broke the German codes in World War II, also expressed his deep resentment at having been circumcised,[65] and the case of W. H. Auden, circumcised at age seven, just before he started boarding school in 1914, is even more suggestive. The precise reasons have not come down to us, but his parents came from precisely the medico-theological formation that regarded circumcision as a wise precaution against boys' picking up "bad habits" from their new schoolmates. Both were children of clergymen, and his mother a nurse who had dreamed of being a missionary; his father was a school medical officer with an interest in child behavior, mental deficiency, and delinquency. The unwanted operation remained an "unpleasant memory," contributed to his sense of being "impaired, damaged and incomplete," and made him both deeply dissatisfied with the condition of his own penis and intensely interested in other men's, especially "the comparison of circumcised with uncircumcised," as he wrote in 1929. Forty years later he commented that it was "men, not women, who suffer most from penis-envy."[66] Like Tom Driberg, his preferred activity was fellatio, receptive role only, a form of sexual expression that provided maximum contact with the contours of his partner's penis and in which the presence or absence of the foreskin would strongly affect the quality of the experience.[67]

That Auden suspected he had been circumcised in order to discourage future or punish past masturbation, and at the instigation of his mother, is suggested by his comments on "the scissor-man" and his construction of mothers in several of his plays as destructive monsters who attack their children. Images of motherhood as malevolent and harmful are central to *The Dog beneath the Skin, The Ascent of F6,* and, much later, the libretto for *The Bassarids,* an operatic version of *The Bacchae.*[68] The scissors-man appears in "The Story of Little Suck-a-Thumb" in Heinrich Hoffman's *Struwwelpeter,* originally published in Germany in 1847 but widely available in English as children's reading of the cautionary variety. In this story little Conrad is prone to thumb sucking, but his mother warns him not to do it while she is out or the "great, long, red-legged scissors-man" will come and cut his thumbs off—which is exactly what happens. Auden later commented that the story was "not about thumb-sucking . . . but about masturbation, which is punished by castration." Perhaps he had been reading too much Freud: when Hoffman published *Struwwelpeter* it was at the height of the onanism scare in Germany, and it is more likely that the punishment with which the Conrads of the time were threatened was circumcision.[69] Auden wrote disapprovingly of Housman's flight from love into death,[70] but he shared some of his sensibility, and his own fascination with ruined industrial machinery and abandoned railway tracks is reminiscent of the other's interest in ancient remains and mutilated texts:

> Deliberately he chose the dry-as-dust,
> Kept his tears like dirty postcards in a drawer;
> Food was his public love, his private lust
> Something to do with violence and the poor.[71]

Did Auden sense that he had more in common with Housman than he was willing to admit?

The failure of circumcision to become universal in Britain (or even routine in the U.S. sense—done automatically in hospitals unless parents objected strenuously and intervened in time) was partly due to class inequality and the public school masturbation scare, but perhaps mainly to the fact that it never commanded the unanimous support of the medical profession. Although they published many articles extolling the advantages of circumcision, the *British Medical Journal* and the *Lancet* remained uncommitted,[72] no medical organization ever issued a statement recommending it as a routine procedure, and there were always skeptics who regarded it as a harmful fad. Two of the most eloquent of these were Elizabeth Blackwell,[73] the first English woman to qualify as a medical practitioner, and Herbert Snow, surgeon to the London cancer hospital, whose heartfelt denunciation of the "barbarity" of circumcision was published in 1890. Blackwell was concerned that it had become fashionable among reputable but "short-sighted" physicians to praise "this unnatural practice" and urge its performance in Christian nations. She detected the quackery inherent in the idea, pointing out that parents' fears "were worked upon by an elaborate but false statement of the evils which would result to the child were this mutilation not performed," and she rejected "the plea that this unnatural practice will lessen the risk of infection to the sensualist in promiscuous intercourse." Overall, it was a vehement denunciation of interference with boys' bodies, based largely on ethical grounds.[74] Herbert Snow's aim was more ambitious: "the abolition of an antiquated practice involving the infliction of very considerable suffering upon helpless infants; and sanctioned, on very questionable grounds, by men of eminent authority." This statement concisely set out the terms of his opposition: circumcision was an antiquated religious custom, not a modern medical therapy; it meant suffering and harm to a class of patients who had not given consent; and the grounds advanced to justify it were spurious. He also implied that the advance of circumcision was an effect of the authority of its promoters, not of the quality of their scientific reasoning. On the first point, Snow rejected hygienic explanations for the origin of ritual circumcision and accepted the argument of anthropologists that it was a sacrifice intended for a deity that obviously required appeasement, and probably an attenuated form of what had once been the sacrifice of something yet more precious, such as the entire genitalia or living children. He took the view that the tribes who practiced circumcision were barbarians whose customs did not warrant emulation by modern Britons. On the second point Snow made the reasonable suggestion that "no sane man who possessed the advantages of a sound and entire prepuce would willingly sacrifice it without just and sufficient cause being shown."[75] He described circumcision as "the abstraction of a structure, not indeed of paramount importance to the organism, but obviously evolved by Nature for wise ends as a protective covering. Were there no necessity for its presence it would not occur; and without overwhelming evidence that such mutilation is unavoidable and beneficial, it must be held ethically criminal thus to lay rough hands upon a perfectly normal organ" (42–43). Snow then argued that the four advantages claimed by the proponents of circumcision did not stand up to scrutiny. He dismissed "enhanced local cleanliness" as trivial and irrelevant in modern conditions, commenting that no one advocated similar tactics like shaving the head or pulling out the toenails. On the argument for greater chastity and "preclusion of immoral personal habits," he agreed about the importance of chastity but considered the evidence to be inconclusive; he countered that plenty of Jews and other circumcised men were known to masturbate, and cited Eugen Levit's desperate and improbable claim that early removal of the prepuce encouraged infantile fondling. On the argument for protection from venereal disease, he found the case "not proven," and he pointed out that even Hutchinson's statistics showed that (circumcised) Jews were more prone to gonorrhea. On the claim for protection against cancer of the penis, Snow replied that this was a rare disease of adults, more likely caused by phimosis and poor hygiene than the foreskin per se (29–35).

Turning to the offensive, Snow then listed the "disadvantages and dangers of circumcision" and devoted several pages (35–42) to a discussion of what are now called "risks and complications"—the most common injuries inflicted during the procedure and some of the longer-term side effects. He commented that the traditional practice of *metsitsah* had been largely discontinued among modern Jewish communities because of its role in transmitting syphilis and tuberculosis. He also warned that infection, hemorrhage, ulceration, and damage to glans, meatus, and shaft were regular occurrences when circumcision was performed in surgical settings, but his case lacked force because he could not produce figures: no one was recording instances even of immediate injury and death, let alone the longer-term problems (such as excessive tissue loss) that might not become apparent until puberty brought the penis to its full size. If official statistics in the 1940s showed sixteen deaths each year from surgical complications,[76] it seems likely that the number of fatalities before antibiotics must have been considerably higher. Snow was rare among medical commentators in showing some regard for the boy being operated on as a subject with his own feelings and opinions, rather than a mere object at the mercy of guardians and doctors: "An American operator . . . speaks of the difficulty of keeping children's knees out of the way after removal of the prepuce, and of the consequent torture to them. Even after healing, contact with flannel napkins and other clothing must long be very painful. There can be little doubt what would be the verdict—could they only give it utterance—upon the immediate results of the operation in question, returned by these inarticulate (if far from mute) victims of hygienic orthodoxy" (42). If Snow was unusual in showing scruples about consent, he was even more radical in admitting that "an objection to circumcision of wholly sentimental character [is] not the less worthy of practical consideration" (42n). Why shouldn't boys be emotional about their penis?

The Barbarity of Circumcision was reviewed cautiously by the *British Medical Journal*, which had reservations about Snow's sweeping rejection of circumcision,[77] and sympathetically by the *Lancet*, which was "inclined to endorse most of what he says." It agreed that circumcision was a relic of primitive man, pointing out that the peoples who still practiced it were "many of the least civilized peoples on the face of the globe." More significantly, it accepted Snow's argument that an operation was rarely necessary "for the relief of congenital phimosis," and it actually proposed that "the prepuce is not the valueless or mischievous appendage that some would have us believe"; although "non-separation of the prepuce from the glans penis is constantly mistaken for phimosis," only genuine cases of the latter required operative treatment. The reviewer did not go so far as to suggest that an adherent prepuce needed no treatment at all, but he supported Snow's view that "forcible retraction" and its "daily repetition for a short time" were all that was required.[78] It is thus clear that Snow was not an isolated voice but equally apparent that the misconceptions about genital anatomy and preputial development that had originally led to the craze for widespread circumcision were very deeply ingrained.

The effectiveness of Snow's intervention was limited by two serious weaknesses. First, he accepted the current medical wisdom that the adherent and nonretractable foreskin was indeed a pathological defect that required speedy correction. Where he differed from most of his colleagues was in his insistence that this could be achieved by manipulation and dressing rather than amputation. It was, however, hard to defend the foreskin by thus conceding the major complaint of its enemies, for it was this very "phimosis" that formed the basis of their charge that it led to childhood masturbation, nervous diseases, and increased susceptibility to syphilis and cancer. Snow argued that all these risks could be managed conservatively, but his methods were a lot of bother, and it is little wonder that many doctors and parents preferred the quick snip. Second, for all the depth of his conviction that possession of one's foreskin was advantageous, Snow was hard-pressed to articulate what those advantages were. The best he could do was cite Dr. Willard (from Keating's *Cyclopaedia of Diseases of Children*) that its functions were "to protect the head of the organ during the years when the penis is but a portion of the urinary apparatus; and later, by its friction over the sensitive corona, to enhance the ejaculatory orgasm." He actually rejected Willard's largely correct echo of *Aristotle's Master-Piece*, that foreskin and glans worked in tandem to generate sexual sensation (though even he emphasized the final orgasm at the expense of the pleasures of getting there). Snow replied with the ignorant majority that "since the prepuce is completely retracted during coition . . . no friction over the corona can well take place."[79] But even if this were true (and there is obviously much variation from one individual to another), the foreskin would still increase sensation by the mere fact that its nerve-rich surfaces were now redeployed along the shaft of the erect penis. All Snow was left with was the rather lame protestation that the foreskin was necessary to protect the glans—a plea that fell easy prey to the sallies of Clifford and Remondino, who simply countered that the protection needed by naked savages leaping over thorn-bushes was no longer essential for civilized men wearing underpants. Without appreciation of the complex innervation and physiological role of the foreskin, and thus awareness that it had significant value in its own right, it was difficult to argue effectively against its dismissal as a redundant scrap of skin. In Britain, however, it was not new appreciation of the role of the adult foreskin that led to the demise of circumcision but concern at the high incidence of injuries, complications, and death; the decline of medical anxiety about infantile sexuality and masturbation, as part of a more general dissolution of the sex-negative culture of the late Victorian age; and the realization that phimosis in male infants and boys was not pathological after all.

By the 1930s what little consensus there might have been on the necessity for circumcision was evaporating. Even in 1920 the *British Medical Journal* recorded a medical society's discussion of the subject under the heading "For and Against Circumcision," and reported one participant as never having been convinced that "the craze" was justified: "According to the law of evolution the foreskin must have been greatly needed by the human race or it would not have persisted. . . . He knew of three fatal cases, one from chloroform. There was often alarming haemorrhage."[80] A protracted debate in the correspondence columns of the *British Medical Journal* in late 1935 showed doctors pretty evenly divided on the merits of circumcision, and that even those who still believed in the malevolence of phimosis were more ready to treat it by dilation than by amputation. The controversy was kicked off by a letter from a doctor concerned at the high rate of complications and death from circumcision, proposing instead his own complicated method of separating foreskin from glans "within the first week," without the need for cutting.[81] This provoked a flood of correspondence, some offering more patent methods for dealing with infantile phimosis; some pointing out that such half-measures often caused recurrent adhesions that required repeated operations and frequently circumcision later; some warning that the manipulations involved in the various stretching regimes might be found pleasurable and thus lead to masturbation; others rehearsing the familiar gamut of ills from which circumcision was supposed to provide protection—masturbation, syphilis, and cancer; and a few striking a quite new note—that it was arrogant and misguided for doctors to interfere so radically with the bodies of children. R. Ainsworth wrote: "The cool assumption of some surgeons that they know better than providence how little boys should be made is laughable and irritating. It is quite time that this horrible mutilation should no longer be regarded as having any sanitary or therapeutic value, and phimosis should be relegated to the list of imaginary diseases. Circumcision is and always was a tribal rite and has no place in surgery."[82] A. H. Williams recalled that it was in "the naughty nineties" that the idea of "promiscuous circumcision began to gain ground." He fell in with the fashion, but was annoyed to see "the healthy progress of the infant . . . interrupted; and still more . . . the lactation of the mother interfered with by worrying over the child."[83] In a revolutionary leap, J. L. Faull dared to suggest that masturbation was harmless and doctors had no business to be concerned with moral issues anyway: "Are doctors to be governed by purely medical reasons or not? Such arguments as those put forward that it lessens the likelihood of masturbation and the sensitivity of the glans penis, that it increases the erotic pleasure of the partner in copulation etc, are scarcely in the realm of medicine, but of morality. Masturbation is a normal and harmless manifestation . . . and it savours of Jovian omniscience to interfere with the naturally provided erotic mechanism." Faull further suggested than the very concept of preemptive amputation was unsound: "Circumcision . . . except when done in the presence of a definite physical lesion . . . is a propitiatory gesture, incapable of justification on surgical grounds."[84] A doctor had finally arrived at the position on male genital surgery that the profession had reached with respect to operations on women back in the 1860s. Ainsworth was equally provocative in suggesting that those who thought circumcision provided protection against venereal disease really meant that circumcised penises were less trouble to treat, and further that there was no need to retract an infant's foreskin: "If I innocently ask why it is so necessary that a baby's prepuce should be retracted at the earliest possible moment I know I shall be met with a sniff and a snort, and be shrivelled up by the magic word 'cleanliness.'" He left a couple of daring questions for those who had time to think: "When does a natural secretion become dirt; and what dreadful thing will happen if a baby's prepuce is left entirely alone?"[85] Had the British Medical Journal not closed the discussion at this point the chorus of doubt might have swelled all the louder. The mood was tending toward the point where an empirical investigation of preputial development was conceivable and feasible, and where a paper debunking infantile phimosis as a myth, and thus rejecting circumcision as a routine procedure, could be accepted with little opposition as the new consensus.

The essential precondition for this transition was the disappearance of medical concern with masturbation. Because it had been the dominant theme in medical discourse on male sexuality for two centuries, the harm of masturbation was an idea that took a long time to die; what is significant about the discourse of masturbation in the twentieth century is the growing divergence between expert medical and popular moralistic opinion. Even after it was realized, at least in advanced circles, that neither organic disease nor madness could be induced by masturbation, uneasiness lingered among educators and the public, though after 1920 it became rare to find reputable authorities seriously claiming that the practice was physically damaging. The impact of nineteenth-century propaganda continued to be felt, however, in the sort of advice manuals that acknowledged that although masturbation "does not permanently injure physical vigour, sexual power or mental capacity," it was still a "bad habit" with "mischievous" psychological effects, and could even prevent a man from attaining "full efficiency and full nervous vigour."[86] This advice from a clergyman was echoed by a urologist who wrote in 1930 that masturbation in the mature male was dangerous only because of "the mental conflict it engenders and the excess that it encourages," though he added that "if practised to excess" by the young, physical health and growth might suffer. Masturbation was "an unpleasant and unsatisfactory practice" that should not be employed as "a source of pleasure."[87] The ghosts of Acton and Paget had not yet been laid to rest, but the 1930s were the decisive decade, as the work of Havelock Ellis, Norman Haire, and other writers of sex manuals exerted influence. Ellis was far from asserting that masturbation was harmless, but his calm and judicious tone did much to allay professional anxieties; his mere invention of the term *auto-erotism*, as Haire remarked, took a lot of heat out of the debate.[88] Although he believed that psychological harm (such as neurasthenia) could arise, Ellis dismissed "the extravagant views . . . concerning the awful results" common in the nineteenth century as the result of "ignorance and false tradition."[89] Norman Haire probably achieved more with his widely read *Encyclopaedia of Sexual Knowledge* (1934), in which he devoted a whole chapter to the sexuality of children and two chapters to masturbation. He went a good deal further than Ellis, reporting that most infants and children masturbated and assuring readers that the practice was "inoffensive and no more dangerous than thumb-sucking," with "no consequences, either physical or psychological." Haire quoted statistics showing that the vast majority of mature males also masturbated without ill effects and concluded that if most people did it, it must be normal. He strongly condemned those who continued to drum up anxiety, such as headmasters and scout leaders, and added that the practice could have no harmful physical effects and that psychological damage could arise only from feelings of guilt.[90] By the 1940s anxiety had receded to the point at which one sex educator could follow his lead in writing that the only harm in masturbation derived from "the mental conflict which may arise from its condemnation."[91] In 1949 the more progressive Eustace Chesser affirmed that masturbation "has no ill-effects, physical or mental" and criticized those who bruised the minds of children by making them feel guilty about the activity.[92] The newly relaxed attitude toward masturbation filtered down into child-care advice. Where the 1928 edition of the *Mothercraft Manual* had warned that "untiring zeal on the part of the mother or the nurse" was the only cure and that it might be "necessary to put the legs in splints," the 1954 edition stated that "parents need no longer look on it as a vice."[93]

It is hard to explain this sudden change of attitude. Doctors and parents had always known that children masturbated, so it cannot have been merely the discovery that the practice was usual; the difference is that it was no longer regarded as harmful. How did this turnaround come about? The answer is not clear, but two vital factors were the appreciation of the real causes of the diseases once attributed to masturbation (especially microorganisms) and the emergence of more positive attitudes toward sexual expression generally—the beginning of the end for Szreter's culture of abstinence. In her study of changing attitudes toward contraception and sexuality, Hera Cook has shown that the perception of sex "as a negative force that had to be restricted and controlled" began to change after the First World War, and that the 1930s were the decisive years for the breakdown of the old antisensualism and the rise of a new paradigm in which sex was constructed positively as a source of mutual pleasure and the genitals as potentially beautiful body parts. Pointing out that no one could learn much about their capacity for sexual pleasure if they were not allowed to explore and fondle their private parts, she writes that "the redefinition of masturbation which took place during the inter-war decades had more impact than any direct challenge to gender relations on sexual practice."[94] There is much evidence to support Cook's scenario, including the surveys on sexual attitudes carried out by Mass Observation in the late 1930s and war years. The study found that "sex for its own sake" was traditionally regarded as "undesirable, perhaps distasteful" and that "this distrust of sex . . . seems to lie behind much of the opposition to birth control and sex education, certainly to prostitution and extra-marital relations." But attitudes were changing: sex education was becoming respectable, and there was wide agreement that "standards" were either declining (44 percent) or much the same (29 percent), meaning that most people thought that sexual rules and behavior were becoming less strict.[95] As a fifty-one-year-old schoolmaster commented, "everything is more open and above board, folk talk sex today. Fifty years ago it was taboo. . . . [Now] boys and girls have more freedom, war always leaves its mark."[96] In his widely read *Psychology of Sex* (1940), Kenneth Walker explained the new freedom as both an effect and a cause of the emerging respectability of contraception: "Whilst methods of limiting childbirth are not entirely new, it is only within the last thirty years that contraceptives have been made reliable and brought within the reach of the masses. This . . . has allowed of the sexual relationship being treated quite differently from how it was treated two or three generations ago."[97] By decoupling sex and reproduction, safe contraception made recreational sex both feasible and morally acceptable. It was in this increasingly liberal atmosphere that Douglas Gairdner revisited the problem of congenital phimosis and concluded that it was a medical myth.

Until the 1940s there had been no scientific study of the anatomy of the foreskin, and when Gairdner turned his attention to the subject he discovered that it developed as a unitary structure with the glans and only separated from it gradually, nearly always after birth. Such separation was a slow and variable process, taking anywhere from a few months to five years to complete; the foreskin of newborn babies was retractable in only 4 percent of cases, and in only 20 percent at six months.[98] At two years of age about 20 percent and at three years 10 percent of boys still had nonretractable prepuces. Much the same observations had been recorded in startled dismay by Sayre, Bland-Sutton, and others, who had interpreted them as meaning that mass circumcision was imperative. What was revolutionary about Gairdner's work was his realization that nonretractability was nothing to worry about: it was natural, normal, and healthy; attempts at correction were harmful; the only care the infant foreskin required was to be left alone, like they always had been until the mid-nineteenth century. Gairdner did not explain how he was able to arrive at this insight, but the clue is provided by the conspicuous absence of masturbation from his later discussion of the reasons normally given for preventive circumcision. By the 1940s masturbation had ceased to be a medical problem, and up-to-date doctors were thus not worried if babies fondled or tugged at their foreskins in the manner that had so alarmed their predecessors, and thus no longer demanded that the foreskin be pulled back each day so that the "secretions" could be scrubbed off. With masturbation no longer seen as a disease or a habit demanding correction, the exorcism of phimosis followed. Gairdner appreciated that any boy's foreskin could be torn from his glans by force but recommended that this not be attempted because it involved tearing two "incompletely separate surfaces," thus causing bleeding and risking infection.

Gairdner made many other significant points in this epoch-making paper, which proved as influential in eliminating circumcision as Hutchinson's observations on syphilis had been in promoting it. He pointed out that circumcision of infants was practiced only in English-speaking countries; that the foreskin performed valuable functions; that injuries and complications were common; and that there was "a surprising variety of reasons why different doctors advise circumcision": some did it "to cure existing pathological conditions . . . [others] to prevent various diseases at a much later date." The most common indication in the first category was "phimosis," but he could now conclude that such a diagnosis in infants was an error arising from ignorance of genital anatomy:

> The commonly performed manipulation known as "stretching the foreskin" by forcibly opening sinus forceps inserted in the preputial orifice cannot be justified on anatomical grounds, besides being painful and traumatising. In spite of the fact that the preputial orifice often appears minute—the so called pin-hole meatus—its effective lumen . . . is almost invariably found to be adequate. . . . Through ignorance of the anatomy of the prepuce . . . mothers and nurses are often instructed to draw the child's foreskin back regularly, on the supposition that stretching . . . is required. I have on three occasions seen young boys with a paraphimosis caused by mothers or nurses who have obediently carried out such instructions.[99]

True or pathological phimosis was a rare condition that could not be diagnosed until the boy was well on his way to maturity. Gairdner further considered the diseases supposedly prevented by circumcision, concluding that there was no proof of protection against venereal disease; that the evidence relating to cervical cancer in women was inconclusive; and that cancer of the penis was a rare condition that could just as easily be prevented by normal hygiene. He made no mention at all of chastity or masturbation. His conclusion marked the end of routine circumcision in Britain: "a conservative attitude to the foreskin is proposed, and a routine for its hygiene is suggested. If adopted this would eliminate the vast majority of the tens of thousands of circumcision operations performed annually in this country, along with their yearly toll of some 16 child deaths."[100] The editorial in the *British Medical Journal*, which accompanied the paper, endorsed Gairdner's view that there was "little medical justification for routine circumcision of the infant" and pointed out that "many doctors" had long been opposed to

> the wholesale and somewhat primitive lopping of the infant foreskins which goes on in some out-patient departments and surgeries. On these occasions the technique of the operation is often deplorable; sacrifice of skin is often too generous, and attendant damage to the glans penis or fraenum is not unknown. . . . it is not easy to find a rational argument for circumcision in most cases, and the operation is more often performed because it is *de rigueur* in certain districts or a habit in some families.[101]

Most remarkably, the *British Medical Journal* overturned a century of contempt by asserting the utility of the foreskin itself: "Of the value of the prepuce in the first two or three years of life there is no doubt, for it has an important function in covering and protecting the glans penis"— though it was to be another forty years before it came be appreciated that the anatomists before the nineteenth century had been right to think that the foreskin did more than that.[102] The editorial sent out an unmistakable message to doctors that they should not encourage, and perhaps not even permit, "a practice which so savours of the barbaric," and it was not long before routine circumcision in Britain became a rare event.

14 · Conclusion

The End of the Culture of Abstinence

Dr. Douglas Gairdner's defence of the foreskin is . . . certainly one of the ablest critical reviews of the barbarous custom of circumcision written in our times. That no one will take the slightest notice of what he says is equally certain. . . . [It is strange] that doctors everywhere do not protest more vigorously . . . at the continuance of this surgico-religious insult to normal physiology—and that in spite of the fact that at least three generations of doctors have sat during their student days at the feet of biologists whose principal function was explain . . . the nature, the wonder and the universality of the relationship in the living world of structure to function.

  GEOFFREY PARKER, *British Medical Journal*, 1950

When the medical profession has realized that circumcision in the first three years of life is an unnecessary operation, the parents will soon be dissuaded from requesting it. . . . If those who teach paediatrics to medical students and those who lecture to midwives would remember to condemn the operation as a treatment for the non-retractable prepuce of the infant, routine circumcision would again be no more than a religious ritual and an anthropological curiosity.

  Editorial, "The Offending Foreskin," *British Medical Journal*, 1952

Routine circumcision in Britain ended with neither a bang nor a whimper, but gradually amid the grumbling of those who still believed in it and the sighs of relief from those who had ceased to regard it as valid medical treatment. Gairdner's intervention inspired a good deal of correspondence in subsequent issues of the *British Medical Journal*, whose evenhanded editors ensured that an equal number of pro and con letters were published. Those in disagreement, most of whom thought that all boys should be routinely circumcised, simply reasserted three of the traditional arguments—prevention of phimosis, syphilis, and cancer—and did not attempt to engage with his reasoned rejection of those grounds.[1] Defending the operation on this basis, C. A. Royde refused to accept the estimate of sixteen deaths annually, suggesting that they were a complication of anesthesia, which could easily be avoided by omitting the anesthetic. He was such a traditionalist that he cited Hutchinson and Wolbarst as his authorities, and such an enthusiast that he commended the opinion of an American urologist that "in addition to complete removal of the prepuce, the urethral meatus should be examined and if any obstruction is found, meatotomy should be performed," all within "a few days after birth."[2] This was indeed the pattern that developed in the United States, but the future of British practice was foreshadowed in the relieved and even joyous letters from correspondents who were grateful to Gairdner "for having aired this most controversial subject which, even among medical men, is hedged about with emotion and prejudice."[3] Gairdner's supporters tended to stress his confirmation of their conviction that there was no valid medical indication for circumcision, to report the frivolous reasons given by parents for wanting it done, and to substantiate his claims of frequent and serious complications. There was general agreement that the most common justification for childhood circumcision was phimosis, but that this was false diagnosis, as Gairdner had shown, arising from ignorance of normal penile anatomy and its development. Better understanding of the foreskin had shown circumcision to be more akin to a folk superstition than an instance of scientific medicine in action. Replying to both his supporters and critics, Gairdner reiterated his arguments on phimosis, venereal disease, and cancer, then replied with dry humor to one who had asserted that circumcision delayed a man's orgasm, thus making sexual intercourse more enjoyable for the woman: "Frenchmen, Swedes and South Americans, to name three different races who are said to take these matters quite seriously, seem to have felt no need to employ circumcision to further their ends." He concluded by hoping that Geoffrey Parker's "sorrowful comment" that his article would be ignored "may prove an overstatement."[4]

And so it turned out. Gairdner's research did not eliminate false misdiagnoses of phimosis because he underestimated the time needed for the foreskin to become retractable in many boys and left the impression that an adherent foreskin after three or four years required treatment. Where he concluded that 92 percent of boys should have a retractable prepuce by age five, more recent research has shown that about 50 percent will have reached this stage by age ten and 99 percent by puberty.[5] Nonetheless, it was a landmark paper: "The Fate of the Foreskin" was a major influence on the decline of routine circumcision in Britain and, after a generation's delay, in the old British dominions. Gairdner's moderate tone was followed in 1953 by a forthright attack on circumcision by a surgeon who described it as a "a stupid and unnecessary operation" that destroyed "a normal mechanism" and exposed "a delicate surface" to air and friction. He stressed not only the harm of circumcision and the high risk of complications, but the valuable purposes of the foreskin itself, and he even achieved a partial recovery of pre-nineteenth-century knowledge about its sexual role. In the uncircumcised, "the penis enters the vagina without any effort, or at any rate without friction, the prepuce unfolding as the penis advances, and each part of it remaining in contact with successive areas of the vaginal walls," thus leading to gentler and more satisfying sex for both parties.[6] We are not quite restored to the world of Aristotle and John Bulwer, but it is clear that the culture of abstinence is not what it was in the days of Jonathan Hutchinson: he could never have defended the foreskin on the ground that it made sexual intercourse more enjoyable; indeed, destruction of the sliding mechanism and exposure of the glans to friction and hardening were the very results he aimed at. This turnaround emphasizes that it was precisely the erotic significance of the foreskin that made it such a pariah during the high tide of Victorian antisensualism. The official seal was placed on this transformation in 1979, when an editorial in the *British Medical Journal*, "The Case against Circumcision," named "Gairdner's important paper" as a significant factor in the decline of the practice from 30 percent in the 1930s to 6 percent in the 1970s.[7] The editorial contrasted the British case with the situation in the United States, where the majority of boys were still routinely circumcised and where doctors defended the procedure with some vehemence. It offered no suggestions as to why the experience of the two leading Anglophone powers should have diverged so sharply after the 1940s, and an explanation is beyond the scope of this study,[8] but a clue may be found in the relatively low incidence of circumcision in Britain and its brief life span: even at the height of its popularity it was still a minority practice, and it lasted scarcely more than two generations. Where the practice reaches an incidence of 80 percent and endures for more than two generations, however, there will soon be few doctors and parents who have any familiarity with the normal penis, and thus know how to manage it, and most fathers, being circumcised themselves, will usually want their sons to be treated likewise. In Britain there were always doctors and relatives who had not lost touch with the way things used to be.

The rise and fall of circumcision in the British dominions (Australia, New Zealand, and Canada) has yet to be studied in detail, but the pattern broadly follows that of the mother country. Circumcision appeared later in the dominions, became far more widespread, and endured longer than in Britain, and in all cases Gairdner's article played a significant role in bringing the routine performance of the operation into doubt and eventually to an end. In Australia the rise of circumcision followed the British example, but the practice endured longer and affected a greater proportion of boys. Since most doctors had been educated in Britain or had received their medical training in Australia from British teachers, it is not surprising that they reproduced the orthodoxies of their colleagues and mentors. In the late nineteenth century circumcision was recommended principally as a cure for spermatorrhea in men and a preventive of masturbation and nervous complaints in the young, but around 1900 the need to treat "congenital phimosis" and provide protection against venereal disease became paramount. The incidence of circumcision rose sharply between 1910 and 1920 as the First World War intensified fears of syphilis, and by the 1920s most doctors and child-care manuals urged early circumcision as the act of a responsible parent. Greater social equality, a less rigid status system, and higher living standards are the social factors that probably explain why this advice was followed by parents across the social spectrum, not principally among the upper classes as in Britain.[9] Where the Australian experience differs most markedly from the British is in the long survival of routine circumcision—which reached its peak incidence at over 80 percent of boys in the 1950s—after Gairdner's debunking of "congenital phimosis." The reasons for this have not been studied, but it may be related to the increased influence of U.S. medical advice (particularly Benjamin Spock's *Baby and Child Care*) as a result of the Second World War, and the substantially higher incidence of the procedure at that point. This meant that there was a higher peak from which to descend, more mothers not knowing how to look after a foreskinned penis and more circumcised fathers not wanting their sons to be different. Although Gairdner's paper was approvingly discussed as early as 1953, it was not until the late 1960s that it really made an impact, and not until 1971 that the Australian Paediatric Association decided to recommend that "male infants should not, as a routine, be circumcised."[10] This policy was cautiously endorsed by the *Medical Journal of Australia*,[11] and the incidence of circumcision then fell steadily to its current low of about 12 percent. The trend was accelerated by a stronger statement issued by the Australian College of Paediatrics in 1983 and slowed down by a weaker and rather equivocal one that mysteriously appeared in 1996. It is likely that the detailed policy issued by the Royal Australasian College of Physicians in 2002, confirming the original stance that there is no justification for routine circumcision, will lead to the resumption of the declining trend.[12] The sequence observed, therefore, is that routine circumcision begins slowly as a doctor-driven innovation; becomes established in the medical repertoire and spreads rapidly; and then declines slowly as doctors cease to recommend it but parents, having absorbed the advice of the generation before and many fathers themselves having been circumcised, continue to ask for it. Even today surveys find that a high proportion of young mothers of British origin, especially those living in rural areas, continue to expect their sons to be circumcised and are resentful when doctors refuse to do it.[13] A significant factor in the decline of circumcision in the 1960s—before the pediatricians took a stand—was the arrival of large numbers of immigrants from noncircumcising European countries, most of whom settled in the cities; a recent study in Western Australia found a higher incidence of circumcision in country areas, with their greater proportion of older Anglo-Celtic stock, than in major urban centers, with their more multicultural and better-educated populations.[14]

The Australian experience, like that of the United States, suggests that routine circumcision has features in common with the discovery of the sorcerer's apprentice, who knew the spell for starting something but not how to stop it. This was surprisingly not the case in New Zealand, where circumcision rose suddenly to near universality and later fell to vanishing point even faster. The procedure was rare before the First World War and became common only in the 1920s, largely to correct supposed "congenital phimosis" when the stretching regime advocated by the influential Frederic Truby King had failed. For reasons not understood, the incidence of the practice rose dramatically during the Second World War (from about 30 to 90 percent), then fell back just as sharply in the 1960s, since which time the procedure has become very rare. McGrath and Young suggest that the expansion of the operation during the 1940s was related to stories about uncircumcised soldiers in the deserts of the Middle East having "problems" with sand under their foreskins (the sand myth), or the idea that venereal disease (always rampant in wartime) could be prevented by circumcision.[15] New Zealand doctors did not have their own organization separate from the British Medical Association until the 1960s, and so they read Gairdner's paper and many subsequent articles critical of circumcision in the *British Medical Journal*. Despite this, circumcision seems to have remained common because parents, remembering the medical advice of the generation before, usually asked for it, and doctors did not yet feel it was their place to refuse. It is not clear why this attitude reversed itself in the 1960s, but quite suddenly doctors took the lead in discouraging the practice, particularly at the new National Women's Hospital in Auckland (established 1962), where the pos-

sibility of circumcision was never mentioned and the operation was effectively banned. New Zealand's small and (until recent times) homogenous
population, and the extreme conformism of its society, may help explain
both the sudden rise of circumcision and its even more rapid disappearance. New Zealand today has one of the lowest rates of circumcision in
the world (less than 2 percent), thus making it, as one wit was heard to
observe, the ideal place for filming a moral epic like *The Lord of the (Preputial) Rings*.

The case of Canada illustrates the importance of cultural and linguis-
tic factors in the spread and decline of circumcision. Although historical
information is hard to find, it appears that the incidence of circumcision
never reached the levels attained in Australia or New Zealand and that
there have been wide variations in the extent of the practice in the different Canadian provinces.[16] Circumcision was always unusual in French-
speaking Quebec, and in 1973 a survey found its incidence to range from
60 percent in Prince Edward Island to only 3 percent in Newfoundland.[17]
It was probably regional disparities like these that prompted the Canadian Paediatric Society to comment in an important statement issued in
1975 that "local customs" were the main influence on the circumcision
decision, and that where the operation was common it was usually done
as a sign of social status or as a consequence of the policy of a large maternity hospital. The CPS followed Australian and U.S. pediatricians in
stating that there was no medical indication for circumcision in the neonatal period, and although it did not cite references, "congenital phimosis" was the first issue it addressed and the one examined in the greatest detail. This emphasis suggests that, as in Britain, misunderstanding of
normal penile anatomy and consequent false diagnoses of phimosis had
been the principal justification for circumcision in the period during
which it had been common, and further implies that Gairdner's article
was exercising delayed influence. This statement was far more detailed
than the Australian documents of 1971 and 1983, and the Canadians
went considerably further in their critique of circumcision, which they
condemned as a "mutilative" and "obsolete" operation that pediatricians
should vigorously discourage.[18] The national incidence of circumcision
had been declining slowly since about 1971, and the result of this policy
was to accelerate the trend—from about 60 percent in the early 1970s to
less than 20 percent in the late 1990s.[19] In 1996 the CPS issued a long
and densely referenced policy concerned largely with assessing the vast
literature on the benefits of circumcision that poured in from the United
States. Despite the bulk of the document, the CPS maintained its conclusion of twenty years before—that circumcision of newborns should
not be routinely performed.[20] According to Dennis Harrison, Canada re-

cruits about 25 percent of its doctors from overseas, particularly Britain, meaning that Canadian policy would be expected to follow the British trend with about a generation's delay. Very few Canadian doctors are trained in the United States, and in recent times more doctors have been recruited from South Africa and (noncircumcising) countries in western Europe, thus reinforcing the tendency for the medical profession to be indifferent or hostile to unnecessary surgeries of this type.[21]

It remains to consider the relation of circumcision to the rise of modern medicine and to summarize the reasons for its emergence. The origins of modern medicine—both in terms of understanding of disease and professional organization—are to be found in the period from the 1860s to the early twentieth century. The triumph of scientific medicine required equally significant advances in therapeutic techniques, and this meant the development of vaccines and antibiotics to deal with the pathogenic microorganism it had discovered, so in this sense its arrival was not complete until the deployment of penicillin in the 1940s.[22] In relation to the rise of routine circumcision, two vital questions must be considered. Was preventive circumcision of male infants and boys the product of the declining old style of "traditional" medicine, or of the rising new style of "scientific" medicine? And if, as I have argued, it was largely the child of the former, how did it survive and prosper following the triumph of the new approach? The short answer for Britain is that it did not: routine male circumcision died out in the 1940s, simultaneous with the consolidation of modern medicine and the development of antibiotics. The issue that still needs to be considered, however, is why it became entrenched just as the acceptance of a correct understanding of disease (microorganisms) drove out prescientific notions, such as the harm caused by masturbation, nervous imbalance, and irritation, which had previously been so important in establishing its legitimacy as a preventive or curative intervention.

Routine circumcision arose from the alignment of four medical errors in the context of a general emphasis on sanitary, preventive, and surgical approaches to disease control and health maximization arising from nerve force theory and the therapeutic stagnation that itself resulted from the final dissolution of Galenic/humoral medicine. The existence of a small but increasingly respected circumcised population (the Jewish community) made it possible for doctors to claim that there was quasi-experimental evidence for the protective value of the therapy they wanted to test. Other necessary elements of the social context were a patriarchal family structure, an authoritarian attitude toward children and no notion that they had rights, a poorly developed sense of medical ethics, and a heavy emphasis on self-control and restraint in sexual matters

(Szreter's "culture of abstinence"). Two of the medical errors involved the ascription of an incorrect etiology to real diseases, and two involved the invention of imaginary diseases.

The misunderstanding of the cause of real diseases concerned masturbation and venereal disease. As to the first of these, under the influence of humoral and then nerve force theory, it was held that many real organic, nervous, and mental diseases were caused by sexual excess, and especially by masturbation. As to VD, because the primary chancre in venereal infections (especially syphilis) was often found on the foreskin, doctors got the idea that excision of that tissue in advance would provide significant protection against syphilis and, by extension, other STDs. The imaginary diseases were spermatorrhea and congenital phimosis. Building on the work of Lallemand and his followers, many nineteenth-century doctors came to believe there was a real disease called spermatorrhea, identified as the involuntary discharge of semen, which could be alleviated or cured by surgical operations intended to reduce the sensitivity of the penis. Combined with the scare over masturbation, this belief created a climate favorable to the idea that preputial secretions, even in infants, had to be scrubbed away, and in the late 1840s the natural condition of the infant penis (adherent and nonretractable) was suddenly characterized as a pathological abnormality in need of urgent surgical correction. In the context of the prevailing conceptions of "filth disease," and following the discovery of germs, it was assumed that subpreputial moisture consisted of harmful or even poisonous secretions that putrefied and either gave rise to zymotic diseases directly or provided an ideal environment in which germs from outside could multiply. It was later expressed as the "cesspool" theory, though it retained traces of the miasmatic theory of disease in that the alleged "stench" of the foreskin proved the pathogenic nature of the matter trapped within it.[23] Muslims and Jews were increasingly cited as models of sanitary wisdom, and their ancient practice of circumcision as a religious rite was reinterpreted in hygienic terms. Circumcision was further justified by the analogy with vaccination, the preventive modification that had proved so successful in controlling smallpox.

If this analysis is correct, it may readily be seen that the rise of circumcision depended first on a serious regression in medical knowledge, including loss of understanding about the normal development of the penis and the pathologization of the normal male sexual function—the production and emission of sperm—as spermatorrhea. It is also apparent that routine circumcision owed something to both the old and the new medicine, particularly acquiring its undeserved status as a preventive health measure from the latter.[24] In a broader sense, the concept of circumcision as a medical therapy, along with the idea of masturbation as a disease agent, may be regarded as a product of the epidemiological confusion that marked the long dissolution, yet persistence, of both Galenic/humoral and nerve force theory, and of the consequent hope that surgery, both fantasy and otherwise, was the field in which new victories in the battle against disease would be won. The long careers of spermatorrhea, masturbatory illness, and circumcision itself show just how easy it is for modern medicine to retain irrational elements from its variegated past.

NOTES

CHAPTER 1. *Introduction*

1. Miller 2002, 501.
2. Darby 2001.
3. Gibbon 1888, 2:231, 156.
4. Burton 1964, 106.
5. Hyam 1990, 75.
6. Lewis 1949; Wallerstein 1980; Romberg 1985; Szasz 1996.
7. Hyam 1990, 74-79.
8. Moscucci 1996, 65.
9. Hodges 1997.
10. Wolbarst 1914, 96.
11. Hodges 1999.
12. Gollaher 2000, 100, 108.
13. Gairdner 1949.
14. Astonishing indifference 2003.
15. Porter 1991, 206-7.
16. Ibid., 208-9, 210.
17. For an example of a text embodying nearly all the tendencies I have tried to avoid, see Miller 1995.
18. Hall 1991, 1.
19. Bynum 1994, 212; Laqueur 1990, 176.
20. Hutchinson 1890a, 267-69; Gay 1984.
21. Shorter 1992, 92-94.
22. Scull and Favreau 1986, 32n49.
23. Circumscisus 1896.
24. Darby 2003a.
25. Laqueur 2003; Rosenman 2003.
26. Smith 1977, 189-90.
27. Knowlton 1877, 47.
28. Ibid., 52-54.
29. Hoppen 1998, 323.
30. Carlile 1828, 11.

31. Malthus 1803, 211-13.
32. Bush 1998, 44-45.
33. Carlile 1828, 38, 42.
34. Owen 1841, 46.
35. Drysdale 1855; Benn 1992.
36. Acton 1865, 133.
37. Acton 1969, 114; Mason 1994b, 217.
38. Parsons 1977, 56-57, 63.
39. Oppenheim 1991, 159.
40. Hall 1991, 3-4.
41. Dunsmuir and Gordon 1999.
42. Rosenman 2003, 399, 371.
43. Darby 2003b; Philo of Alexandria 1937, 7:105.
44. Maimonides 1963, pt. 3, chap. 49, 609.
45. John Scoffern, *The London Surgical Home and Modern Surgical Psychology,* as quoted in Dally 1991. Dally takes the book at face value and does not seem to appreciate that it is a satirical spoof. There is a copy in the British Library. John Scoffern (1814-1882) wrote several works on botany and chemistry.
46. Dally 1991, 157-58.
47. Penicillin, discovered by chance in 1928, was brought into effective clinical use and mass production around 1941.
48. Le Fanu 1999, 210-11.
49. Ibid., 3.
50. Szreter 1988; Wilson 1990.
51. Dally 1996, 1, 10-11.
52. Ibid., 111.
53. Worboys 2004.
54. Thompson 1968, 13.
55. Circumcision 2002, 50.

321

1. Trumbach 1998 is a good introduction.
2. Porter and Hall 1995, 53.
3. Ibid., chaps. 1 and 2; Porter 1987, 1994; Hitchcock 1997, 49-51.
4. Walter 1888, 30, 19.
5. Venette 1712, 4.
6. *Aristotle's complete masterpiece* 1749, 13.
7. Da Carpi 1959, 72-73.
8. Bulwer 1650, 212-14; Sharp 1671, 19-20, 31-32.
9. Hunter 1786, 221-22.
10. Venette 1712, 16; *Aristotle's complete masterpiece* 1749, 24.
11. Laqueur 1990.
12. Comfort 1967, 17; Hodges 2001; Schleiner 1995, 135-37.
13. Harvey 1964, 211.
14. Hodges 2001.
15. James 1743-45, vol. 3, s.v. "Phimosis."
16. Ibid., s.v. "Paraphimosis."
17. Hunter 1786, 221, 235.
18. Ibid., 222.
19. Porter 1994, 150.
20. Marten 1709, 68-69, as quoted and discussed in Porter 1994, 147.
21. Trumbach 1998, 62, 157, 202.
22. Hitchcock 1997, 38-40.
23. Ibid., 30-33.
24. Stone 1977, 553ff.
25. Ibid., 566ff.
26. Ibid., 57-58.
27. Rowlandson 1969, pl. 38.
28. Shoemaker 1998; Cook 2004.
29. Venette 1712, 6.
30. Ibid., 29, 470.
31. Harvey 1964, 185.
32. Cleland 1748, 63.
33. Hitchcock 1997, 22, 8.
34. Ibid., 29.
35. *Onania*, ca. 1716, 64.
36. Walter 1888, 27-28. Hereafter, page references are given in the text.
37. Gibson 2001.
38. Hodges 2001.
39. Quoted in Steinberg 1996, 53-54.
40. Proceedings of the Council of Florence, 1438-45.
41. Steinberg 1996, 54, 166-67, 71.
42. Gibbon 1903, chap. 52.
43. Vitkus 2001, 36; 2000, 5-6, 236-37.
44. Dalrymple 2002, 24.

45. Colley 2002, 288.
46. Bristow, as quoted in Lawrence 1929, 35.
47. Dalrymple 2002, 28; Colley 2002, 289.
48. Shapiro 1996, 25.
49. Bulwer 1650, 213-14.
50. Sharp 1671, 31-32.
51. Evelyn 1955, 2:293-94.
52. Shapiro 1996, chaps. 3 and 4, esp. 105 and 111.
53. Ibid., 121.
54. Quoted ibid., 209.
55. Ibid., 197.
56. Wolper 1982, 24.
57. Shapiro 1996, 214ff.
58. Ibid., 217.
59. Wolper 1982, 33.
60. Buchan 1772, xvii-xxi.
61. Conrad et al. 1995, 380.
62. Temkin 1973; Hitchcock 1997, 42-43; Conrad et al. 1995, 58, 141, 255ff.
63. Conrad et al. 1995, 415, 417, 423-24.
64. Ibid., 393-95; Pearn 2001, 12; Risse 1992.
65. Shorter 1992, 19.
66. Bynum 1994, 17.
67. Risse 1992, 165.
68. Shorter 1992, 21.
69. Stone 1977, 485-86; Conrad et al. 1995, 462.
70. James 1743-45, vol. 2, s.v. "Infans."
71. Conrad et al. 1995, 406.
72. Ibid., 424-25.
73. Ibid., 403, 443.
74. Lawrence 1992a, 5.
75. Hitchcock 1997, 47.
76. Conrad et al. 1995, 475.
77. Laqueur 1990, 143.
78. Hitchcock 1997, 44.
79. *Aristotle's book of problems* 1776, 62.
80. Stone 1977, 495.
81. James 1743-45, vol. 2, s.v. "Generatio."
82. Ibid., vol. 3, s.v. "Phimosis."
83. Ibid., vol. 2, s.v. "Circumcisio."
84. Weiss 1997; Morris 1999; Van Howe 1998.
85. It is a sad comment on the reluctance of the medical profession to study what they were so vigorously condemning that the content of subpreputial moisture was not

analyzed until the 1990s. It was then found to consist of water; shed skin cells; secretions from the prostate, seminal vesicle, and urethral glands; various sterols and fatty acids that protect skin surfaces in other contexts; and a variety of benign bacteria. See Cold and Taylor 1999, 39-40.

86. Hodges 2001.
87. Steinberg 1996, 62-64, 165-66, 167.
88. Cleland 1748, 63.
89. Hitchcock 1997, 2, 24-28.
90. Shoemaker 1998, 60.
91. Porter 1982b.
92. A charivari (or shivaree, according to *Webster's Eleventh Collegiate Dictionary*) is a ritual demonstration in which the community would single out and humiliate individuals who had violated local norms, particularly in the sexual arena. See Thompson 1991, 467-531.

CHAPTER 3. *Pathologizing Male Sexuality*

1. Biale 1992, 28-29.
2. Preuss 1911, 111; Biale 1992, 56-57.
3. Philo of Alexandria 1937, 105.
4. Preuss 1911, 489.
5. Szasz 1996, 141.
6. Spitz 1952, 493.
7. Stengers and van Neck 2001, 24.
8. Stevenson 2000, 227.
9. Crawford 1994, 88-89.
10. Stengers and van Neck 2001, 32.
11. Venette 1712, 475.
12. Stengers and van Neck 2001, 30, 26; Schleiner 1995, 129-32. Patrick Singy (2003, 347) quotes a seventeenth-century theologian as stating that masturbation was "neither allowed for health, nor for life, nor for any other end. Therefore physicians seriously sin when they advise this practice for the sake of health, and those who obey them are not immune to mortal sin."
13. Quoted in Stengers and van Neck 2001, 36, 197n86.
14. Stevenson 2000, 229.
15. Ryerson 1961, esp. 310.
16. Hitchcock 1997, 54.
17. Stengers and van Neck 2001, 194n68.
18. Stolberg 2000a, 48-49.
19. Ibid., 44-45; Hitchcock 1997, 54.
20. Its full title was *Onania: Or the Heinous Sin of Self Pollution and All Its Frightful Consequences in Both Sexes Considered, with Spiritual and Physical Advice to Those Who Have Already Injured Themselves by This Abominable Practice*. Hereafter, page references are given in the text.
21. Stolberg 2000a, 39-43.
22. Ibid., 49-50.
23. Quoted ibid., 50.
24. Marten 1708, 68-69.
25. Ibid., 392-93.
26. Ibid., 370-71, 373; Marten 1709, 12.
27. Marten 1708, 370.
28. Marten 1709, 20.
29. Stolberg 2000a; Donat 2001; Laqueur 2003, 32. Singy 2003, 2004. As we have seen, Marten's own work exhibits much the same combination of medical warning and moral exhortation as *Onania*, and they both sold quack remedies, so the matter remains unsettled.
30. Singy 2003, 346.
31. Gladstone 1968, 1:250, diary entry of 13 July 1829; Hall 1904, 1:432.
32. Stengers and van Neck 2001, 67.
33. Tissot 1974, vi. Hereafter, page references are given in the text.
34. Stone 1977, 495. Abu ibn Sina (980-1037) was a Persian physician who sought to systematize the teachings of Hippocrates, Galen, and Aristotle.
35. Stolberg 2000a, 57-58.
36. Porter and Hall 1995, 329n86.
37. *Onania*, 111-12.
38. Jordanova 1987, 71, 73.
39. Hitchcock 1997, 56.
40. Porter and Hall 1995, 89.
41. Porter 1982a, 17.
42. Porter and Hall 1995, 89.
43. Quoted in Comfort 1967, 81-82.
44. Porter and Hall 1995, 120.
45. Pankhurst 1913, 61.
46. Hunter 1786, 200.
47. Ibid., 200-201.
48. Hunter 1810, 293.
49. Stengers and van Neck 2001, 53-54.
50. Drysdale 1855, 91-92; Benn 1992, 38-39, 46.
51. *Encyclopaedia Britannica* 1797, 12:213-14, s.v. "Onanism."

52. Gay 1984, 309.

53. Stone 1977, 515.

54. Porter and Hall 1995, 118–19; Bouce 1980, 182–83.

55. Szasz 1971, 213.

56. Gilbert 1974.

57. Neuman 1975, 8–9.

58. Spitz 1952, 501.

59. Crawford 1994, 98.

60. Allen 1998, 445–47.

61. Biale 1992, 291n27.

62. This perspective is also argued persuasively in recent articles by Patrick Singy.

63. Wagner 1988, 16.

64. Wagner 1983, 179.

65. Stolberg 2000b, 6.

66. Lawson Tait, 1888, as quoted in Engelhardt 1974, 239.

67. Stolberg 2000b, 5–7, 10.

68. Ibid., 9.

69. The commission was established by Louis XVI and included Antoine Lavoisier and Benjamin Franklin. Their conclusion (that mesmerism was a fraud) in *Report of the Commissioners Charged by the King to Examine Animal Magnetism,* is described by Stephen Jay Gould (1992, 189) as "a key document in the history of human reason."

70. Stolberg 2000b, 56.

71. Except in the United States, where some doctors claimed to identify a specific form of adolescent insanity, caused by masturbation, which they called hebephrenia (Hare 1962, 8; Neuman 1978).

72. Szasz 1971, 210.

73. Ellis 1936, 249; Ellis blamed Voltaire because of an entry ascribed to his *Philosophical Dictionary.* Only Frederick Hodges (1997) has given Lallemand his due.

74. Webster 1995.

75. Lallemand 1858, 34. Hereafter, page references are given in the text.

76. See chap. 8 for further details.

77. The leading French medical dictionary from the period defines *marasme* as a drying up, withering, and emaciation of the body, often associated with decrepitude and senility. It was not a disease in itself but an effect of diseases such as dysentery or consumption. Lallemand's distance from the medical orthodoxy of his day may be judged from the comment that *marasme* had many causes, but "excessive losses of semen and other fluids" was not one of them unless prolonged beyond a critical point (*Dictionnaire des sciences medicales* 1812–22, 31:1–4). Lallemand ploughed an even lonelier furrow on the question of circumcision. The same dictionary (5:223–27) described "cette operation bizarre" as having few surgical justifications. It was a procedure known in ancient times but rarely practiced for medical reasons; its performance was nearly always based on religious or political motives, such as the idea that if a man sacrificed part of the organ that meant most to him, it would enhance his prospects in the life hereafter. The entry added that in infants and young boys, the foreskin was naturally long, tight, and difficult to draw back, and that this condition did not normally cause any problems.

78. Note that Lallemand does not regard the penis and foreskin as two separate organs: the penis is a single unit, consisting of an erectile portion and a nonerectile portion (the foreskin). The conceptual error by which the foreskin came to be classified as extraneous to the penis, and thus that its removal could be seen as the removal of something from the penis, not the removal of part of the penis itself, had not yet developed.

79. Gollaher 1994; 2000, chap. 4.

80. Morris 1999, 61–62.

CHAPTER 4 . *The Shadow of Parson Malthus*

1. Szreter 1996a, 397.

2. Peterson 1986, 569–70.

3. Szreter 1996a, 1996b; Cook 2004, esp. 106.

4. Smith 1977; Stearns and Stearns 1985.

5. Mason 1994b, 3.

6. Stone 1977, 545.

7. Weeks 1981, 23, 73.

8. Szreter 1996b; Baldwin 1999, 495; Cook 2004, 67.

9. Cook 2004, 183.

10. Porter and Hall 1995, 127–28.

11. Drysdale 1855; Benn 1992; Mason 1994b, 189–213.

12. Malthus 1803, 211–13, 23, 218.

13. Mason 1994a, 258–88.

14. Porter 1982a, 21; Porter and Hall 1995, 27–28.

15. Stone 1977, 673.

16. Mason 1994a, 20–26.

17. Weeks 1981, 27.

18. Laqueur 1990, 201.

19. Porter 2000, 158.

20. Hunt 1999, 86.

21. Gilman 1989, 2.

22. Hull 1973, 87ff.; Carpenter 1853, 942.

23. Haley 1978, 40–41.

24. Ibid., 41.

25. Cominos 1963, 23.

26. Carpenter 1853, 956.

27. Pratt 1872, 17.

28. Cominos 1963, 23.

29. *Times* 1857, as quoted in the introduction to Nield 1973; Acton 1860, 197; *British and Foreign Medico-Chirurgical Review* 1857, 117.

30. Hall 1904, vol. 1, chap. 6.

31. Szreter 1996a, 416.

32. Cook 2004, 95.

33. Hunt 1998, 589.

34. Oppenheim 1991, 159.

35. Tait 1889, 61.

36. Tosh 1991, 46.

37. Tosh 1999, 189.

38. Hyam 1990, 71.

39. Hunt 1999, 86.

40. Szreter 1996a, 1; Cook 15, 107.

41. Szreter 1996a, chap. 8.

42. Stone 1977, 645.

43. Cook 2004, 15.

44. Ibid., 103.

45. I am certainly not suggesting that circumcision was seen as a means of birth control. Quite the contrary, it was seen as a means of discouraging sexual activities other than intercourse and thus promoting fertility. The frequent claim that the foreskin hindered conception was another reason to cut it off. In a sense, the doctors were hoping that circumcision might undo some of the effects of the sexual restraint they regularly urged.

46. Beisel 1997. For a more extended discussion, see chap. 13.

47. Bristow 1977, 2, 3, 41, 44–47.

48. Hunt 1999, 78–79, 98–100.

49. Baldwin 1999, chaps. 1 and 5, esp. 483–509.

50. Mason 1994b, 212–13.

51. Baldwin 1999, 457, 466–68.

52. Davenport-Hines 1990, 197.

53. Smith 1976.

54. Orwell 1998, 12:539.

55. Mason 1994b, 211.

56. Hynes 1968, 281, 283, 285–86, 294, 215.

57. Quoted in Weeks 1981, 29.

58. Stone 1977, 667–69.

59. Tosh 1991, 54–55; 1999.

60. Stone 1977, 671; "The Innocence of Reginald," in Munro 1930, 40.

61. Neuman 1975, 1978.

62. Neuman 1978, 25; see the next chapter.

63. *Aristotle's complete masterpiece* 1749, 29; Venette 1712, 91–94.

64. Oppenheim 1991, 249, 259.

65. Ibid., 239, 259.

66. Aronson 1994.

67. Hall 1904, 1:441, 446.

68. Oppenheim 1991, 251.

69. Pratt 1872, 6, 10.

70. Jones 1999, 26–27.

71. Cook (2004, 101, 169–70) argues that sexual ignorance increased throughout the late Victorian and Edwardian periods because sexual knowledge was regarded as a danger from which children had to be protected, and that this ignorance was a significant factor in sexual inexpressiveness. See also Szreter 1996b, 143–44.

72. Oppenheim 1991, 261.

73. Sexual ignorance 1885. According to Bartrip (1990, 166–67), the proposal "sank like a lead balloon."

74. Lyttelton 1900, 10–11. Hereafter, page references are given in the text.

75. A doctor, ca. 1900.

76. Arthur ca. 1900a, 12.

77. Worsley 1967, 123.

78. Lewis 1991, 174, 178.

79. Tuke 1892, 998.

80. Weisse 1904, 706.

81. Symonds 1984, 62, 94.

82. Daley 1986, 22–23.

83. Lehmann 1985, 10, 14.

84. Ackerley 1968, 70–72; Driberg 1977, 7, 12–16.

85. Ellis 1936, 1:230 (pt. 3).

86. Gay 1984, 290.

87. Gebhard and Johnson 1979, table 102.

CHAPTER 5. *The Priests of the Body*

1. Haley 1978, 3.
2. Wohl 1983, 118.
3. Szreter 1988, 18-19.
4. Wohl 1983, 10, 21-23.
5. Ibid., 35.
6. That the implications about germs took a long time to be appreciated is demonstrated vividly by Michael Worboys (2004) in the case of gonorrhea.
7. Gaw 1999.
8. Lawrence and Dixey 1992; Granshaw 1992.
9. Pelling 1993, 310.
10. Worboys 2000, 36-37.
11. Nichols 1873, 95-96, 179.
12. Worboys 2000, 39.
13. Ibid., 37.
14. Bynum 1994, 72.
15. Chadwick 1965, 422-23.
16. Crellin 1968; Worboys 2000, 130.
17. Szreter 1988, 7, 13-15, 18.
18. Schwartz 1986, 129; Dally 1996, 111.
19. Szreter 1988, 26; Wilson 1990.
20. Wohl 1983, 124; Bynum 1994, 79-81.
21. Wohl 1983, 132.
22. Worboys 2000, 57; Bynum 1994, 154.
23. Remondino 1891, chap. 16. Given their resistance to compulsory vaccination (Durbach 2000), one can imagine how the working class would have reacted to any attempt to make circumcision mandatory.
24. Worboys 2000, 41.
25. Malthus 1803, 209.
26. Stevenson 1955, 14; Bynum 1994, 59.
27. Pelling 1993, 327.
28. Mort 1987, xvii.
29. Townsend 1999, 20.
30. Hunt 1998, 1999.
31. Chadwick 1965, 423-25.
32. For details see *Dictionary of Scientific Biography* 1971, 3:87-89.
33. Haley 1978, 37.
34. Acton (1862) was not alone in his concern. In his study of modern diseases, B. W. Richardson (1878, 190-92) also covered the harmful effects of rail travel on the nerves.
35. Carpenter 1853, chap. 18, and 941-92.
36. Handfield Jones 1867, 1.
37. Oppenheim 1991, 80.
38. Ibid., 87.
39. Ibid., 88-89.
40. Ibid., 85.
41. Shorter 1992, 25-39; Oppenheim 1991, 94.
42. Shorter 1992, 40.
43. Ibid., 45-46; Gollaher 2000, chap. 4.
44. Quain 1894, 634-35.
45. Shorter 1992, 221.
46. Oppenheim 1991, 92-100.
47. Shorter 1992, 220-32.
48. Beard 1884, 793-805, 888-89.
49. Quoted in Miller 2002, 527; and see Thomson 2001.
50. Parry and Parry 1976, chap. 6; and more generally Peterson 1978; Digby 1994.
51. Bynum 1992, 150.
52. Parry and Parry 1976, 125.
53. Peterson 1978, chap. 6.
54. Parry and Parry 1976, 131.
55. Townsend 1999, 167-68.
56. Davenport-Hines 1990, 159.
57. Shorter 1992, 34.
58. Acton 1865, 146.
59. Porter 1993, 180.
60. Parry and Parry 1976, 119; Peterson 1978, 34-37.
61. Oppenheim 1991, 163-64.
62. Rosenman (2003, 384) comments that "the boundary between quackery and legitimate medicine was . . . hazy" and that there were few differences between "legitimate and illegitimate" pamphlets on sexual problems such as masturbation and spermatorrhea.
63. Spencer 1895, 908.
64. Mason 1994b, 187-88.
65. Davenport-Hines 1990, 256.
66. Rosenman 2003, 376-81.
67. Provincial FRCP 1866, 478.
68. Lay criticism 1898, 1344-45.
69. Townsend 1999, 170-72.
70. Quoted ibid., 172-74.
71. Laqueur 1990, 215; Peterson 1978, 198, 291.
72. Acton 1865, 25.
73. Gilbert 1975, 221.
74. Continence versus syphilis 1889, 1042.
75. Scull and Favreau 1986, 13.
76. Shettle 1867, 98.
77. Aberrations 1867, 141-42, 146.

78. Sexual ignorance 1885.

79. Ellis 1936, 2:119 (pt. 1).

80. Marshall 1910, 262.

81. Porter and Hall 1995, 169, 209.

82. *British Medical Journal*, cited in Porter and Hall 1995, 162.

83. *Lancet* 1837, 20,

84. Youngson 1979, 17.

85. Acton 1851, 33; 1969, 92.

86. Quoted in Worboys 2004, 44.

87. Townsend 1999, 193.

88. Doyle 1934, 4-5.

89. Bynum 1994, 109-14; Worboys 2000, 14-15, 151; Gay 1984, 294.

90. Bynum 1994, 140.

91. Ibid., 226; see also Shryock 1948, chap. 13; Digby 1996, 97.

92. Lawrence 1985, 504.

93. Winter 1997.

94. Shortt 1983, 59.

95. Peterson 1978, 60, 41.

96. Gaw 1999, 115.

97. Oldroyd 1983, 197; Milton 1873, 6.

98. Browne 2002, 422.

99. Shortt 1983, 62.

100. Peterson 1978, 4.

101. Lawrence 1985, 504-5.

102. Shryock 1948, chap. 14; Keele 1968; Temkin 1973, 191.

103. Quoted in Keele 1968, 8.

104. Lane 1873, 11, 36-37, 1, 35, 22.

105. Le Fanu 1999, 207.

106. Szasz 1971, 220.

107. Dally 1996; Shorter 1994, 41-55.

108. Holt 1913; Darby 2003d.

109. Royde 1950, 182.

110. Gallop 1950, 123.

111. Morris 1897.

112. Keynes 1981, 111.

113. Shryock 1948, 275; Digby 1994, 95-97.

114. Digby 1994, 279, 286.

115. Cooter 1992, 11.

116. Hall 2001a, 284.

117. Newman 1932, 238.

118. Worboys 2000, 28-29.

119. Youngson 1979, 29.

120. Bynum 1994, 222.

121. Brieger 1992, 227-29.

122. Ibid., 219.

123. Lawrence 1992a, 25.

124. Freeland 1900, 1869.

CHAPTER 6 . *A Source of Serious Mischief*

1. Acton 1851, 77.

2. Galen 1968, 628-29; Laqueur 1990, 45.

3. Laqueur 1990, 94, 97-98, 133.

4. Ibid., 14-15.

5. Sharp 1671, 43.

6. Ibid., 42.

7. *Encyclopaedia Britannica*, 3rd ed., vol. 5, s.v. "Circumcision."

8. Carpenter 1853, 956, 501.

9. Cold and Taylor 1999; McGrath 2001.

10. Da Carpi 1959, 72-73.

11. Laqueur 1989, 129n80; Comfort 1967, 17; Schleiner 1995, 137.

12. *Geneanthropeiae* (1642), as quoted in Comfort 1967, 26. Similar comments were made by Jane Sharp, John Bulwer, and John Marten.

13. Acton 1865, 114-15; 1903, 180.

14. Carpenter 1853, 956.

15. Laqueur 1989, 97-98.

16. Ellis 1936, 2:129 (pt. 1).

17. Acton 1865, 153n1; 1903, 77. Hereafter, references to *Functions and Disorders* are given in the text. The third edition is cited (1865) unless otherwise noted.

18. Laqueur 1989, 92.

19. Marcus 1966, 2-3, Crozier 2000b; Lesley Hall, entry on Acton, in *New Dictionary of National Biography*. I am grateful to Hall for sending me an advance copy of her contribution.

20. The publication details for *Functions and Disorders* are as follows: 1st ed., 1857; 2nd ed., 1858; 3rd ed., 1862; 4th ed., 1865; 5th ed., 1871; 6th ed., 1875. See the checklist of Acton's publications in the appendix to Peter Fryer's edition of *Prostitution*. I have used the third edition (published in Philadelphia in 1865) and the sixth edition (reprinted in London in 1903) of *Functions and Disorders*.

21. As Miriam Benn (1992, 41) comments, Acton was "at pains to deny any arguments found in the *Elements* without mentioning the book by name."

22. Ivan Crozier (2000b, 12) implies that Acton meant moderate sexual activity when he used the term *continence*.

23. *Lancet* 1862, 518.

24. The General Confession as given in

the *Book of Common Prayer* reads: "We acknowledge and bewail our manifold sins and wickedness, Which we, from time to time, most grievously have committed, By thought, word, and deed, Against thy Divine majesty."

25. Acton 1851, 236.

26. Since Acton accepted that it was the circulation of the semen within the body that maintained masculine characteristics (193–94), this policy would appear to expose boys to the risk of eunuchism, but the thought does not seem to have occurred to him.

27. Acton 1851, 249.

28. Carpenter 1853, 956–57; quoted in Acton 1851, 237.

29. Carpenter 1853, 944n2.

30. Ibid., 943–44n2.

31. Tissot 1974, 46–52.

32. Carpenter 1846, 448–49.

33. Venette 1712, 162–70.

34. Acton 1851, 69–70.

35. The most likely place for Ricord to have expressed approval of circumcision was during his course Lectures on Venereal and Other Diseases Arising from Sexual Intercourse, delivered at the Hôpital du Midi in the summer of 1847. All twenty-eight lectures were published in the *Lancet* between July 1847 and June 1848. Nothing resembling Acton's quotation appears in any of them, and in lecture 5, on treatments for phimosis, he showed himself very reluctant to perform circumcisions even in cases of venereal infections on the penis and severe phimosis in adults, and he warned against excising "too much of the preputial substance" if it really had to be done. In cases of balano-posthitis (infections affecting both glans and prepuce) there were the options of circumcision or conservative therapies, and he preferred the latter: "The rule formerly was to operate at once; but the illustrious Cullerier very justly opposed this practice; for phimosis which is the accidental result of balano-posthitis generally disappears when the inflammation has been subdued; and under such circumstances it would be worse than useless to perform an operation" (Ricord 1847, 570). In lecture 28, a recapitulation, he described the appropriate treatment of "preputial complications" involving chancres and buboes: "Phi-

mosis: Inject between the glans and prepuce the aromatic wine with opium . . . and use emollient and sedative applications; if gangrene be imminent, operate. Paraphimosis: Keep the organ raised and surround it with cold compresses. Bland diet, refreshing drinks; endeavour to reduce or free the constriction by an incision, according to circumstances" (Ricord 1848, 682).

Ricord was no more favorably disposed toward circumcision in his *Treatise on Venereal Diseases* (1838). He made no mention of the operation in a section on prophylactic measures against syphilis (Ricord 1842, 216–19), and in his description of the procedure for treating severe phimosis in adult men he described circumcision as a mutilation: "Permanent phimosis, with too great a length of prepuce, or with indurations on the margin . . . requires circumcision if it be desired to cure one deformity by producing another" (ibid., 321). Ricord understood that syphilis was communicated by intercourse and that it entered the male through the skin of the penis, but he did not single out the largest section of that covering as being particularly vulnerable (ibid., 50). Far from regarding the foreskin as an encumbrance and its removal as a liberation, Ricord's reluctance to circumcise even in cases of serious organic disease (and only if gangrene was likely) suggests that he placed a high valuation on that complex tissue, saw its loss as a serious misfortune, and regarded the duty of physicians to do all they could to save it from harm.

36. Marcus 1966, 13.

37. The reviewer agreed with Acton that "irritation of the glans penis, from the non-removal of the smegma preputii, is one of the commonest of the exciting causes of the genital organs. . . . We believe that . . . the use of cold water, in which the penis is inserted while the foreskin is withdrawn, together with . . . a sponge . . . will prevent all excitement of the child's sexual feelings" (Acton on the reproductive organs 1862, 142). Note that the cleanliness is intended to prevent sexual arousal, not disease.

38. Acton 1851, 75.

39. Ibid., 77.

40. A similar view was expressed by the American William Hammond (1887, 272–

73), who also wrote that "circumcision, when performed in early life, generally lessens the voluptuous sensations of sexual intercourse."

41. Hunt 1998; Stall 1904, 81, 93–96; Lyttelton 1887, 9.

42. Quoted in Hall 1994, 351.

43. Smith 1977; Peterson 1986.

44. Porter and Hall 1995, 141–45.

45. Crozier 2000b.

46. Marcus 1966, 2, 28, 17, 18.

47. Hall 2001a.

48. Priestley, *Considerations for the use of young men* (1776), as quoted in Mason 1994a, 7.

49. Quoted ibid., 13.

50. Quoted ibid., 9.

51. Pankhurst 1913, 57.

52. Quoted ibid., 55.

53. West 1874, 713–14. West's textbook, *Lectures on the Diseases of Infancy and Child-*

hood, was based on lectures given in 1847 and first published as a book in 1848. It went through many editions, but the only one I have been able to examine is the sixth edition (1874). I do not know if this passage was included in the original lectures, and if not, when it was added.

54. Forster 1855, 491–92.

55. H. Hutchinson 1946.

56. J. Hutchinson 1855.

57. Curling 1856, 403.

58. Copland 1858, 3:442–445, s.v. "Pollution."

59. Circumcision in Tangiers 1851, 241.

60. Johnson 1860.

61. Fowler 1860, 382.

62. *Lancet* 1860, 436.

63. Acton 1865, 165–66; Epilepsy for thirty-two years 1859.

64. Heckford 1865.

65. Cases of epilepsy 1867.

CHAPTER 7. *A Compromising and Unpublishable Mutilation*

1. The Giovanni Sinibaldi text in the first epigraph was quoted by Thomas Littleton (1866, 537) in the original Latin. I am grateful to Chris Cudabec, a graduate student in classics at the University of North Carolina for the translation.

2. Carlile 1828, 20; Mason 1994b, 195–200.

3. Daniell 1847.

4. Shorter 1992, 82.

5. Dally 1991, 161.

6. Thomas 1816, 619, as quoted in Shorter 1992, 82. There were many editions of *Practice of Physic* between 1807 and 1853.

7. *British Medical Journal*, 2 June 1866, 593, as quoted in Shorter 1992, 81–82.

8. Gilman 1993, 65.

9. Other accounts of the affair are given in Fleming 1960; Dally 1991, chaps. 9, 10; Moscucci 1996; and Sheehan 1997. I analyze the incident from a different angle and seek to place it in the context of nerve force theory and the wider vogue for behavior-altering surgery in both males and females.

10. Operations on the internal organs are a different matter: the craze for ovariectomy and hysterectomy was only just beginning,

facilitated (and probably driven) by advances in aseptic surgery: see Moscucci 1991; Scull and Favreau 1986.

11. Burton 1964, 107.

12. Moscucci 1996.

13. *Lancet* 1873.

14. Brown-Sequard 1858.

15. Brown 1866a, v–vi.

16. Brown 1861, x, 233–34.

17. The volume had a long title: *On the Curability of Certain Forms of Insanity, Epilepsy, Catalepsy and Hysteria in Females.*

18. Brown 1866a, 7, 5–6, 8.

19. Ibid., 9.

20. *British Medical Journal* 1866b, 456.

21. Ibid., 438–40.

22. *Lancet* 1866c, 485–86.

23. Tanner 1866.

24. Littleton 1866.

25. *British Medical Journal* 1866a.

26. *Lancet* 1866b, 699.

27. Operation of excision 1866, 697.

28. Routh 1867, 28–29.

29. Shettle 1867, 98.

30. See, e.g., the letter from "A provincial FRCP" (1866, 478).

31. The 1864 edition of West 1879, quoted in Brown 1866c.

32. Brown 1866c.

33. West 1866.

34. Brown 1866b, 675-76.

35. *Lancet* 1866a, 689; see also Clitoridectomy 1866, 664; *Lancet* 1867, 29.

36. Greenhalgh 1866, 730.

37. Greenhalgh 1867, 42.

38. Brown was supported in this by a letter from some of his allies, which stated that Greenhalgh's written report of what he had said at the discussion of Dr. Tanner's paper "differed materially" from what he had actually said (*Lancet* 1866b, 710).

39. There were four major editorials in medical journals critical of Baker Brown. Three were published in the *Medical Times and Gazette:* "A Gloomy Rite" (1866); "The Obstetrical Society and Mr. Brown" (1867); and "Clitoridectomy and Medical Ethics" (1867). The fourth, published in *Lancet,* was "The Operation of Excision of the Clitoris" (1866).

40. Clitoridectomy 1866, 664.

41. Operation of excision 1866, 698.

42. William Heberden (1710-1801) was an English physician and author of many publications on disease. I have not been able to find the source of the *mulier frigida.*

43. A gloomy rite 1866, 642.

44. Coote 1866, 705.

45. Maudsley 1866, 617.

46. Ibid., 705.

47. *Lancet* 1866b, 52.

48. Greenhalgh 1867, 28, 42.

49. Bantock 1866, 663.

50. *British Medical Journal* 1867b, 401. Hereinafter, page references to this meeting report are given in the text. A report of the meeting was also published in *Medical Times and Gazette* 1867b.

51. Shettle 1867, 98; Bantock 1866, 663.

52. Obstetrical Society 1867, 356-59.

53. Laqueur 1990, 163, 188.

54. Mason 1994b, 196-97.

55. Tait 1889, 59-61.

56. Acton on the reproductive organs 1862, 145.

57. In "Of the Character of Women": "A very heathen in the carnal part / Yet still a sad, good Christian at her heart." Quoted in Moscucci 1991, 105-6.

58. Gay 1984, 85.

59. Mason 1994b, 198, 200-202.

60. Picktop 1866, 52; Greenhalgh 1866, 730, 729.

61. Moscucci 1991, 113-17; Crozier 2000b.

62. O'Hara and O'Hara 1999 argues that it has a significant adverse effect.

63. Rosenman 2003 suggests this is one reason why surgeons were keen to treat spermatorrhea with invasive procedures on the penis.

64. Clitoridectomy and medical ethics 1867, 392.

65. Ibid.

66. *British Medical Journal* 1866b, 77.

67. Clitoridectomy 1866, 665.

68. *British Medical Journal* 1867a, 61.

69. Brown 1866c.

70. Doctors simply did not know where desire came from. Lawson Tait (1889, 57) wrote: "the sexual appetite is not situated in the ovaries of women . . . [nor] in the testicles of men. Nor is it in the clitoris. It is chiefly mental, and the sexual organs are only contributory to its indulgence."

71. Hammond 1999.

72. Peterson 2001.

73. Clitoridectomy and medical ethics 1867, 391.

74. Hutchinson 1893, 380.

75. West 1879, 652-53.

76. Tait 1889, 63.

CHAPTER 8 . *One of the Most Grievous Diseases of Humanity*

1. Royal Australasian College of Physicians 2002.

2. Cold and Taylor 1999, 34.

3. *British Medical Journal* 1907, 117.

4. Bland-Sutton 1907, 1410.

5. In 1894 German researchers using the newly invented aesthesiometer discovered that the glans was quite insensitive, and their findings were confirmed by the English neurologist Henry Head in 1908. In his *Studies in Neurology* (1920) Head reported that the glans was about as sensitive as the heel of the foot. Other German researchers had established the rich and complex innervation of the prepuce in a study published in 1893, but there was no

further work on the subject until the 1930s. I am grateful to Ken McGrath, Auckland University of Technology, for these references.

6. Moses 1871, 370; *Medical Press* 1900, 304.

7. *British Medical Journal* 1907, 860.

8. New South Wales Supreme Court 1916.

9. Foster 1891, 4:1510-11.

10. Kellogg 1888, 79.

11. Bland-Sutton 1907, 1410.

12. Remondino 1891, 8-9. Hereinafter, page references are given in the text.

13. Where Remondino found his atrophied "climbing muscle" is not clear, but it was not from Charles Darwin. In *The Descent of Man* Darwin discusses vestigial or rudimentary organs, including several facial and cranial muscles, and the "ischio-pubic" muscle, thought by Prof. Vlacovich to have once aided the male "in the act of reproduction." But there is no mention of any climbing muscle (Darwin 2004, chaps. 1, 2, esp. 60).

14. *British Medical Journal* 1892, 391-92.

15. Wolbarst 1914, 95.

16. Peterson 1978, 244n.

17. Mason 1994b, 211, 214.

18. Porter and Hall 1995, 139-45.

19. Crozier 2000b, 16-20.

20. Rosenman 2003.

21. Mason 1994b, 211.

22. Courtenay 1882, 1.

23. Marten 1709, 385-86, 392-95.

24. See the first epigraph to chap. 3. Quoted in James 1743-45, vol. 2, s.v. "Gonorrhoea (1)"; also in Aretaeus 1856, 346-47.

25. Hunter 1786, 206-8.

26. Mason 1994b, 297-98.

27. Crozier 2000b, 7.

28. Wehrbein 1935, 492, 496; Rosebury 1971, 21; Oriel 1994, 104; Hirsch 1930, 419.

29. Acton 1851, 89n; Buchan 1796, 43-44.

30. Oriel 1994, 121-22; Childs 1842-43, 646.

31. Bynum 1987, 18, 11.

32. Wilson 1856, 643 (pt. 4).

33. Acton 1851, 88-91, 102-3, 255-56.

34. *Lancet* 1882, 513.

35. Phillips 1842-43, 451.

36. Phillips 1845, 17-19.

37. Phillips 1847, 177.

38. Phillips 1848, 489-93.

39. Thompson 1852, 89.

40. Wilson 1856, 216 (pt. 1). Rosenman (2003, 368) rather charitably suggests that the surgeons saw spermatorrhea as a two-stage disease. In the first the body was overactive in its production of sperm, with frequent nocturnal emissions, premature ejaculation, and emissions at stool or when horse riding. In the second exhaustion set in: the testicles shrank; semen (or something) dribbled with neither erection nor sensation, or escaped with the urine; and the patients complained of depression and languor. Assuming these observations were true, much of it could simply have been the usual transition from young and horny to old and losing it as a man aged—again emphasizing the extent to which spermatorrhea was little more than normal male sexuality.

41. Wilson, 1856, 215-16 (pt. 1).

42. Milton 1854, 245, 244 (pt. 1).

43. Milton 1852, 241-42.

44. Porter and Hall 1995, 144; Comfort 1967, 97, 103, 105 (illustration).

45. Spitz 1952, 503; Wallerstein 1980, 38.

46. Dawson 1852, 13, 26-27.

47. Drysdale 1855, 102-3.

48. Acton 1969, 11.

49. Acton 1851, 222-58, 224, 236.

50. Acton 1865, 206, 207-10.

51. Ibid., 212. Acton was not a lone voice: B. W. Richardson (1878, 402-3) listed clergyman's throat among his occupational diseases as a well-known syndrome, in 90 percent of cases caused by "exhaustion of nervous energy."

52. Acton on the reproductive organs 1862, 147.

53. Acton 1865, 219-29.

54. Drysdale 1855, 93-94; Benn 1992, chap. 6.

55. Symonds 1984, 64.

56. Symonds was case 17 in Havelock Ellis's *Sexual Inversion*, published in 1897 (Ellis 1936, vol. 1, pt. 4).

57. Symonds 1984, 154.

58. Ibid., 287.

59. Acton 1851, 233.

60. Courtenay 1882.

61. *Medical Press and Circular,* 1871, 541.

62. Chambers 1861, 637.

63. Quotations in this and the next few paragraphs are from Gascoyen 1872.

64. But not so strongly as would justify Jeanne Peterson (1986) calling him "Mr Acton's enemy." A careful reading of her principal source for this view, his lecture "Sexual Hypochondriasis" (Paget 1879, 268-91), reveals that he agreed with Acton on nine points and disagreed on seven. The most important of these was his outright denial, most unusual for his time and profession, that masturbation caused organic disease or insanity.

65. Paget 1879, 276-77.

66. Ibid., 279, 280.

67. Marr 1998, 171-76.

68. Worboys 2004.

69. Maguire 1885, 167-71.

70. Quain 1894, 787-88.

71. Ibid., v.

CHAPTER 9. *The Besetting Trial of Our Boys*

1. Pusey 1866, 4b, 12d.

2. Beale 1866, 681.

3. Meadows 1867, 16.

4. Pusey 1867, 126.

5. Hunt 1998, 593.

6. Aberrations of the sexual instinct 1867, 142.

7. Pratt 1872.

8. Sexual disorders 1870, 159-60.

9. Davidson 1889, 356.

10. Solomons 1920, 768.

11. Taylor 2000, 34.

12. Bristow 1977, 133-34.

13. Parkin 1898, 2:155, 160, 161.

14. Orwell 1998, 19:372.

15. Ellis 1936, 1:233 (pt. 3).

16. Hunt 1998, 585-86n38; Davenport-Hines 1995, 38.

17. Bristow 1977, 134.

18. Davenport-Hines 1990, 208.

19. Haley 1978, 164-67; Parker 1987, 80.

20. Almond 1893, 902-3.

21. Parker 1987, 61.

22. Lyttelton 1987, 5. Hereafter, page references are given in the text.

23. Tait 1889, 61.

24. Milton 1852, 242.

25. Hilton 1863, 123.

26. Porter and Hall 1995, 145-48; Comfort 1967, 104-5; Stengers and van Neck 2001, chap. 7; Spitz 1952; Hare 1962.

27. *British Medical Journal* 1889, 1315.

28. Gathorne-Hardy 1972, 270.

29. Clark and Clark 1899, 838.

30. Hamilton 1903, 206.

31. Acton 1865, 232.

32. Hutchinson 1890a, 268.

33. Hamowy 1977; Hodges 1997; Hall 1904, 1:428-30; Gilbert 1915, 608-10. Gilbert describes in great, almost pornographic, detail how he circumcised a pre-pubescent boy for persistent masturbation and then castrated him when that had been found to fail.

34. *Onania* ca. 1716, 80.

35. James 1743-45, vol. 2, s.v. "Infibulatio."

36. Yellowlees 1876.

37. Schultheiss, Mattelaer, and Hodges 2003, 761.

38. Hamowy 1977; Schultheiss, Mattelaer, and Hodges 2003.

39. Yellowlees 1892, 785.

40. Jordan 1997, 52.

41. Spratling 1895, 442-43.

42. *Medical Times and Gazette* 1867, 79. The surgeon was probably Jonathan Hutchinson: there were many Jews in his practice in East London in the 1850s, and the expression "long been inclined" recalls a similar phrase in his article on syphilis of 1855, in which the example of the Jews was again pressed into service as a reason for mass circumcision.

43. Soper 1867, 133.

44. Acton 1903, 7.

45. Cadell 1873, 750.

46. *British Medical Journal* 1874, 727, 759.

47. Jacobi 1876, 177.

48. Little 1883, 417

49. Hutchinson 1890b, 15; 1890c, 769.

50. Clifford 1893, 7.

51. Holt 1897, 696, 698.

52. Owen 1897, 281-82.

53. Stall ca. 1900, 279-80.

54. Hall 1904, 1:467.

55. Corner 1910, 225-27.

56. Cockshutt 1935, 764.

57. Hutchinson 1890a, 267.

58. Hutchinson 1893, 279.

59. Hutchinson 1900, 641.

60. A Jewish surgeon 1874, 856.

61. *Lancet* 1876, 509.

62. Biale 1992, 39, 90-95.

63. Snow 1890, 11.

64. Probably J. J. Virey, author of *Histoire naturelle du genre humain* (Paris, 1824).

65. Davenport 1875, 181. John Davenport (1789-1877) was a businessman and amateur scholar of erotic subjects. Publication of his book was financed by Henry Spencer Ashbee. See Gibson 2001, 24, 54.

66. Remondino 1891, 224.

67. Ibid., 201.

68. Beugnies 1902, 271-72.

69. Burton 1885, 10:233 (terminal essay).

70. See Immerman and Mackey 1997, 1998.

71. Dr. Peachey 1890, 116.

72. Dr. Beevor 1890, 1240.

73. *British Medical Journal* 1901, 938.

74. Consultant to the Children's Hospital 1901, 1023-24.

75. For details see Darby 2001, 187-88.

76. Hall 1992, 312; 1991, 134; additional letters kindly sent by Lesley Hall.

77. Kinsey, Pomeroy, and Martin 1948, 159.

78. Ibid., 176.

79. Friedrich et al. 2000

80. Ibid., 124, table 4.

81. Roth 1969, 18, 167.

82. Steinberg 1996, 257-58.

83. Immerman and Mackey 1997, 1998.

84. Yellowlees 1892, 784-85.

85. In a careful examination of Ellis's case studies, Ivan Crozier could find no evidence that a questionnaire had been used,

and he takes the view that the histories are generally reliable—that is, factual rather than fantasies. See Crozier 2000a, esp. 138n51. The sexual histories in Ellis 1936 appear as follows: vol. 1, pt. 2, "Analysis of the Sexual Impulse" (278-341), contains 19 cases histories; pt. 3, "Sexual Selection in Man" (223-59), contains 3 case histories; pt. 4, "Sexual Inversion" (92-194), contains 33 case histories; and vol. 2, pt. 1, "Erotic Symbolism" (231-73), contains 5 case histories.

86. Ellis 1936, 1:224 (pt. 3).

87. Ibid., 333 (pt. 2).

88. Ibid., 230 (pt. 3).

89. Ibid., 144-56 (pt. 4). The respondent does not state that he was circumcised, but he reports that his father was Jewish, so it seems highly likely that he was.

90. Ibid., 130-32 (pt. 4).

91. A modern authority on child development such as Ernest Borneman takes it for granted that most males masturbate from early infancy onward, but all his data are from modern Austria, Germany, and Switzerland, where circumcision is practically unknown (Borneman 1994).

92. Ellis 1936: 2:249 (pt. 1).

93. See the revealing French drawing of a male/female couple masturbating each other in Bayley 2001, 116. The facilitating role of the foreskin is very apparent.

94. O'Hara and O'Hara 1999.

95. Eagle 1986, 134.

96. Johnson 2001.

CHAPTER 10. *This Unyielding Tube of Flesh*

1. Rickwood 1999; Spilsbury et al. 2003a, 2003b.

2. Rickwood 1999.

3. Hodges 1999, 38-39.

4. Hodges 2001, 396-97.

5. Laqueur 1990, 129n80; Schleiner 1995, 137-40; W. Harvey 1964, 211.

6. Marten 1709, 13-22.

7. *Three treatises* 1985.

8. James 1743-45, vol. 3, s.v. "Paraphimosis."

9. Buchan is not saying he cut anything but is using the subjunctive: he would have needed to amputate three inches to permanently expose the glans.

10. Buchan 1796, 83.

11. Ibid., 85.

12. Ibid., 92.

13. Hodges 1999, 40.

14. Contraction of the prepuce 1846, 553.

15. Kempe 1878.

16. West 1874, 714.

17. Roberton 1999, 378-79.

18. Forster 1855, 491-92.

19. Dixon 1845. I am grateful to Dr. Leonard Glick for this reference; I have not been able to consult the book.

20. Morris 1999.

21. Gollaher 1994; 2000, chap. 4.

22. Wolbarst 1914; Ravich 1973. It is now known that penile and cervical cancer are both caused by papilloma (wart) viruses,

though it is not clear what activates them. Smoking seems to be one of the main risk factors.

23. Gollaher 2000, 73–79, including the quotations by Sayre and the unnamed doctor.

24. Remondino 1891, 255.

25. Jacobi 1876, 177.

26. Bryant 1863.

27. Erichsen 1877, 2:930, 931.

28. Joseph Francois Malgaigne (1806–65) was a French surgeon and authority on bones and fractures.

29. Kempe 1878.

30. Owen 1880, 514.

31. Fenwick 1890, 201. Sayre gave a paper on his miraculous cures to the International Medical Congress in 1887, and his book, *On the Deleterious Results of a Narrow Prepuce*, was briefly reviewed in the *Lancet* (1888).

32. Snow 1890, 22.

33. Davidson 1889, 351–52.

34. Jackson 1891.

35. Teale 1883, 720; Morris 1895, 2:1009–10.

36. *British Medical Journal* 1907, 303.

37. *Medical Annual* 1905, 259–60.

38. Langmead 1913, 222–23.

39. Parker 1879, 86–87.

40. Whitfield 1927, 187.

41. *British Medical Journal* 1927, 1043.

42. Owen 1897, 280.

43. *British Medical Journal* 1944, 876.

44. *British Medical Journal* 1894, 1044.

45. Hutchinson 1852, 415; Remondino 1891, 235, 211.

46. Parker 1879, 86–87; Jacobi 1876, 177.

47. Remondino 1891, 210, 218–21.

48. Snow 1890, 44.

49. Owen 1897, 280.

50. Mathews Duncan, as quoted in Bett 1956, 21. See also Moscucci 1991, 173; and the obituary for Bland-Sutton, in *Lancet* 1936. Bland-Sutton was a disciple of Lawson Tait, himself an advocate of ovariectomy, hysterectomy, and clitoridectomy for many diseases in women. Bett (1956, 24) comments that he had a reputation as a "surgical swashbuckler whose wholesale spaying of women discredited the profession."

51. Bland-Sutton 1907, 1410.

52. Ibid., 1411.

53. Corner 1910, 390

54. Ibid., 387–88, 390.

55. Ibid., 394–95.

56. Ibid., 395–96.

57. Ibid., 394.

58. Acton 1865, 161, 174.

59. Hutchinson 1900, 641.

60. Clifford 1893, 6–8.

61. King 1931, 123.

62. Benjamin 1944, 88.

63. Robinson 1915:390.

64. Ellis 1936, 1:332 (pt. 2).

65. Connolly 1935, 359.

66. Booysen 1935, 472; Ainsworth 1935, 472.

67. Gautier-Smith 1935, 642.

68. *British Medical Journal* 1935, 763.

69. Ainsworth 1935, 877.

70. *British Medical Journal* 1944, 585.

71. Sawday 1944, 876.

CHAPTER 11. *Prevention Is Better Than Cure*

1. Freeland 1900.

2. Cadell 1873, 752–73.

3. *Edinburgh Medical Journal* 1908, 3–5; Watson 1860.

4. Remondino 1891, 206.

5. Wolbarst 1914, 97.

6. Hardy 1993, 193; *Bleak House,* chap. 22.

7. *Bleak House,* chap. 46.

8. Hardy 1993, 218.

9. Hamlin 1985, 389.

10. Another preventative was bathing newborn babies' eyes with a solution of silver nitrate to kill gonorrhea (the cause of ophthalmia neonatum, usually leading to

blindness) in those born of infected mothers. The Royal Commission on the Blind, Deaf, and Mute (1889) recommended that such washing be made a routine, and this was endorsed by obstetricians. They were already adopting the procedure as part of a goal to reduce puerperal infection and their campaign to control childbirth by displacing midwives (Worboys 2004, 53). Such routine swabbing was an example of a precaution that was indeed valuable where gonococcal infection existed and usually harmless where it did not.

11. Crellin 1968; Richardson 1878, 88.

12. Hamlin 1985, 389, 405.
13. Crellin 1968, 66.
14. Malthus 1803, 209.
15. Hamlin 1985, 384-86.
16. Fergus 1879, 219.
17. Hamlin 1985, 383, 388.
18. Corfield 1870, 645-46.
19. Worboys 2000, 142.
20. Corfield 1870, 617.
21. Fergus 1879, 217. The idea of quarantining the sick was a contagionist rather than sanitarian approach, suggesting that the lineup of contagionists versus sanitarians was not hard and fast, and that zymotic theory could be used equally by both factions. See also Baldwin 1999, 7-8.
22. Worboys 2000, 57, 238.
23. Feldman 1994, 1-2; Lipman 1990, 11.
24. Hart remained there as editor except for a brief interruption in 1869-70, when the post was held by Jonathan Hutchinson. Hart himself did not care to draw attention to his background and always insisted on the primacy of scientific fact. See Bartrip 1990, 63-69.
25. Feldman 1994, 2-3.
26. Lipman 1990, 3, 38, 81.
27. Copland 1844-58, 3:445.
28. Corfield 1870, 617-18.
29. Gibbon 1876, 465; Sheppard 1876, 518.
30. Hart 1877.
31. See Glick 2001.
32. Kellogg 1888, 106-7. Kellogg added that circumcision of women was carried out by some cultures for the same reasons: "In some countries females are also circumcised by removal of the nymphae. The object is the same as that of circumcision in the male. The same evils result from inattention to local cleanliness, and the same measure of prevention, daily cleansing, is necessitated by a similar secretion."
33. Davidson 1889, 356.
34. Hardy 1993, 286.
35. Ibid., 287-88.
36. Wohl 1983, 331-32; Hyam 1990, 77.
37. Interdepartmental Committee on Physical Deterioration 1904, Q[uestion] 10356. Hereafter, references to this report are given in the text.
38. Wohl 1983, 27-32.
39. Maurice 1903, 56.
40. Hart 1877, 199.

41. Newman 1932, 44-45, 47-48. As Anna Russell said of the plot of *Der Ring des Nibelungen*, "I'm not making this up, you know."
42. Feldman 1994, 169-71; Szreter 1996a, 1, 470ff.
43. Remondino 1891, 201; Bland-Sutton 1907, 1409.
44. Curtis 1916, 101.
45. Hall 1904, 1:467.
46. Pratt 1872, 18.
47. Haire, Costler, and Wiley 1934, 32, 466.
48. Wear 1993, 1300-1303.
49. Benn 1992, 118.
50. Granshaw 1992, 17-18, 20, 45.
51. Lawrence and Dixey 1992, 180.
52. Ibid., 164.
53. Simon 1874; Worboys 2000, 130.
54. Worboys 2000, 79.
55. Ibid., 185.
56. Dally 1996, 70.
57. Ibid., chap. 3, esp. 67-68.
58. Schwartz 1986, 129.
59. Dally 1996, 111, 169, 73.
60. Shorter 1994, 42-45.
61. Hunter 1911, 83.
62. Daniel 1910, 121, 125.
63. Bolande 1969.
64. Glick 2001, 29.
65. Forster 1855, 492.
66. Foott 1903, 448.
67. Connolly 1935, 822.
68. Musalman 1903, 1028.
69. Wolbarst 1914, 93, 96.
70. Haire, *Birth control methods* (1936), as quoted in Cook 2004, 146.
71. Remondino 1891, 175-77, 177-78.
72. Richardson 1878, 23-24. Richardson also considered the various explanations for the supposed superior health of the "Jewish race." He made no reference to circumcision at all but explained their health in terms of "soberness of life": Jewish people drank less, ate better food, married earlier, and took better care of their children (19-25).
73. Remondino 1891, 195.
74. Ibid., 180, 195.
75. Brown 1897, 124-25.
76. Howe 1887, 94-95.
77. Ibid., 19, 147 (quotation), 147-52.
78. Hutchinson 1852, 415.
79. Hutchinson 1882, 5.
80. Remondino 1891, 227, 232-33.

81. Wallerstein 1980, chap. 10; Hodges 1997; Gollaher 2000, chap. 6.

82. Allen 1909. Quotations throughout the rest of the chapter are taken from this article.

83. Most South African tribes perform circumcision at around the age of eighteen, with such a high rate of injury and mortal- ity even today that, after the death of 25 initiates, and the admission of 92 to hospi- tal, 16 of whom required the amputation of what was left of their penis, the *South African Medical Journal* (vol. 93, August 2003) condemned the practice as "bar- baric" and called for action to "stop the carnage."

CHAPTER 12. *The Purity Movement and the Social Evil*

1. Beugnies 1902, 272.

2. Cadell 1873.

3. Beier 1992, 78.

4. Oriel 1994, 118.

5. Baldwin (1999, 451-52) notes that sev- eral observers entertained the possibility that circumcision provided some protection against syphilis and believed that Jews and Muslims were less affected than Christians and Hindus; one such observer was Fallop- pio, who was probably the first to suggest the condom as an even more effective pre- caution. But Baldwin points out that while these connections were speculative, there was no doubt that unhygienic surgical prac- tices, such as the Jewish *metsitsah* (the suck- ing of the wound following the cutting of the foreskin), certainly did spread disease and that several governments banned the practice. In Paris, Ricord was able to per- suade the Jewish community to abandon this phase of the rite.

6. Harvey 1672, 64; James 1743-45, vol. 3, s.v. "Phimosis."

7. Bynum comments that it would be re- garded "as a nuisance but not a stigma" (1987, 6). See also Trumbach 1998, chaps. 1 and 7.

8. Acton 1860, 197. Additional comments from 1850 and 1904, quoted in Davenport- Hines 1990, 162-63.

9. Drysdale 1855, 137, 135-36, 155-56.

10. Hutchinson 1855, 542-43.

11. See Darby 2003d.

12. Hutchinson 1855, 542-43.

13. *Oxford Companion to Medicine* 1:569, s.v. "Hutchinson." The signs were intersti- tial keratitis in the cornea of the eyes, nerve deafness, and notched teeth. See also 2:1428, s.v. "Venereology." Oriel 1994; Worboys 2000, 14-15, 151.

14. Hutchinson 1946, 222, 28-30.

15. Sykes 1995, 87; Townsend 1999, 179-82.

16. Hutchinson 1946, 30.

17. Hutchinson 1887, 545; Copland 1844-58, 3:442, 445, s.v. "Pollution."

18. Hutchinson 1946, 200.

19. Townsend 1999, 66.

20. A good survey is Hall 2001b and Roger Davidson's introduction to Davidson and Hall 2001.

21. Walkowitz 1980 49-50.

22. *British Medical Journal*, 26 April 1862, quoted in Townsend 1999, 162; Chapman 1869, 180.

23. Acton 1969, 32.

24. Walkowitz 1980, 42.

25. Acton 1860, 196-98. According to Baldwin (1999, 510-11) the incidence of VD among soldiers in 1860 was 369 per 1,000 in Britain, 70 per 1,000 in France, and 34 per 1,000 in Prussia. He explains this in social and behavioral terms as an effect of the differing conditions of military service, particularly the contrast between the British system of a volunteer army drawn from the lower classes, with long terms of service and leave and relatively high pay, and the Continental system of general conscription, short terms of service, less leave, and low pay—the upshot being more opportunity for the British to play around and get infected.

26. Acton 1969, 21.

27. Ibid., 22.

28. Laisser faire and its results 1870, 193.

29. Acton 1860.

30. E.g., see Peter Fryer's introduction to Acton 1969, 7.

31. Acton 1860.

32. Control of prostitution 1870, 631.

33. McHugh 1980, 39-41.

34. Bartrip 1990, 93-98.
35. Control of prostitution 1870, 630-32.
36. Acton 1851, 21.
37. Mort 1987, 89, 93.
38. Pankhurst 1913.
39. Townsend 1999, 113.
40. Pankhurst 1913, 50, 59.
41. Baldwin 1999, 485, 282.
42. Ibid., 486-87, 493.
43. Ibid., 502.
44. Hall 2001b, 123; see also Porter and Hall 1995, chap. 10, esp. 226; Gilman 1989, 238ff.
45. Dock 1910, 138-40; Hall 1992, 299, 302.
46. Townsend 1999, 255.
47. Dock 1910, 138, 139.
48. Henry 1898, chap. 8, 69-76.
49. Ibid., 70-71, 74.
50. Mort 1987, 119-26.
51. Hopkins 1902, 47.
52. Greg, in *Westminster Review,* as quoted in Walkowitz 1980, 43.
53. Worboys 2000, 124.
54. Acton 1860, 197.
55. Oriel 1994, 9.
56. Townsend 1999, 67-68.
57. Oriel 1994, 58.
58. Hutchinson 1876, 291, 535.
59. Granshaw 1992, 38.
60. Dock 1910, 32-34.
61. *Lancet* 1876b, 542-43.
62. Hutchinson 1895, 1:387.
63. For a contemporary perspective, see Donovan 2000.
64. Though washing after intercourse certainly helped if it was done promptly.
65. *Lancet* 1876a, 636.
66. Bristowe 1884, 263.
67. Townsend 1999, 111-12.
68. Baldwin 1999, 461-68.
69. Himes 1963, 186-206; Mason 1994a, 184.
70. McLaren 1991, 184.
71. Drysdale 1855, 155-56.
72. Szreter 1996a, 398-99, 435-36, 513, 559.
73. Bland 1994, 197.
74. Hutchinson 1890b, 15.
75. Hutchinson 1893, 379-80.
76. Hutchinson 1900, 641-42.
77. Circumcision and VD 1947, 31.

78. Snow 1890, 32.
79. Cadell 1873, 750-53.
80. *Edinburgh Medical Journal* 1874, 282.
81. Little 1883, 417; Clifford 1893, 4-5, 8.
82. *British Medical Journal* 1900, 1562.
83. Foott 1903, 448.
84. Remondino 1891, 179, 191-92.
85. Ibid., 194-95.
86. Freeland 1900, 1869.
87. Sedi boys are Indian sailors from the Mumbai region.
88. Hunter 1786, 221.
89. Buchan 1796, 71.
90. Drysdale 1855, 139.
91. Freeland 1900, 1870.
92. Wolbarst, 1914, 94.
93. Ibid., 93.
94. Ibid., 94.
95. O'Donnell 2001, 2. O'Donnell based his calculations on U.S. census data and figures on historical circumcision rates given in Wallerstein 1980, 216-17. See also Bollinger 2004.
96. *Medical Annual* 1915, 450. Royde 1950, 182. Gairdner (1950, 440) described Wolbarst's figures as "much quoted."
97. Harvey 1672, 64.
98. This is taken for granted by modern scholars such as Wallerstein (1980, 12-13).
99. Drysdale 1874, 399.
100. Snow 1890, 32-33.
101. Powell 1901, 1409.
102. For a more detailed discussion of the debate, see Darby 2003d.
103. Hutchinson 1946.
104. Hutchinson 1887.
105. Royal Commission on Venereal Diseases 1916, 19.
106. Fiaschi 1922, 92.
107. F.G. 1935, 560; Gautier-Smith 1935, 642.
108. Hanschell 1935, 642.
109. Lloyd and Lloyd 1935, 642.
110. Lloyd and Lloyd 1934.
111. Hall 2001b, 127ff.
112. For details on circumcision as a prophylactic, see Darby 2003d. Van Howe 1999, 59.
113. Reynolds et al. 2004, 1039-40. See also my reply, Darby 2004a, which points out that studies such as these are always compromised by confounding.

1. Circumcision specialist 1894, 1043–44.
2. Gollaher 2000, 100.
3. *Medical Press* 1900, 304.
4. *Harmsworth's home doctor* ca. 1926, 1057–58.
5. Bland-Sutton 1907, 1412.
6. O'Farrell 1888.
7. Glover 1929, 91–92.
8. MacCarthy, Douglas, and Mogford 1952, 756; Snow 1890, 25.
9. Osmond 1953.
10. Carne 1956.
11. Hyam 1990, 78.
12. Gairdner 1949, 1435.
13. Hoggart 1988, 134.
14. MacCarthy, Douglas, and Mogford 1952, 756.
15. Comfort 1950, 304
16. *British Medical Journal* 1950, 375.
17. Beisel 1997, 4–5.
18. Hunt 1999, 98–100.
19. Stall 1909, 114.
20. Beisel 1997, 55–56, 59–60.
21. Ibid., 199.
22. Morris 1892, 296.
23. Owen 1897, 283.
24. Gollaher 2000, 100.
25. Corner 1910, 390.
26. Snow 1890, 29n.
27. Macleod 1883, 807–88.
28. *Edinburgh Medical Journal* 1883, 855.
29. Sinclair 1889.
30. Atkins 1936, 610.
31. Yellen 1935.
32. Wan (2002) reports that the Gomco clamp can exert up to "20,000 pounds of hemostatic force against the prepuce" and describes it as "a noteworthy urologic invention because of its longevity and functional elegance." He wonders about the ethics of a doctor patenting an invention, but not about whether it is ethical to amputate healthy body parts from nonconsenting minors. For a less starry-eyed account, see www.infocirc.org/methods.htm.
33. Cited in Snow 1890, 27.
34. Freeland 1900, 1871.
35. Fullerton 1881, 140; Snow 1890, 29n.
36. Hutchinson 1893, 380.
37. Royde 1950, 182.
38. Fullerton 1881, 139; Owen 1897, 284.

39. Ellis 1936, 2:245, 251 (pt. 1).
40. *Medical Annual* 1895, 175.
41. Hutchinson 1893.
42. Clifford 1893, 3–4, 2.
43. Morris 1895, 1010.
44. Bland-Sutton 1907, 1411. For further details see Holt 1913; Darby 2003d.
45. Curtis 1916.
46. *British Medical Journal* 1950, 181.
47. Gairdner 1949, 1436.
48. Hall 1992, 134.
49. Graves 1979, 21–22.
50. Ibid., 28–30; Housman 1997, 199.
51. Graves 1979, 21.
52. Housman 1997 30–31.
53. Ibid., 48–49.
54. Davenport-Hines 1995, 31.
55. Davis 1998, 4.
56. Epigraph to Housman's last collection, *More Poems* (Housman 1997, 113).
57. Housman to Maurice Pollet, 5 February 1933, in Maas 329.
58. Skidelsky 1983, 66.
59. E-mail from Lord Skidelsky, 28 August 2002.
60. Keynes 1981, 22–23.
61. There is an account of what is represented as a true story of such a punishment at www.bmezine.com, a website devoted to stories and true experiences of body modifications of various types. Modern authorities on child development report that pissing competitions are very common among boys in the six- to nine-year-old age group (Borneman 1994, 162, 208).
62. Keynes 1981, 105, 151, 255.
63. Davenport-Hines 1995, 31.
64. Driberg 1977, 144. J. R. Ackerley (1968, 110) was unusual in preferring his rough trade cut and complained that the condition was rare among the policemen, sailors, and laborers he encountered.
65. Hodges 1984, 77.
66. Davenport-Hines 1995, 7–9, 32.
67. Ibid., 59, 105, 212.
68. Ibid., 312–14.
69. Stengers and van Neck 2001, 104. The *Struwwelpeter* stories were widely translated: see "The Story of Little Suck-a-Thumb," in *A Book of Nonsense* (London: Dent, 1927), 157–58.

70. "Jehovah Housman and Satan Housman," *New Verse* (January 1938), in Auden 1977.

71. "A. E. Housman" (1938), in Auden 1977, 238.

72. Earnest Hart, the editor of the *British Medical Journal* for much of the decisive period, was even skeptical of claims that masturbation induced organic disease and dismissed Maudsley's demonstration that it caused insanity (Bartrip 1990, 163-64). Such a cool attitude probably meant that the journal was also far less committed to promoting circumcision than it would have been had Hutchinson remained as editor.

73. Elizabeth Blackwell (1821-1910) was born in Britain and became the first woman in the United States to take a medical degree. See *American National Biography* (1999), vol. 2, s.v. "Blackwell."

74. Blackwell 1894, 35-36.

75. Snow 1890, 41. Hereafter, page references are given in the text.

76. Gairdner 1949, 1435.

77. *British Medical Journal* 1891, 1078.

78. *Lancet* 1891, 1386.

79. Snow 1890, 16.

80. For and against circumcision 1920, 768.

81. *British Medical Journal* 1935, 359.

82. Ainsworth 1935, 472.

83. Williams 1935, 822.

84. Faull 1935, 876.

85. Ainsworth 1935, 877.

86. A. Herbert Gray, *Sex Teaching* (1920s), as quoted in Hall 1992, 306.

87. Kenneth Walker, *Male Disorders of Sex* (1930), as quoted in Hall 1992, 306.

88. Haire, Costler, and Wiley 1934, 77.

89. Ellis 1936, 1:259 (pt. 1).

90. Haire, Costler, and Wiley 1934, 43, 79-82.

91. Cyril Bibby, *Sex Education* (1946), as quoted in Hall 1992, 308.

92. Eustace Chesser, *Love without Fear* (1942) and *Grow up and Live* (1949), as quoted in Hall 1992, 308.

93. Comfort 1967, 113.

94. Cook 2004, 207ff.

95. Stanley 1995, 72-73, 86-87, 166.

96. Ibid., 172.

97. As quoted in Cook 2004, 193.

98. We now know that it can take even longer, and that in some boys separation is not complete until puberty. See Hill 2003.

99. Gairdner 1949, 1435.

100. Ibid., 1437.

101. Ritual operation 1949, 1458.

102. Cold and Taylor 1999.

CHAPTER 14. *Conclusion*

1. None was so traditional as to mention masturbation.

2. Royde 1950, 182.

3. *British Medical Journal* 1950, 375.

4. Gairdner 1950, 440.

5. Hill 2003.

6. Whiddon 1953.

7. Case against circumcision 1979.

8. For pioneering research see Hodges 1997; Gollaher 2000; Miller 2002.

9. Darby 2001.

10. Begg 1953; Wright 1967; Leitch 1970; Australian Paediatric Association 1971, 1148.

11. Circumcision as a hygiene measure 1971.

12. The various statements are most readily accessible at http://www.cirp.org/library/statements.

13. Watters and Carroll 2003.

14. Spilsbury et al. 2003b.

15. McGrath and Young 2001.

16. There is a brief chronology of circumcision in Canada, with a heavy emphasis post-1975, at http://www.courtchallenge.com/refs/history0.html.

17. Wirth 1980.

18. Canadian Paediatric Society 1975.

19. Mayer et al. 2003.

20. Canadian Paediatric Society 1996.

21. E-mail from Dennis Harrison, Vancouver, 11 December 2003.

22. Le Fanu 1999.

23. Morris (1999, 31) states that uncircumcised men need "several showers a day" to keep down the smell.

24. Szasz 1996.

REFERENCES

Aberrations of the sexual instinct. 1867. Editorial. *Medical Times and Gazette,* 9 February, 141–46.

Ackerley, J. R. 1968. *My father and myself.* New York: Penguin, 1971.

Acton, William. 1851. *A practical treatise on the diseases of the urinary and generative organs in both sexes.* 2nd ed. London: Churchill.

———. 1860. On the rarity and mildness of syphilis amongst the Belgian troops quartered at Brussels, as compared with its prevalence and severity amongst the footguards in London. *Lancet,* 25 February, 196–98.

———. 1862. Personal experiences of an habitual traveller. *Lancet,* 22 February, 210–11.

———. 1865. *The functions and disorders of the reproductive organs in childhood, youth, adult age and advanced life.* Reprint of 3rd London ed. (1862). Philadelphia: Lindsay and Blakiston.

———. 1903. *The functions and disorders of the reproductive organs in childhood, youth, adult age and advanced life.* 6th ed. London: J. and A. Churchill. (Orig. pub. 1875.)

———. 1969. *Prostitution.* 2nd ed. Ed. and with an introduction by Peter Fryer. New York: Praeger. (Orig. pub. 1857, 2nd ed. 1870.)

Acton on the reproductive organs. 1862. Review of Acton, *Functions and disorders,* 3rd ed. *London Medical Review,* 3 September, 141–47.

A doctor. Ca. 1900. *A talk to a boy.* Purity Series, no. 8. Sydney: Australasian White Cross League.

Ainsworth, R. 1935. Letters. *British Medical Journal,* 7 September, 472; 2 November, 877.

Aldeeb Abu-Sahlieh, Sami A. 2001. *Male and female circumcision among Jews, Christians and Muslims: Religious, medical, social and legal debate.* Marco Polo Monographs, no. 5. Warren, PA: Shangri-La Publications.

Allen, James. 1909. Bilharzia haematoba and circumcision. *Lancet,* 8 May, 1317–20.

Allen, William R. 1998. Mercantilism. In *New Palgrave dictionary of economics,* ed. John Eatwell et al., 445–47. New York: Macmillan.

Almond, Hutchinson. 1893. Football as a moral agent. *Nineteenth Century* 34 (December): 899–911.

Antiseptic surgery. 1879. *British Medical Journal,* 20 December, 1000–1005.

Aretaeus. 1856. *The extant works of Aretaeus the Cappadocian.* London. Reprint, Boston: Milford House, 1972.

Aristotle's book of problems. 1776. Facsimile of the 30th London ed. New York: Garland, 1986.

Aristotle's complete masterpiece, in three parts, displaying the secrets of nature in the generation of man. 1749. Facsimile of the 23rd London ed. New York: Garland, 1986.

Aristotle's master-piece. 1690. London.

Aronson, Theo. 1994. *Prince Eddy and the homosexual underworld.* London: John Murray.

Arthur, Richard. Ca. 1900a. *The moral training of children.* Papers for Men, no. 15. London: White Cross League.

———. Ca. 1900b. *Purity and impurity.* Sydney: Australian White Cross League.

———. Ca. 1900c. *The training of children in purity: A booklet for parents.* Sydney: George Robertson.

Astonishing indifference to deaths due to botched ritual circumcision. 2003. Editorial. *South African Medical Journal* 93 (August).

Atkins, H. J. B. 1936. Special circumcision forceps. *Lancet,* 14 March, 610.

Auden, W. H. 1977. *The English Auden: Poems, essays and dramatic writings, 1927-39.* Ed. Edward Mendelson. London: Faber.

Australian College of Paediatrics. 1983. Statement on circumcision. Standing Committee on Perinatal Medicine. Available at http://www.circinfo.org/previous_statements.html.

———. 1996. Position statement: Routine circumcision of normal male infants and boys.

Australian Paediatric Association. 1971. Letter. *Medical Journal of Australia,* 22 May, 1148.

Baldwin, Peter. 1999. *Contagion and the state in Europe.* Cambridge: Cambridge University Press.

Bantock, Granville. 1866. Letter. *Lancet,* 16 June, 663.

Barton, Mary. 1936. A minor operation for phimosis. *Lancet,* 19 December, 1463.

Bartrip, W. J. 1990. *Mirror of medicine: A history of the British Medical Journal.* Oxford: *British Medical Journal* and Oxford University Press.

Bayley, Stephen, ed. 2001. *Sex: The erotic review.* London: Cassell.

Beale, Lionel. 1866. Letter. *Medical Times and Gazette,* 22 December, 681.

Beard, George. 1884. *The new cyclopaedia of family medicine—Our home physician: A popular guide to the art of preserving health and treating disease.* Sydney: McNeil and Coffee.

Beevor, Dr. 1890. Letter. *British Medical Journal,* 29 November, 1240.

Begg, John D. 1953. Why circumcise? *Medical Journal of Australia,* 25 April, 603-4.

Beier, Lucinda McCray. 1992. Seventeenth-century English surgery: The casebook of Joseph Binns. In *Medical theory, surgical practice: Studies in the history of medicine,* ed. Christopher Lawrence. London: Routledge.

Beisel, Nicola. 1997. Imperilled innocents: Anthony Comstock and family reproduction in Victorian America.

Benjamin, Zoe. 1944. *The young child,* vol. 1 of *You and your children.* Sydney: Gayle Publishing.

Benn, J. Miriam. 1992. *Predicaments of love.* London: Pluto Press.

Bennett, Paula, and Vernon A. Rosario, eds. 1995. *Solitary pleasures: The historical, literary and artistic discourses of autoeroticism.* New York and London: Routledge.

Bertwistle, A. P. 1936. Juvenile circumcision: A plea for a standardised technique. *Lancet,* 12 January, 85-86.

Bett, W. R. 1956. *Sir John Bland-Sutton.* Edinburgh: E. & S. Livingstone.

[Beugnies, Dr.]. 1902. The hygiene value of circumcision. *British Medical Journal,* 26 July, 271-72.

Biale, David. 1992. *Eros and the Jews: From biblical Israel to contemporary America.* New York: Basic Books.

Billings, John S. 1891. Vital statistics of the Jews. *North American Review* 152: 70-84.

Blackwell, Elizabeth. 1894. *The human element in sex: Being a medical enquiry into the relation of sexual physiology to Christian morality.* 2nd ed. London: Churchill.

Bland, Lucy. 1994. *Banishing the beast: English feminism and sexual morality, 1885-1914.* Harmondsworth: Penguin.

Bland-Sutton, John. 1907. Circumcision as a rite and as a surgical operation. *British Medical Journal,* 15 June, 1408-12.

Bolande, Robert. 1969. Ritualistic surgery: Circumcision and tonsillectomy. *New England Journal of Medicine* 280 (3 March): 591-96.

Bollinger, Dan. 2004. Normal versus circumcised: U.S. neonatal male genital ratio. http://www.cirp.org/library/statistics/bollinger2004.

Booysen, Cecile. 1935. Letter. *British Medical Journal,* 7 September, 472.

Borneman, Ernest. 1994. *Childhood phases of maturity.* Trans. Michael Lombardi-Nash. New York: Prometheus Books.

Bouce, Paul-Gabriel. 1980. Aspects of sexual tolerance and intolerance in eighteenth-century England. *British Journal for Eighteenth Century Studies* 3: 173-91.

Brandt, Alan M. 1993. Sexually transmitted diseases. In *Companion encyclopaedia to the history of medicine,* ed. W. F. Bynum and Roy Porter. London: Routledge.

Brieger, Gert. 1992. From conservative to radical surgery in late nineteenth-century America. In *Medical theory, surgical practice: Studies in the history of medicine,* ed. Christopher Lawrence, 216-31. London: Routledge.

Bristow, Edward J. 1977. *Vice and vigilance: Purity movements in Britain since 1700.* London: Gill and Macmillan.

Bristowe, John Syer. 1884. *A treatise on the theory and practice of medicine.* 5th ed. London: Smith Elder.

British and Foreign Medico-Chirurgical Review. 1857. Review of Acton, *Functions and disorders.* No. 39 (July): 176-77.

British Medical Journal. 1866a. Letter. 16 June, 654.

———. 1866b. Reviews of Baker Brown, On the curability of certain forms of insanity, epilepsy, catalepsy and hysteria in females. 20 January, 77; 28 April, 438-40, 456.

———. 1867a. Editorial. 19 January, 61.

———. 1867b. Report of the meeting on 3 April 1867 of the Obstetrical Society to consider the expulsion of Baker Brown. 6 April, 395-409.

———. 1874. Letters. 5 December, 727; 12 December, 759.

———. 1889. Advertisement. 7 December, 1315.

———. 1891. Review of Snow, *Barbarity of circumcision.* 16 May, 1078.

———. 1892. Review of Remondino, *History of circumcision.* 20 February, 391-92.

———. 1894. Letter. 12 May, 1044.

———. 1900. Letter. 23 June, 1562.

———. 1901. Reply to letter. 28 September, 938.

———. 1907. Letters. 13 July, 117; 3 August, 303; 28 September, 860.

———. 1927. Letter. 4 June, 1043.

———. 1935. Letters. 24 August, 359; 19 October, 763.

———. 1944. Letters. 28 October, 585; 30 December, 876.

———. 1950. Letters. 21 January 1950, 181; 11 February, 375.

Brown, Isaac Baker. 1861. *On surgical diseases of women.* 2nd ed., rev. and enlarged. London: John Davies.

———. 1866a. *On the curability of certain forms of insanity, epilepsy, catalepsy and hysteria in females.* London: Robert Hardwicke.

———. 1866b. Letter. *British Medical Journal*, 15 December, 675–76.

———. 1866c. Reply to critics. *Lancet*, 3 November, 495.

Brown, S. G. A. 1897. A plea for circumcision. *Medical World* 15: 124–25.

Brown-Sequard, E. 1858. Course of lectures on the physiology and pathology of the central nervous system. *Lancet*, July–December (twelve lectures).

Browne, Janet. 2002. *Charles Darwin: The power of place*. New York: Knopf.

Bryant, Thomas. 1863. *The surgical diseases of children: Being the Lettsomian lectures delivered before the medical Society of London, 1863*. London: Churchill.

Bryk, Felix. 1934. *Circumcision in man and woman: Its history, psychology and ethnology*. New York: American Ethnological Press.

Buchan, William. 1772. *Domestic medicine, or a treatise on the prevention and cure of diseases by regimen and simple medicines*. Facsimile reprint of the 2nd ed. New York: Garland, 1985.

———. 1796. *Observations concerning the prevention and cure of venereal disease*. Facsimile reprint. New York: Garland, 1985.

Bulwer, John. 1650. *Anthropometamorphosis, man transform'd, or the artificial changeling*. London: printed for J. Hardesty.

Burton, Richard, trans. 1885. *A plain and literal translation of the Arabian nights' entertainments, now entitled "The book of the thousand nights and a night."* 10 vols. London: Burton Club.

———. 1964. *Love, war and fancy: The customs and manners of the East from writings on the Arabian Nights*. Ed. Kenneth Walker. London: William Kimber.

Bush, M. L. 1998. *What is love? Richard Carlile's philosophy of sex*. London: Verso.

Bynum, W. F. 1987. Treating the wages of sin: Venereal disease and specialism in eighteenth-century Britain. In *Medical fringe and medical orthodoxy, 1750–1850*, ed. W. F. Bynum and Roy Porter. London: Croom Helm.

———. 1992. Medical values in a commercial age. *Proceedings of the British Academy* 78: 149–63.

———. 1994. *Science and the practice of medicine in the nineteenth century*. Cambridge: Cambridge University Press.

Bynum, W. F., and Roy Porter, eds. 1993. *Companion encyclopaedia to the history of medicine*. 2 vols. London: Routledge.

[Cadell, Francis]. 1873. The advantages of circumcision from a surgical point of view. Paper given to the Medico-Chirurgical Society of Edinburgh, 20 November 1872. *Edinburgh Medical Journal* 18 (February): 750–53.

Canadian Paediatric Society. 1975. Circumcision in the newborn period. *CPS News Bulletin* (suppl.) 8: 1–2.

———. 1996. Neonatal circumcision revisited. *Canadian Medical Association Journal* 154: 769–80.

Carlile, Richard. 1828. *Every woman's book; or, What is love?* London.

Carne, Stuart. 1956. Incidence of tonsillectomy, circumcision and appendicectomy among RAF recruits. *British Medical Journal*, 7 July, 19–23.

Carpenter, W. B. 1846. *Elements of physiology, including physiological anatomy for the use of the medical student*. Philadelphia: Lea and Blanchard.

———. 1853. *Principles of human physiology, with their chief applications to psychology, pathology, therapeutics, hygiene and forensic medicine*. 5th American ed., from 4th London ed. Philadelphia: Blanchard and Lea.

———. 1856. *A manual of physiology, including physiological anatomy*. 3rd ed. London: Churchill.

The case against circumcision. 1979. Editorial. *British Medical Journal*, 5 May, 1163–64.

Cases of epilepsy with complications. 1867. *Lancet*, 16 February, 208–9.

Chadwick, Edwin. 1965. *Report on the sanitary condition of the labouring population of Great Britain.* Ed. M. W. Flinn. Edinburgh: Edinburgh University Press. (Orig. pub. 1842.)

Chambers, Thomas K. 1861. Gonorrhoea and imaginary spermatorrhoea. *Lancet* 1 (29 June): 635–37.

Chapman, John. 1869. Prostitution in relation to the national health. *Westminster Review,* n.s., 36. In *Prostitution in the Victorian age: Debates on the issue from nineteenth-century critical journals,* ed. Keith Nield. Westmead, U.K.: Gregg International, 1973.

Childs, G. B. 1842–43. Treatment of gonorrhoea by superficial cauterisation of the urethra. *London Medical Gazette,* n.s., 2: 646–47.

Circumcision: Foreskin or against. 2002. *Practical Parenting* (Sydney, Australia), June, 48–50.

Circumcision and VD. 1947. *Newsweek,* 21 July, 31.

Circumcision as a hygiene measure. 1971. Editorial. *Medical Journal of Australia,* 24 July, 175.

Circumcision as a preventive of venereal disease. 1901. *Medical Record* 59 (6 April): 541.

Circumcision in Tangiers. 1851. *Lancet* 1: 241.

A circumcision specialist. 1894. *British Medical Journal,* 12 May, 1043–44.

Circumscisus [*sic*]. 1896. *Medical Record* 49 (21 March): 430.

Clark, A. Campbell, and Henry E. Clark. 1899. Neurectomy, a preventive of masturbation. *Lancet,* 23 September, 838.

Cleland, John. 1748. *Fanny Hill; or, Memoirs of a woman of pleasure.* Ed. Peter Wagner. New York: Penguin, 1985.

Clifford, M. 1893. *Circumcision: Its advantages and how to perform it.* London: Churchill.

Clitoridectomy. 1866. Editorial. *British Medical Journal,* 15 December, 664–65.

Clitoridectomy and medical ethics. 1867. *Medical Times and Gazette,* 13 April, 391–92.

Cockshutt, R. W. 1935. Circumcision. *British Medical Journal,* 19 October, 764.

Cold, C. J., and K. A. McGrath. 1999. Anatomy and histology of the penile and clitoral prepuce in primates: Evolutionary perspective of specialised sensory tissue in the external genitalia. In *Male and female circumcision: Medical, legal and ethical considerations in pediatric practice,* ed. George C. Denniston, Frederick Hodges, and Marilyn Milos. New York: Kluwer Academic/Plenum Publishers.

Cold, C. J., and J. R. Taylor. 1999. The prepuce. *BJU International* 83 (suppl. 1) (January): 34–44.

Colley, Linda. 2000. Going native, telling tales: Captivity, collaboration and the Empire. *Past and Present,* no. 168 (August): 170–93.

———. 2002. *Captives.* New York: Pantheon.

Collini, Stefan. 1985. The idea of character in Victorian political thought. *Transactions of the Royal Historical Society,* ser. 5, 35: 29–50.

Comfort, Alex. 1950. Informal survey. *British Medical Journal,* 4 February, 304.

———. 1967. *The anxiety makers: Some curious preoccupations of the medical profession.* London: Nelson.

Cominos, Peter. 1963. Late Victorian respectability and the social system. *International Review of Social History* 8: 18–48, 216–50.

Connolly, D. I. 1935. Letters. *British Medical Journal,* 24 August, 359; 26 October 1935, 822.

Conrad, Lawrence I., Michael Neve, Vivian Nutton, Roy Porter, and Andrew Wear. 1995. *The Western medical tradition, 800 BC–AD 1800.* Cambridge: Cambridge University Press.

Consultant to the Children's Hospital. 1901. Letter. *British Medical Journal,* 5 October, 1023–24.

Continence versus syphilis. 1889. *Lancet,* 25 May, 1042–43.

Contraction of the prepuce. 1846. *Lancet,* 16 May, 553.

The control of prostitution. 1870. *British Medical Journal*, 18 June, 630-32.

Cook, Hera. 2004. *The long sexual revolution: English women, sex and contraception, 1800–1975.* Oxford: Oxford University Press.

Coote, Holmes. 1866. Letter. *British Medical Journal*, 22 December, 705.

Cooter, Roger, ed. 1992. *In the name of the child: Health and welfare, 1880-1940.* London: Routledge.

Copland, James. 1844-58. *A dictionary of practical medicine.* 4 vols. London: Longmans.

Corfield, W. H. 1870. Introductory lecture . . . on hygiene and public health. *British Medical Journal*, 18 June, 617-19; 25 June, 645-46.

Corner, Edred M. 1910. *Male diseases in general practice: An introduction to andrology.* London: Oxford University Press.

Courtenay, F. B. Ca. 1860. *Revelations of quacks and quackery.* London: N.p.

———. 1882. *On spermatorrhoea and certain functional derangements and debilities of the generative system: Their nature, treatment and cure.* 12th ed. London: Bailliere, Tindall.

Crawford, Patricia. 1994. Sexual knowledge in England, 1500-1750. In *Sexual knowledge, sexual science: The history of attitudes to sexuality,* ed. Roy Porter and Mikulas Teich. Cambridge: Cambridge University Press.

Crellin, J. K. 1968. The dawn of germ theory: Particles, infection and biology. In *Medicine and science in the 1860s,* ed. F. N. L. Poynter. London: Wellcome Institute for the History of Medicine.

Crozier, Ivan. 2000a. Havelock Ellis, eonism and the patient's discourse: Or, writing a book about sex. *History of Psychiatry* 11: 125-54.

———. 2000b. William Acton and the history of sexuality: The medical and professional context. *Journal of Victorian Culture* 5: 1-27.

———. 2001. "Rough winds do shake the darling buds of May": A note on William Acton and the sexuality of the male child. *Journal of Family History* 26: 411-20.

Curling, T. B. 1856. *A practical treatise on the diseases of the testis and of the spermatic cord and scrotum.* 2nd ed. London: Churchill.

Curtis, Henry. 1916. A new method of bloodless circumcision. *Practitioner* 97: 101-5.

da Carpi, Jacopo Berengario. 1959. *A short introduction to anatomy.* Trans L. R. Lind. Chicago: University of Chicago Press.

Daley, Harry. 1986. *This small cloud: A personal memoir.* London: Weidenfeld and Nicolson.

Dally, Ann. 1991. *Women under the knife: A history of surgery.* New York: Routledge.

———. 1996. *Fantasy surgery, 1880-1930: With special reference to Sir William Arbuthnot Lane.* Amsterdam: Rodopi.

Dalrymple, William. 2002. *White mughals: Love and betrayal in eighteenth-century India.* London: Harper Collins.

Dampier-Bennett, Arthur G. 1907. The origins of circumcision. *British Medical Journal*, 27 July, 243-44.

Daniel, Peter. 1910. Diseases of the orifices of the body. *British Medical Journal*, 15 January, 121-25.

Daniell, W. F. 1847. On the circumcision of females in western Africa. *London Medical Gazette*, n.s., 5: 374-78.

Darby, Robert. 2001. "A source of serious mischief": The demonisation of the foreskin and the rise of preventive circumcision in Australia. In *Understanding circumcision: A multidisciplinary approach to a multi-dimensional problem,* ed. George C. Denniston, Frederick Hodges, and Marilyn Milos. New York: Kluwer Academic/Plenum Press.

———. 2003a. Circumcision as a preventive of masturbation: A review of the historiography. *Journal of Social History* 36 (Spring): 737-58.

———. 2003b. Medical history and medical practice: Persistent myths about the foreskin. *Medical Journal of Australia* 178 (17 February): 178–79.

———. 2003c. "An oblique and slovenly initiation": The circumcision episode in *Tristram Shandy. Eighteenth-Century Life* 27 (Winter): 72–84.

———. 2003d. Where doctors differ: The debate on circumcision as a protection against syphilis, 1855–1914. *Social History of Medicine* 16: 57–78.

———. 2004a. Male circumcision and risk of HIV-1 infection. *Lancet,* 12 June, 1997.

———. 2004b. A post-modernist theory of wanking. Review of Thomas Laqueur, *Solitary Sex. Journal of Social History* 38 (Fall).

Darwin, Charles. 2004. *The descent of man.* Ed. James Moore and Adrian Desmond. New York: Penguin. (Orig. pub. 1871–79.)

Davenport, John. 1875. *Curiositates eroticae physiologiae, or tabooed subjects freely treated.* London: privately printed. Reprinted as *Aphrodisiacs and love stimulants, with other chapters on the secrets of Venus.* Ed. Henry Hull Walton. London: Luxor Press, 1965.

Davenport-Hines, Richard. 1990. *Sex, death and punishment: Attitudes to sex and sexuality in Britain since the Renaissance.* London: Collins.

———. 1995. *Auden.* New York: Pantheon.

Davidson, Alexander. 1889. Genital irritation in boys. *Practitioner* 42: 350–56.

Davidson, Roger, and Lesley Hall, eds. 2001. *Sex, sin and suffering: Venereal disease and European society since 1870.* London: Routledge.

Davis, Dick. 1998. Blue remembered hills. *Times Literary Supplement,* 5 June, 4.

Dawson, Richard. 1852. *An essay on spermatorrhoea and urinary deposits.* 6th ed. London: Aylott and Jones.

De Mause, Lloyd. 1974. The evolution of childhood. *History of Childhood Quarterly* 1: 503–74.

Dictionary of Scientific Biography. 1971. New York: Scribner.

Dictionnaire des sciences medicales. 1812–22. Ed. Charles Panckoucke. Paris. http://www.bium.univ-paris5.fr/histmed/medica/panckoucke.htm (19 June 2004).

Diderot, Denis. 1966. Letter on the blind. In *Diderot's selected writings,* ed. Lester G. Crocker. New York: Macmillan.

Digby, Anne. 1994. *Making a medical living: Doctors and patients in the English market for medicine, 1720–1911.* Cambridge: Cambridge University Press.

Dixon, Edward. 1845. *A treatise on diseases of the sexual organs.* New York.

Dock, Lavinia. 1910. *Hygiene and morality.* New York.

Donat, James G. 2001. The Rev. John Wesley's extractions from Dr. Tissot: A Methodist imprimatur. *History of Science* 39: 285–98.

Donovan, Basil. 2000. The repertoire of human efforts to avoid sexually transmissible diseases. *Sexually Transmitted Infections* 76: 7–12, 88–93.

Douglas, Mary. 1966. *Purity and danger: An analysis of concepts of pollution and taboo.* New York: Pelican, 1970.

Doyle, Arthur Conan. 1934. *Round the red lamp: Being facts and fancies of medical life.* London: John Murray. (Orig. pub. 1894.)

Driberg, Tom. 1977. *Ruling passions.* London: Jonathan Cape.

Drysdale, C. R. 1874. Report on syphilis. *Medical Press and Circular,* 13 May, 399–400.

Drysdale, George. 1855. *The elements of social science, or physical, sexual and natural religion.* 35th ed. enlarged. London: G. Standring, 1905.

Dunsmuir, W. D., and E. M. Gordon. 1999. The history of circumcision. *BJU International* 83 (suppl. 1) (January): 1–12.

Durbach, Nadia. 2000. "They might as well brand us": Working-class resistance to compulsory vaccination in Victorian England. *Social History of Medicine* 13: 45–62.

Eagle, Chester. 1986. *Play together dark blue twenty*. Melbourne: McPhee Gribble.

Edinburgh Medical Journal. 1874. Review of Aissa Hamdy, *De la circoncision*. Vol. 20 (September): 282.

———. 1883. Comment. Vol. 28 (March): 855.

———. 1908. Obituary for Patrick Heron Watson. N.s., 23: 3–5.

Efron, John M. 2001. *Medicine and the German Jews: A history*. New Haven: Yale University Press.

Ellis, Havelock. 1936. *Studies in the psychology of sex*. 2 vols. Modern Library ed. New York: Random House.

Encyclopaedia Britannica. 1781 (2nd ed.);1797 (3rd ed.); 1853–60 (8th ed.); 1876 (9th ed.); 1910 (11th ed.); 1929 (14th ed.).

Engelhardt, H. Tristram. 1974. The disease of masturbation: Values and the concept of disease. *Bulletin of the History of Medicine* 48 (2): 234–48.

Epilepsy for thirty-two years in a man, aged forty-four, with discolouration of the skin from nitrate of silver; operation of castration. 1859. *Lancet*, 22 January, 81–82.

Erichsen, John. 1877. *The science and art of surgery, being a treatise on surgical injuries, diseases and operations*. 7th ed. 2 vols. London: Longmans Green.

Evelyn, John. 1955. *The diary of John Evelyn*. Ed. E. S. de Beer. 6 vols. Oxford: Clarendon Press.

Faull, J. L. 1935. Letter. *British Medical Journal*, 2 November, 876.

Feldman, David. 1994. *Englishmen and Jews: Social relations and political culture, 1840–1914*. New Haven: Yale University Press.

Fenwick, E. Hurry. 1890. Circumcision. *Medical Annual*, 201–2.

Fergus, Andrew. 1879. Address on public medicine: Preventative or state medicine. *British Medical Journal*, 9 August, 217–22.

F.G. 1935. Letter. *British Medical Journal*, 21 September, 560.

Fiaschi, P. 1922. The prophylaxis of venereal diseases. *Medical Journal of Australia*, 28 January, 85–94.

Fleming, J. B. 1960. Clitoridectomy: The disastrous downfall of Isaac Baker Brown FRCS (1867). *Journal of Obstetrics and Gynaecology of the British Empire* 67: 1017–34.

Foott, R. E. 1903. Letter. *British Medical Journal*, 29 August, 448.

For and against circumcision. 1920. *British Medical Journal*, 5 June, 768.

Forster, J. Cooper. 1855. A few remarks on the surgical disease of children. I. Congenital phimosis. *Medical Times and Gazette*, n.s., 2 (November): 491–92.

Foster, Michael. 1891. *A textbook of physiology*. 5th ed. 4 vols. London: Macmillan.

Foucault, Michel. 1981. *A history of sexuality: An introduction*. New York: Penguin. (Orig. pub. 1976.)

Fowler, Dr. Robert. 1860. Letter. *Lancet*, 14 April, 382.

Freeland, E. Harding. 1900. Circumcision as a preventive of syphilis and other disorders. *Lancet*, 29 December, 1869–71.

Friedrich, William, Theo Sandfort, Jacqueline Oostveen, and Peggy Cohen-Kettenis. 2000. Cultural differences in sexual behaviour: 2–6 year old Dutch and American children. In *Childhood sexuality: Normal sexual behaviour and development*, ed. Theo Sandfort and Jany Rademakers. New York: Haworth Press.

Fullerton, George. 1881. *The family medical guide, with plain directions for the treatment of every case*. 4th ed. Sydney: William Maddock.

Gairdner, Douglas. 1949. The fate of the foreskin: A study of circumcision. *British Medical Journal*, 24 December, 1433–37.

———. 1950. Fate of the foreskin [Reply to correspondence]. *British Medical Journal*, 18 February, 439–40.

Galen. 1968. *Galen on the usefulness of the parts of the body*. Trans. from the Greek with introduction and commentary by Margaret Tallmadge May. Ithaca, NY: Cornell University Press.

Gallop, E. 1950. Letter. *British Medical Journal*, 14 January, 123.

Garton, Stephen. 1984. Insanity in New South Wales: Some aspects of its social history, 1878–1958. PhD diss., University of Sydney.

Gascoyen, George. 1872. On spermatorrhoea and its treatment. *British Medical Journal*, 20 January, 67–69; 27 January, 95–96.

Gathorne-Hardy, Jonathan. 1972. *The rise and fall of the British nanny*. London: Hodder and Stoughton.

Gautier-Smith, C. E. 1935. Letter. *British Medical Journal*, 5 October, 642.

Gaw, Jerry L. 1999. *A time to heal: The diffusion of Listerism in Victorian Britain*. Philadelphia: American Philosophical Society.

Gay, Peter. 1984. *Education of the senses*. The bourgeois experience—Victoria to Freud. New York: Oxford University Press.

Gebhard, Paul H., and Alan B. Johnson. 1979. *The Kinsey data: Marginal tabulations of the 1938–1963 interviews*. Bloomington: Indiana University Press.

Gibbon, Dr. 1876. Letter. *Lancet*, 25 March, 465.

Gibbon, Edward. 1903. *The history of the decline and fall of the Roman Empire*. Ed. Dean Milman, M. Guizot, and Sir William Smith. 8 vols. London: John Murray.

Gibson, Ian. 1978. *The English vice: Beating, sex and shame in Victorian England and after*. London: Duckworth.

Gibson, Ian. 2001. *The erotomaniac: The secret life of Henry Spencer Ashbee*. New York: Da Capo Press.

Gilbert, Allen. 1915. An unusual case of masturbation. *Medical Record* 88: 608–10.

Gilbert, Arthur N. 1975. Doctor, patient, and onanist diseases in the nineteenth century. *Journal of the History of Medicine and Allied Sciences* 30: 217–34.

Gilman, Sander L. 1989. *Sexuality: An illustrated history*. New York: Wiley.

———. 1993. *Freud, race, and gender*. Princeton, NJ: Princeton University Press.

Gladstone, William. 1968. *The Gladstone diaries*. Ed. M. R. D. Foott. Oxford: Clarendon Press.

Glick, Leonard. 2001. Jewish circumcision: An enigma in historical perspective. In *Understanding circumcision: A multi-disciplinary approach to a multi-dimensional problem*, ed. George C. Denniston, Frederick Hodges, and Marilyn Milos. New York: Kluwer Academic/ Plenum Press.

A gloomy rite. 1866. Editorial. *Medical Times and Gazette*, 15 December, 641–42.

Glover, Edward. 1929. The screening function of traumatic memories. *International Journal of Psychoanalysis* 10: 90–93.

Gollaher, David L. 1994. From ritual to science: The medical transformation of circumcision in America. *Journal of Social History* 28: 5–36.

———. 2000. *Circumcision: A history of the world's most controversial surgery*. New York: Basic Books.

Gould, Steven Jay. 1992. The chain of reason and the chain of thumbs. In *Bully for brontosaurus*, 182–97. New York: Penguin.

Granshaw, Lindsay. 1992. "Upon this principle I have based a practice": The development and reception of antisepsis in Britain, 1867–90. In *Medical innovations in historical perspective*, ed. John Pickard, 17–46. New York: St. Martin's Press.

A grave social problem. 1881. Editorial. *British Medical Journal*, 3 December, 904-5.

Graves, Richard Percival. 1979. *A. E. Housman: The scholar poet.* London: Routledge and Kegan Paul.

Greenhalgh, Robert. 1866. Letter. *British Medical Journal*, 29 December, 730.

——. 1867. Letters. *Lancet*, 5 January, 28; *British Medical Journal*, 12 January, 42.

Grosskurth, Phyllis. 1980. *Havelock Ellis: A biography.* New York: Knopf.

Haire, Norman, A. Costler, and A. Wiley. 1934. *Encyclopaedia of sexual knowledge.* London: Encyclopaedic Press.

Haley, Bruce. 1978. *The healthy body in Victorian culture.* Cambridge: Harvard University Press.

Hall, G. Stanley. 1904. *Adolescence: Its psychology and its relations to physiology, anthropology, sociology, sex, crime, religion and education.* 2 vols. New York: D. Appleton.

Hall, Lesley. 1991. *Hidden anxieties: Male sexuality, 1900-1950.* Cambridge, MA: Polity Press.

——. 1992. Forbidden by god, despised by men: Masturbation, medical warnings, moral panic and manhood in Great Britain, 1850-1950. In *Forbidden history: The state, society and the regulation of sexuality in modern Europe*, ed. John C. Fout. Chicago: University of Chicago Press.

——. 1994. "The English have hot water bottles": The morganatic marriage between sexology and medicine in Britain since William Acton. In *Sexual knowledge, sexual science: The history of attitudes to sexuality*, ed. Roy Porter and Mikulas Teich. Cambridge: Cambridge University Press.

——. 2001a. Masturbation. In *Encyclopedia of European Social History, 1350-2000*, ed. Peter Stearns, 4:279-90. New York: Scribner.

——. 2001b. Venereal diseases and society in Britain, from the contagious Diseases Acts to the National Health Service. In *Sex, sin, and suffering: Venereal disease and European society since 1870*, ed. Roger Davidson and Lesley Hall, 120-36. London: Routledge.

Hamilton, J. A. G. 1903. Treatment of nymphomania by division of branches of internal pudic and inferior pudendal nerves. *Australasian Medical Gazette* 22 (20 May): 205-6.

Hamlin, Christopher. 1985. Providence and putrefaction: Victorian sanitarians and the natural theology of health and disease. *Victorian Studies* 28: 381-411.

Hammond, Tim. 1999. A preliminary poll of men circumcised in infancy or childhood. *BJU International* 83 (suppl. 1) (January): 85-92.

Hammond, William A. 1887. *Sexual impotence in the male and female.* Facsimile reprint. New York: Arno, 1974.

Hamowy, Ronald. 1977. Medicine and the crimination of sin: "Self-abuse" in nineteenth-century America. *Journal of Libertarian Studies* 1: 229-70.

Handfield Jones, C. 1867. *Clinical observations on functional nervous disorders.* 4th ed. Philadelphia: Blanchard and Lea.

Hanschell, H. M. 1935. Letter. *British Medical Journal*, 5 October, 642.

Hardy, Anne. 1993. *The epidemic streets: Infectious disease and the rise of preventive medicine.* Oxford: Oxford University Press.

Hare, E. H. 1962. Masturbatory insanity: The history of an idea. *Journal of Mental Science* 108 (January): 2-25.

Harmsworth's home doctor and encyclopaedia of good health. Ca. 1926. London: Educational Book Co.

Hart, Ernest. 1877. The mosaic code of sanitation. *Sanitary Record* 6: 181-83, 197-99.

Harvey, Gideon. 1672. *Great Venus unmasked; or, A more exact discovery of the venereal evil.* London: printed for Nath. Brook.

Harvey, William. 1964. *The anatomical lectures of William Harvey*. Ed. and trans. Gweneth Williams. Edinburgh: E. and S. Livingstone for RCP.

Heckford, N. 1865. Circumcision as a remedial measure in certain cases of epilepsy, chorea etc. *Clinical lectures and reports by the medical and surgical staff of London Hospital* 2: 58-64.

Henry, Mrs. S. M. I. 1898. *Confidential talks on home and child life*. Edinburgh: Oliphant, Anderson and Ferrier.

Hill, George. 2003. Circumcision for phimosis. *Medical Journal of Australia* 178: 587.

Hilton, John. 1863. A course of lectures on pain. Lecture 5, pt. 3. *Lancet*, 1 August, 122-24.

Himes, Norman E. 1963. *Medical history of contraception*. New York: Gamut Press. (Orig. pub. 1936.)

Hirsch, Edwin. 1930. An historical survey of gonorrhoea. *Annals of Medical History*, n.s., 2.

Hitchcock, Tim. 1997. *English sexualities, 1700-1800*. New York: St. Martin's Press.

Hodges, Andrew. 1984. *Alan Turing: The enigma*. New York: Simon and Schuster.

Hodges, Frederick. 1997. A short history of the institutionalization of involuntary sexual mutilation in the United States. In *Sexual mutilations: A human tragedy*, ed. George C. Denniston and Marilyn Milos. New York: Plenum Press.

———. 1999. The history of phimosis from antiquity to the present. In *Male and female circumcision: Medical, legal and ethical considerations in pediatric practice*, ed. George C. Denniston, Frederick Hodges, and Marilyn Milos. New York: Kluwer Academic/Plenum Publishers.

———. 2001. The ideal prepuce in Ancient Greece and Rome: Male genital aesthetics and their relation to lipodermos, circumcision, foreskin restoration and the Kinodesme. *Bulletin of the History of Medicine* 75: 375-405.

Hoffman, Lawrence. 1996. *Covenant of blood: Circumcision and gender in rabbinic Judaism*. Chicago: University of Chicago Press.

Hoggart, Richard. 1988. *A local habitation*, vol. 1 (1918-40) of *Life and times*. London: Chatto and Windus.

Holt, L. Emmett. 1897. *The diseases of infancy and childhood, for the use of students and practitioners of medicine*. New York and London: Appleton.

———. 1913. Tuberculosis acquired through ritual circumcision. *Journal of the American Medical Association* 61 (12 July): 99-102.

Hopkins, Ellice. 1902. *The power of womanhood; or, Mothers and sons. A book for parents and those in loco parentis*. 7th ed. Melbourne: George Robertson.

Hoppen, K. Theodore. 1998. *The mid-Victorian generation, 1846-1886*. Oxford: Clarendon Press.

Housman, A. E. 1997. *The poems of A. E. Housman*. Ed. Archie Burnett. Oxford: Oxford University Press.

Howe, Joseph W. 1887. *Excessive venery, masturbation and continence*. New York.

Hull, David L. 1973. *Darwin and his critics: The reception of Darwin's theory of evolution by the scientific community*. Cambridge: Harvard University Press.

Humphries, Stephen. 1988. *A secret world of sex: Forbidden fruit—The British experience, 1900-1950*. London: Sidgwick and Jackson.

Hunt, Alan. 1998. The great masturbation panic and the discourse of moral regulation in nineteenth- and early twentieth-century Britain. *Journal of the History of Sexuality* 8: 575-615.

———. 1999. *Governing morals: A social history of moral regulation*. Cambridge: Cambridge University Press.

Hunter, John. 1786. *A treatise on the venereal disease*. London.

———. 1810. *A treatise on the venereal disease*. Rev. ed., with an introduction and commentary by Joseph Adams, M.D. London.

Hunter, William. 1911. The role of sepsis and antisepsis in medicine. *Lancet*, 14 January, 79–86.

Hutchinson, Herbert. 1946. *Jonathan Hutchison: His life and letters.* London: Heinemann.

Hutchinson, Jonathan [?]. 1852. Epithelial cancer of the penis—Amputation and recovery. *Medical Times and Gazette*, 23 October, 415–16.

———. 1855. On the influence of circumcision in preventing syphilis. *Medical Times and Gazette*, n.s., 2 (1 December): 542–43.

———. 1876. Notes on syphilis. *Lancet*, 5 February, 291; 8 April, 535.

———. 1882. The pre-cancerous stage of cancer and the importance of early operations. *British Medical Journal*, 7 January, 5–6.

———. 1887. *Syphilis.* London: Cassell.

———. 1890a. On circumcision as a preventive of masturbation. *Archives of Surgery* 2: 267–69.

———. 1890b. A plea for circumcision. *Archives of Surgery* 2: 15.

———. 1890c. A plea for circumcision. *British Medical Journal*, 27 September, 769.

———. 1893. On circumcision. *Archives of Surgery* 4: 379–80.

———. 1895. Syphilis. In *A system of surgery*, ed. Frederick Treves, 385–432. London: Cassell.

———. 1900. The advantages of circumcision. *Medical Review* 3: 641–42.

Hyam, Ronald. 1990. *Empire and sexuality: The British experience.* Manchester, UK: Manchester University Press.

Hygienic value of circumcision. *British Medical Journal*, 26 July 1902, 271–72.

Hynes, Samuel. 1968. *The Edwardian turn of mind.* London: Pimlico, 1991.

Immerman, Ronald S., and Wade C. Mackey. 1997. A biocultural analysis of circumcision. *Social Biology* 44: 265–75.

———. 1998. A proposed relationship between circumcision and neural reorganisation. *Journal of Genetic Psychology* 159: 367–78.

Indications for circumcision. 1901. *British Medical Journal*, 5 October, 1023–24.

Interdepartmental Committee on Physical Deterioration. 1904. *Report of the Interdepartmental Committee on Physical Deterioration.* Parliamentary Papers, vol. 32. Great Britain.

Jackson, Arthur. 1891. A few notes on foreskins. *British Medical Journal*, 18 April, 861.

Jacobi, Abraham. 1876. Dr. Jacobi on masturbation in children. *Medical Times and Gazette*, 12 February, 177.

James, Robert. 1743–45. *A medicinal dictionary: Including physic, surgery, anatomy, chymistry, and botany, in all their branches relative to medicine.* 3 vols. London: T. Osborne.

A Jewish surgeon. 1874. Letter. *Lancet*, 12 December, 856.

Johnson, Athol W. 1860. On an injurious habit occasionally met with in infancy and early childhood. *Lancet*, 7 April, 344–45.

Johnson, Michael. 2001. Submission to ACP/RACP review of policy on routine circumcision of normal male infants and boys. Sydney.

Jones, Nigel. 1999. *Rupert Brooke: Life, death and myth.* London: Richard Cohen Books.

Jordan, Mark. 1997. *The invention of sodomy in Christian theology.* Chicago: University of Chicago Press.

Jordanova, Ludmilla. 1987. The popularization of medicine: Tissot on onanism. *Textual Practice* 1: 68–80.

Keele, K. D. 1968. Clinical medicine. In *Medicine and science in the 1860s*, ed. F. N. L. Poynter. London: Wellcome Institute for the History of Medicine.

Kellogg, J. H. 1888. *Plain facts for young and old: Embracing the natural history of hygiene and organic life.* Facsimile reprint of the 2nd ed. (Burlington, IA). New York: Arno, 1974.

Kempe, J. Arthur. 1878. Phimosis as a cause of rupture in children. *Lancet*, 27 July, 119–20.

Keynes, Geoffrey, ed., 1966. *The complete writings of William Blake*. Oxford: Oxford University Press.

———. 1981. *The gates of memory*. Oxford: Clarendon Press.

King, F. Truby. 1930. *The expectant mother and baby's first months*. London: Macmillan.

———. 1931. *Feeding and care of baby*. London: Macmillan.

Kinsey, Alfred, Wardell Pomeroy, and Clyde Martin. 1948. *Sexual behavior in the human male*. Philadelphia: W. B. Saunders.

Kiple, Kenneth, ed. 1993. *Cambridge world history of human disease*. Cambridge: Cambridge University Press.

Kistler, S. L. 1910. Rapid bloodless circumcision. *Journal of the American Medical Association* 54 (28 May): 1782–83.

Knott, John. 1906. Literary notes: John Knott on circumcision. *British Medical Journal*, 25 August, 441.

Knowlton, Charles. 1877. *Fruits of philosophy: An essay on the population question*. 2nd new ed., with introduction by Charles Bradlaugh and Annie Besant. London: Freethought Publishing.

Kolmer, John A. 1912. Diphtheroid bacilli of the penis, with report of two cases of diphtheria following circumcision. *Archives of Paediatrics* 19: 94–101.

Laisser faire and its results. 1870. Editorial. *British Medical Journal*, 20 August, 193–95.

Lallemand, Claude-François. 1858. *A practical treatise on the causes, symptoms and treatment of spermatorrhoea*. Trans. and ed. Henry J. McDougall. 3rd American ed. Philadelphia: Blanchard and Lea.

Lancet. 1837. Editorial. 30 September, 20.

———. 1860. Letter. 28 April, 436.

———. 1862. Review of Acton, *Functions and disorders*, 3rd ed. 17 May, 518.

———. 1866a. Editorial. 8 December, 689.

———. 1866b. Letters. 23 June, 699; 14 July, 52; 22 December, 710.

———. 1866c. Review of Baker Brown, *On the curability of certain forms of insanity, epilepsy, catalepsy and hysteria in females*. 5 May, 485–86.

———. 1867. Letter. 5 January, 29.

———. 1873. Obituary of Isaac Baker Brown. 8 February, 222–23.

———. 1876a. Debate on syphilis. 8 April 1876, 636.

———. 1876b. Editorials. 1 April, 509; 8 April, 542–43.

———. 1882. Survey of doctors. 23 September, 513.

———. 1888. Review of Sayre, *On the deleterious results of a narrow prepuce*. 22 December, 1401.

———. 1891. Review of Snow, *Barbarity of circumcision*. 20 June, 1386.

———. 1936. Obituary of John Bland-Sutton. 26 December, 1546–47.

Lane, E. W. 1873. *Old medicine and new*. London: Churchill.

Langmead, Frederick. 1913. Enuresis nocturna. *Medical Annual*, 222–25.

Laqueur, Thomas. 1987. Orgasm, generation and the politics of reproductive biology. In *The making of the modern body: Sexuality and society in the nineteenth century*, ed. Catherine Gallagher and Thomas Laqueur. Berkeley: University of California Press.

———. 1989. Amor veneris, vel dulcedo appeletur. In *Fragments for a history of the human body*, ed. Michel Feher, with Ramona Naddaff and Nadia Tazi, vol. 3. New York: Zone.

———. 1990. *Making sex: Body and gender from the Greeks to Freud*. Cambridge: Harvard University Press.

———. 2003. *Solitary sex: A cultural history of masturbation*. New York: Zone Books.

Lawrence, A. W., ed. 1929. *Captives of Tipu: Survivors' narratives*. London: Jonathan Cape.

Lawrence, Christopher. 1985. Incommunicable knowledge: Science, technology and the clinical art in Britain, 1850-1914. *Journal of Contemporary History* 20: 503-20.

——. 1992a. Democratic, divine and heroic: The story and historiography of surgery. In *Medical theory, surgical practice: Studies in the history of medicine*, ed. Christopher Lawrence. London: Routledge.

——, ed. 1992b. *Medical theory, surgical practice: Studies in the history of medicine*. London: Routledge.

Lawrence, Christopher, and Richard Dixey. 1992. Practising on principle: Joseph Lister and the germ theories of disease. In *Medical theory, surgical practice: Studies in the history of medicine*, ed. Christopher Lawrence, 153-215. London: Routledge.

Lay criticism of medical affairs. 1898. *Lancet*, 19 November, 1344-45.

Le Fanu, James. 1999. *The rise and fall of modern medicine*. Boston: Little Brown.

Lehmann, John. 1985. *In the purely pagan sense*. London: Gay Men's Press. (Orig. pub. 1976.)

Leitch, I. O. W. 1970. Circumcision: A continuing enigma. *Australian Paediatric Journal* 6: 59-65.

Lewis, Joseph. 1949. *In the name of humanity*. New York: Freethought Press.

Lewis, Milton. 1998. *Thorns on the rose: The history of sexually transmitted diseases in Australia in international perspective*. Canberra: Australian Government Publishing Service.

Lewis, Peter. 1991. Mummy, matron and the maids: Feminine presence and absence in male institutions, 1934-63. In *Manful assertions: Masculinities in Britain since 1800*, ed. Michael Roper and John Tosh. London: Routledge.

Lipman, V. D. 1990. *A history of the Jews in Britain since 1858*. Leicester, UK: Leicester University Press.

Little, Fletcher. 1883. Letter. *British Medical Journal*, 3 March, 417.

Littleton, Thomas. 1866. Letter. *British Medical Journal*, 19 May, 537.

Lloyd, V. E., and N. L. Lloyd. 1934. Circumcision and syphilis. *British Medical Journal*, 27 January, 144-46.

——. 1935. Letter. *British Medical Journal*, 5 October, 642.

London Infirmary for Epilepsy and Paralysis. 1867. Cases of epilepsy with complications; Remarks upon treatment. *Lancet* 1 (16 February): 208.

Lord, Alexandra M. 2001. Puberty. In *Encyclopedia of European Social History, 1350-2000*, ed. Peter Stearns, 4:269-78. New York: Scribner.

Lorence, Bogna W. 1974. Parents and children in eighteenth-century Europe. *History of Childhood Quarterly* 2: 1-30.

Lyttelton, Edward. 1887. *The causes and prevention of immorality in schools*. London: privately printed; copies distributed by Rev. R. A. Bullen, St. Margaret's Westminster.

——. 1900. *Training of the young in laws of sex*. London: Longmans.

Maas, Henry, ed. 1971. *The letters of A. E. Housman*. London.

MacCarthy, D., J. W. B. Douglas, and C. Mogford. 1952. Circumcision in a national sample of four-year-old children. *British Medical Journal*, 4 October, 755-56.

MacDonald, Robert H. 1967. The frightful consequences of onanism: Notes on the history of a delusion. *Journal of the History of Ideas* 28: 423-31.

Macleod, Neil. 1883. An improved method of circumcision for congenital phimosis. *Edinburgh Medical Journal* 28: 807-8.

Maguire, Robert. 1885. *A practical treatise on urinary and renal disorders*. London: Smith Elder.

Maimonides, Moses ben Maimon. 1963. *Guide for the perplexed*. Trans. Shlomo Pines. Chicago: University of Chicago Press.

Malthus, Thomas. 1803. *An essay on the principle of population*. Ed. Donald Winch. Cambridge: Cambridge University Press, 1992.

Mangan, J. A., and James Walvin, eds. 1987. *Manliness and morality: Middle-class masculinity in Britain and America, 1800-1940*. Manchester, UK: Manchester University Press.

Marcus, Steven. 1966. *The other Victorians: A study of sexuality and pornography in mid-nineteenth-century England*. London: Weidenfeld and Nicolson.

Marr, Lisa. 1998. *Sexually transmitted diseases*. Baltimore: Johns Hopkins University Press.

Marshall, F. H. A. 1910. *The physiology of reproduction*. London: Longmans Green.

Marten, John. 1708. *A treatise of all the degrees and symptoms of the venereal disease, in both sexes*. Facsimile reprint of the 6th London ed. New York: Garland, 1985.

———. 1709. *Gonosologium novum: Or a new system of all the secret infirmities and diseases, natural, accidental and venereal in men and women*. Facsimile reprint of London ed. New York: Garland, 1985.

Mason, Michael. 1994a. *The making of Victorian sexual attitudes*. Oxford: Oxford University Press.

———. 1994b. *The making of Victorian sexuality*. Oxford: Oxford University Press.

Masturbation in a child. 1901. *British Medical Journal*, 20 April, 1000.

Maudsley, Henry. 1866. Letters. *Lancet*, 1 December, 617; *British Medical Journal*, 22 December, 705.

Maurice, Sir Frederick. 1903. National health: A soldier's study. *Contemporary Review* 83: 41-56.

Mayer, E., D. J. Caruso, M. Ankem, et al. 2003. Anatomic variants associated with newborn circumcision complications. *Canadian Journal of Urology* 10: 2013-16.

McGrath, Ken. 2001. The frenular delta: A new preputial structure. In *Understanding circumcision: A multi-disciplinary approach to a multi-dimensional problem*, ed. George C. Denniston, Frederick Hodges, and Marilyn Milos. New York: Kluwer Academic/Plenum Press.

McGrath, Ken, and Hugh Young. 2001. A review of circumcision in New Zealand. In *Understanding circumcision: A multi-disciplinary approach to a multi-dimensional problem*, ed. George C. Denniston, Frederick Hodges, and Marilyn Milos. New York: Kluwer Academic/Plenum Press.

McHugh, Paul. 1980. *Prostitution and Victorian social reform*. London: Croom Helm.

McLaren, Angus. 1984. *Reproductive rituals: The perception of fertility in England*. London: Methuen.

———. 1991. *A history of contraception: From antiquity to the present*. Oxford: Blackwell.

Meadows, Alfred. 1867. Letter. *Medical Times and Gazette*, 5 January, 16.

Medical Annual. 1895, 1905, 1915. London.

Medical Press. 1900. Editorial. 19 September, 304.

Medical Press and Circular. 1871. Review of F. B. Courtenay, *On Spermatorrhoea*. 21 June, 541.

Medical Times and Gazette. 1867a. Letter. 19 January, 79.

———. 1867b. Report of the meeting on 3 April 1867 of the Obstetrical Society to consider the expulsion of Baker Brown. 6 April, 366-78.

Miller, Albert. 1899. The evils of the ritual practice of circumcision. *Medical Record* 56 (26 August): 302-3.

Miller, Geoffrey. 2002. Circumcision: Cultural-legal analysis. *Virginia Journal of Social Policy and the Law* 9: 497-585.

Miller, Toby. 1995. A short history of the penis. *Social Text* 43: 1-26.

Milton, John L. 1852. Spermatorrhoea. *Medical Times and Gazette*, n.s., 4: 241-42.

———. 1854. On the nature and treatment of spermatorrhoea. *Lancet* 1: 243-46, 269-70, 467-68, 595-96.

———. 1873. Some remarks on the history and origin of syphilis. *Edinburgh Medical Journal* 19 (July): 1–15.

Money, Angel. 1887. *Treatment of disease in children.* London: H. K. Lewis.

Morris, Brian. 1999. *In favour of circumcision.* Sydney: New South Wales University Press.

Morris, Henry. 1895. Injuries and diseases of the testes, scrotum and penis. In *A system of surgery,* ed. Frederick Treves, 956–1017. London: Cassell.

Morris, Malcolm. 1897. The progress of medicine during the Queen's reign. *Nineteenth Century* 49: 739–58.

Morris, Robert T. 1892. Is evolution trying to do away with the clitoris? *Transactions of the American Association of Obstetricians and Gynaecologists* 5: 288–302.

Mort, Frank. 1987. *Dangerous sexualities: Medico-moral politics in England since 1830.* London: Routledge.

Moscucci, Ornella. 1991. *The science of woman: Gynaecology and gender in England, 1800–1929.* Cambridge: Cambridge University Press.

———. 1996. Clitoridectomy, circumcision and the politics of sexual pleasure in mid-Victorian Britain. In *Sexualities in Victorian Britain,* ed. Andrew H. Miller and James Eli Adams. Bloomington: Indiana University Press.

Moses, M. J. 1871. The value of circumcision as a hygienic and therapeutic measure. *New York Medical Journal* 14 (October): 368–74.

Munro, Hector. 1930. *The short stories of Saki.* London: Bodley Head.

Musalman [pseud.]. 1903. Letter. *British Medical Journal,* 17 October, 1028.

Neuman, R. 1975. Masturbation, madness and the modern concepts of childhood and adolescence. *Journal of Social History* 8: 1–27.

———. 1978. The priests of the body and masturbatory insanity in the late nineteenth century. *Psychohistory Review* 6: 21–32.

Newman, Sir George. 1932. *The rise of preventive medicine.* London: Oxford University Press.

New South Wales Supreme Court. 1916. Testimony of A. A. Palmer, Chief Medical Officer of New South Wales, at the hearing of William Chidley's appeal against committal for insanity. May–June. State Records of New South Wales, Court Reporting Office. Transcripts of Evidence, 1899–1960, 6/1041, p. 538.

Nichols, T. L. 1873. *Esoteric anthropology: The mysteries of man.* London: Dr. Nichols at the Hygienic Institute.

Nield, Keith, ed. 1973. *Prostitution in the Victorian age: Debates on the issue from nineteenth-century critical journals.* Westmead, U.K.: Gregg International.

The Obstetrical Society and Mr. Baker Brown. 1867. Editorial. *Medical Times and Gazette,* 6 April, 356–59.

O'Donnell, Hugh. 2001. A century of circumcision in America. Paper. Sydney. Available at http://www.historyofcircumcision.net.

O'Farrell, Charles. 1888. Circumcision in enuresis. *Lancet,* 2 July, 112.

The offending foreskin. 1952. Editorial. *British Medical Journal,* 4 October, 766.

O'Hara, K., and J. O'Hara. 1999. The effect of circumcision on the sexual enjoyment of the female partner. *BJU International* 83 (suppl. 1) (January): 79–84.

Oldroyd, D. R. 1983. *Darwinian impacts: An introduction to the Darwinian revolution.* 2nd ed. Sydney: New South Wales University Press.

Onania: Or the heinous sin of self pollution and all its frightful consequences considered, with spiritual and physical advice to those who have already injured themselves by this abominable practice. Ca. 1716. Facsimile reprint of the 1724 Boston ed. In *The secret vice exposed: Some arguments against masturbation.* New York: Arno, 1974.

The operation of excision of the clitoris. 1866. Editorial. *Lancet,* 22 December, 697–98.

Oppenheim, Janet. 1991. *Shattered nerves: Doctors, patients and depression in Victorian England*. New York: Oxford University Press.

Oriel, J. D. 1994. *Scars of Venus: A history of venereology*. London: Springer.

Origins of circumcision. *British Medical Journal*, 24 December 1904, 1704–5.

Orwell, George. 1998. *The complete works of George Orwell*. 20 vols. Ed. Peter Davison. London: Secker and Warburg.

Osmond, T. E. 1953. Is routine circumcision desirable? *Journal of the Royal Army Medical Corps* 99: 253–54.

Owen, Edmund. 1880. Certain practical points in connection with the surgery of childhood. *British Medical Journal*, 28 February, 313–14.

———. 1897. *The surgical diseases of children*. 3rd ed. London: Cassell.

Owen, Robert Dale. 1841. *Moral physiology: Or a plain and brief treatise on the population question*. 5th ed. London: J. Watson.

Paget, James. 1879. Sexual hypochondriasis. In *Clinical lectures and essays*, 2nd ed., ed. Howard March. London: Longmans.

Pankhurst, Christabel. 1913. *The great scourge and how to end it*. London: the author.

Parker, Geoffrey. 1950. Letter. *British Medical Journal*, 21 January, 181.

Parker, Peter. 1987. *The old lie: The Great War and the public school ethos*. London: Constable.

Parker, Robert. 1879. Dilatation of the prepuce versus circumcision. *British Medical Journal*, 19 July, 86–87.

Parkin, George. 1898. *Edward Thring: Headmaster of Uppingham School: Diary and letters*. 2 vols. London: Macmillan. Microfiche, Canadian Institute for Historical Reproductions, 1981.

Parry, Noel, and José Parry. 1976. *The rise of the medical profession: A study of collective social mobility*. London: Croom Helm.

Parsons, Gail Pat. 1977. Equal treatment for all: American medical remedies for male sexual problems, 1850–1900. *Journal of the History of Medicine and Allied Sciences* 32: 55–71.

Peachey, Dr. 1890. Letter. *British Medical Journal*, 11 January 1890, 116.

Pearn, John. 2001. The final common path: Muscle action and the evolution of knowledge concerning neuro-muscular disease. Meryon Lecture, Worcester College, Oxford.

Pelling, Margaret. 1993. Contagion/germ theory/specificity. In *Companion encyclopaedia to the history of medicine*, ed. W. F. Bynum and Roy Porter. London: Routledge.

Peterson, M. Jeanne. 1978. *The medical profession in mid-Victorian London*. Berkeley: University of California Press.

———. 1986. Dr. Acton's enemy: Medicine, sex, and society in Victorian England. *Victorian Studies* 29: 569–90.

Peterson, Shane. 2001. Assaulted and mutilated: A personal account of circumcision trauma. In *Understanding circumcision: A multi-disciplinary approach to a multi-dimensional problem*, ed. George C. Denniston, Frederick Hodges, and Marilyn Milos. New York: Kluwer Academic/Plenum Press.

Phillips, Benjamin. 1842–43. Observations on seminal and other discharges from the urethra. *London Medical Gazette*, n.s., 1: 451–56, 584–88.

———. 1845. Further remarks on spermatic discharges. *London Medical Gazette*, n.s., 1: 17–19.

———. 1847. Clinical observations . . . on urethral affections. *London Medical Gazette*, n.s., 4: 177–81.

———. 1848. Further observations on spermatic discharges. *London Medical Gazette*, n.s., 6: 489–93.

Philo of Alexandria. 1937. Of the special laws. In *Works of Philo*, trans. F. H. Colson, 1:2. Loeb Classical Library, vol. 7.

Pickop, John. 1866. Letter. *Lancet*, 14 July, 52.

Plumb, J. H. 1975. The new world of children in eighteenth-century England. *Past and Present*, no. 67, 64–93.

Porter, Roy. 1982a. Mixed feelings: The Enlightenment and sexuality in eighteenth-century Britain. In *Sexuality in eighteenth-century Britain*, ed. Paul-Gabriel Bouce. Manchester, UK: Manchester University Press.

———. 1982b. Was there a medical enlightenment in eighteenth-century England? *British Journal for Eighteenth Century Studies* 5: 49–63.

———. 1987. "The secrets of generation display'd": *Aristotle's master-piece* in eighteenth-century England. In *"Tis nature's fault": Unauthorised sexuality during the Enlightenment*, ed. Robert MacCubbin. Cambridge: Cambridge University Press.

———. 1991. History of the body. In *New Perspectives on historical writing*, ed. Peter Burke, 203–32. Cambridge, MA: Polity Press.

———. 1993. The rise of the physical examination. In *Medicine and the five senses*, ed. W. F. Bynum and Roy Porter. Cambridge: Cambridge University Press.

———. 1994. The literature of sexual advice before 1800. In *Sexual knowledge, sexual science: The history of attitudes to sexuality*, ed. Roy Porter and Mikulas Teich. Cambridge: Cambridge University Press.

———. 2000. *Enlightenment: Britain and the creation of the modern world*. London: Allen Lane.

Porter, Roy, and Lesley Hall. 1995. *The facts of life: Sexual knowledge in Britain, 1650–1950*. New Haven: Yale University Press.

Porter, Roy, and Mikulas Teich, eds. 1994. *Sexual knowledge, sexual science: The history of attitudes to sexuality*. Cambridge: Cambridge University Press.

Powell, Arthur. 1901. The comparative frequency of syphilis among the circumcised and uncircumcised. *British Medical Journal*, 9 November, 1409.

Poynter, F. N. L., ed. 1968. *Medicine and science in the 1860s*. London: Wellcome Institute for the History of Medicine.

Pratt, William. 1872. *A physician's sermon to young men*. London: Bailliere, Tindall and Cox.

Preuss, Julius. 1911. *Biblical and Talmudic medicine*. Trans. Fred Rosner. Northvale, NJ: Jason Aronson Inc., 1993.

Proceedings of the Council of Florence. 1438–45. Available at http://www.ewtn.com/library/councils/Florence.htm.

A provincial FRCP. 1866. *British Medical Journal*, 5 May, 478.

Pusey, E. B. 1866. Letters. *Times*, 11 December, 4b; 15 December 1866, 12d.

———. 1867. Letter. *Medical Times and Gazette*, 2 February, 126.

Quaife, W. F. 1896. Tinnitus connected with onanism. *Australasian Medical Gazette* 15 (20 January): 20–22.

Quain, Richard. 1894. *A dictionary of medicine*. 3rd ed. 2 vols. London: Longmans Green.

Ravich, Abraham. 1973. *Preventing VD and cancer by circumcision*. New York: Philosophical Library.

Recent works on venereal diseases. 1860–61. *Edinburgh Medical Journal* 6: 635–50, 911–35.

Remondino, P. C. 1891. *History of circumcision from the earliest times to the present: Moral and physical reasons for its performance*. Philadelphia: F. A. Davis.

Reynolds, S. J., M. E. Shepherd, A. R. Risbud, et al. 2004. Male circumcision and risk of HIV-1 and other sexually transmitted diseases in India. *Lancet* 363: 1039–40.

Richardson, Benjamin Ward. 1878. *Disease of modern life*. 5th ed. London: Macmillan.

Rickwood, A. M. K. 1999. Indications for paediatric circumcision. *BJU International* 83 (supp. 1) (January): 45–51.

Ricord, Philippe. 1842. *A practical treatise on venereal diseases*. Trans. from the French. New York: Gordon. Reprint, Birmingham, AL: Gryphon Editions, 1988.

———. 1847. Lecture V: Remarks on the treatment of blenorrhagia . . . operations for phimosis and paraphimosis. *Lancet* (2): 570.

———. 1847–48. Lectures on venereal and other diseases arising from sexual intercourse. *Lancet* 2 (1847); 1 (1848).

———. 1848. Lecture XXVIII: Recapitulation. *Lancet* (1): 682.

Risse, Gunter B. 1992. Medicine in the age of Enlightenment. In *Medicine in society: Historical essays*, ed. Andrew Wear. Cambridge: Cambridge University Press.

Ritual circumcision. 1874. *Lancet*, 5 December, 823.

A ritual operation. 1949. Editorial. *British Medical Journal*, 24 December, 1458.

Roberton, N. R. C. 1999. Care of the normal term newborn baby. In *Textbook of neonatology*, ed. Janet M. Rennie and N. R. C. Roberton. 3rd ed. Edinburgh: Churchill Livingston.

Robinson, Fred Byron. 1893. The intimate nervous connection of the genito-urinary organs with the cerebro-spinal and sympathetic systems. *New York Medical Journal*, 11 March, 261–64.

Robinson, William J. 1915. Circumcision and masturbation. *Medical World*: 390.

Romberg, Rosemary. 1985. *Circumcision: The painful dilemma.* South Hadley, MA: Bergin and Garvey.

Roper, Michael, and John Tosh, eds. 1991. *Manful assertions: Masculinities in Britain since 1800.* London: Routledge.

Rosebury, Theodor. 1971. *Microbes and morals: The strange story of venereal disease.* London: Secker and Warburg.

Rosenman, Ellen Bayuk. 2003. Body doubles: The spermatorrhoea panic. *Journal of the History of Sexuality* 12: 365–99.

Roth, Philip. 1969. *Portnoy's complaint.* New York: Penguin, 1970.

Routh, Dr. 1867. Letter. *Lancet*, 5 January, 28–29.

Rowlandson, Thomas. 1969. *The amorous illustrations of Thomas Rowlandson.* Ed. Gert Schiff. New York: Cythera Press.

Royal Australasian College of Physicians [RACP]. 2002. Policy statement on circumcision. Sydney: Royal Australasian College of Physicians. September. Available at http://www .racp.edu.au/hpu/paed/circumcision/index.htm.

Royal Commission on Venereal Diseases. 1916. *Final report of the commissioners.* Parliamentary Papers, vol. 16. Great Britain.

Royde, C. A. 1950. Letter. *British Medical Journal*, 21 January, 182.

Rutherford, Jonathan. 1997. *Forever England: Reflections on masculinity and empire.* London: Lawrence and Wishart.

Ryerson, Alice. 1961. Medical advice on child rearing, 1550–1900. *Harvard Educational Review* 31: 302–23.

Sawday, Ernest. 1944. Letter. *British Medical Journal*, 30 December, 876.

Scheper-Hughes, Nancy. 1991. Virgin territory: The male discovers the clitoris. *Medical Anthropology Quarterly* 5: 25–28.

Schleiner, Winfried. 1995. *Medical ethics in the Renaissance.* Washington, DC: Georgetown University Press.

Schultheiss, D., J. J. Mattelaer, and F. M. Hodges. 2003. Preputial infibulation: From ancient medicine to modern genital piercing. *BJU International* 92: 758–63.

Schwartz, Hillel. 1986. *Never satisfied: A cultural history of diets, fantasies and fat.* New York: Free Press.

Scull, A., and D. Favreau. 1986. A chance to cut is a chance to cure: Sexual surgery for psychosis in three nineteenth-century societies. *Research in Law, Deviance and Social Control* 8: 3–39.

Sexual disorders. 1870. Editorial. *Lancet*, 30 July, 159-60.

Sexual ignorance. 1885. Editorial. *British Medical Journal*, 15 August, 303-4.

Shapiro, James. 1996. *Shakespeare and the Jews*. New York: Columbia University Press.

Sharp, Jane. 1671. *The midwives' book: Or the whole art of midwifery discovered*. Facsimile reprint. New York: Garland, 1985.

Sheehan, Elizabeth A. 1997. Victorian clitoridectomy: Isaac Baker Brown and his harmless operation. In *The gender/sexuality reader: Culture, history, political economy*, ed. Roger N. Lancaster and Micaela di Leonardo. London: Routledge.

Sheppard, Edgar. Letter. *Lancet*, 1 April, 518.

Shettle, R. C. 1867. Letter. *Lancet*, 19 January, 98.

Shoemaker, Robert. 1998. *Gender in English society: The emergence of separate spheres?* London: Longmans.

Shorter, Edward. 1992. *From paralysis to fatigue: A history of psychosomatic illness in the modern era*. New York: Free Press.

———. 1994. *From the mind to the body: The cultural origins of psychosomatic symptoms*. New York: Free Press.

Shortt, S. E. D. 1983. Physicians, science, and status: Issues in the professionalization of Anglo-American medicine in the nineteenth century. *Medical History* 27: 51-68.

Shryock, R. H. 1948. *The development of modern medicine*. London: Gollancz.

Simon, John. 1874. Filth diseases and their prevention. Report of the Medical Officer of the Privy Council and Local Government Board. Parliamentary Papers. Great Britain.

Sinclair, W. W. 1889. On circumcision. *Lancet*, 20 April, 783.

Singy, Patrick. 2003. Friction of the genitals and secularization of morality. *Journal of the History of Sexuality* 12: 345-64.

———. 2004. The history of masturbation. Review of Thomas Laqueur, *Solitary sex*. *Journal of the History of Medicine and Allied Sciences* 59: 112-21.

Skidelsky, Robert. 1983. *John Maynard Keynes: A biography*. Vol. 1, Hopes betrayed, 1883-1920. London: Macmillan.

Smith, F. B. 1976. Labouchere's amendment to the Criminal Law Amendment Bill. *Historical Studies* 17: 165-76.

———. 1977. Sexuality in Britain, 1800-1900: Some suggested revisions. In *A widening sphere: Changing roles of Victorian women*, ed. Martha Vicinus. Bloomington: Indiana University Press.

———. 1979. *The people's health, 1830-1910*. Canberra: Australian National University Press.

Snow, Herbert. 1890. *The barbarity of circumcision as a remedy for congenital abnormality*. London: Churchill.

Solomons, Dr. 1920. Letter. *British Medical Journal* 5 June, 768.

Somerville, Margaret A. 2000. Altering baby boys' bodies: The ethics of infant male circumcision. In *The ethical canary: Science, society and the human spirit*. Toronto: Viking/Penguin.

Soper, William. 1867. Letter. *Medical Times and Gazette*, 2 February, 133.

Spencer, Herbert. 1895. Professional institutions. II. Physician and surgeon. *Contemporary Review* 67 (June): 898-908.

Spilsbury, K., J. B. Semmens, Z. S. Wisniewski, and C. D. Holman. 2003a. Circumcision for phimosis and other medical indications in Western Australian boys. *Medical Journal of Australia* 178 (17 February): 155-58.

———. 2003b. Routine circumcision practice in Western Australia, 1981-1999. *ANZ Journal of Surgery* 73: 610-14.

Spitz, René A. 1952. Authority and masturbation: Some remarks on a bibliographical investigation. *Psychoanalytic Quarterly* 21: 490-527.

Spratling, Edgar. 1895. Masturbation in the adult. *Medical Record* 48: 442-43.

Springhall, John. 1987. Building character in the British boy: The attempt to extend Christian manliness to working class adolescents, 1880-1914. In *Manliness and morality: Middle-class masculinity in Britain and America, 1800-1940*, ed. J. A. Mangan and James Walvin. Manchester, UK: Manchester University Press.

Springthorpe, John. 1884. On the psychological aspect of the sexual appetite. *Australasian Medical Gazette* 4 (October): 8-13.

Stall, Sylvanus, D.D. Ca. 1900. *What a young husband ought to know.* Philadelphia, London, and Toronto: Vir Publishing.

———. 1904. *What a young man ought to know.* Philadelphia, London, and Toronto: Vir Publishing. (Orig. pub. 1897.)

———. 1909. *What a young boy ought to know.* Philadelphia, London, and Toronto: Vir Publishing. (Orig. pub. 1897.)

Stanley, Liz, ed. 1995. *Sex surveyed, 1949-1994: From Mass Observation's Little Kinsey to the National Survey and the Hite reports.* London: Taylor and Francis.

Stearns, Carol, and Peter Stearns. 1985. Victorian sexuality: Can historians do it better? *Journal of Social History* 18: 625-34.

Steinberg, Leo. 1996. *The sexuality of Christ in renaissance art and in later oblivion.* 2nd ed. Chicago: University of Chicago Press. (Orig. pub. 1984.)

Stengers, Jean, and Anne van Neck. 2001. *Masturbation: The history of a great terror.* New York: Palgrave.

Stevenson, David. 2000. Recording the unspeakable: Masturbation in the diary of William Drummond, 1657-1659. *Journal of the History of Sexuality* 9: 223-39.

Stevenson, Lloyd. 1955. Science down the drain: On the hostility of certain sanitarians to animal experimentation, bacteriology, and immunology. *Bulletin of the History of Medicine* 29: 1-26.

Stolberg, Michael. 2000a. Self-pollution, moral reform and the venereal trade: Notes on the sources and historical context of *Onania. Journal of the History of Sexuality* 9: 37-61.

———. 2000b. An unmanly vice: Self-pollution, anxiety and the body in the eighteenth century. *Social History of Medicine* 13: 1-21.

Stone, Lawrence. 1977. *The family, sex and marriage in England, 1500-1800.* New York: Harper and Row.

Sykes, Alan H. 1995. *The doctors in Vanity Fair.* London: the author.

Symonds, J. A. 1984. *The memoirs of John Addington Symonds.* Ed. Phyllis Grosskurth. London: Hutchinson.

Szasz, Thomas. 1971. *The manufacture of madness.* London: Paladin.

———. 1996. Neonatal circumcision: Symbol of the birth of the therapeutic state. *Journal of Medicine and Philosophy* 21: 137-48.

Szreter, Simon. 1988. The importance of social intervention in Britain's mortality decline, ca. 1850-1914: A reinterpretation of the role of public health. *Social History of Medicine* 1: 1-37.

———. 1996a. *Fertility, class, and gender in Britain, 1860-1940.* Cambridge: Cambridge University Press.

———. 1996b. Victorian Britain, 1837-1963: Towards a social history of sexuality. *Journal of Victorian Culture* 1: 136-47.

Tait, Lawson. 1889. *Diseases of women and abdominal surgery.* Leicester, UK: Richardson and Co.

Tanner, T. Hawkes. 1866. On excision of the clitoris as a cure for hysteria etc. *British Medical Journal*, 15 December, 672-75.

Taylor, D. J. 2000. *Thackeray: The life of a literary man*. London: Pimlico.

Taylor, H. Coupland. 1883. The treatment of spermatorrhoea. *British Medical Journal,* 24 March, 562.

Taylor, J. R., A. P. Lockwood, and A. J. Taylor. 1996. The prepuce: Specialized mucosa of the penis and its loss to circumcision. *British Journal of Urology* 77: 291-95.

Taylor, R. W. 1873. On the question of the transmission of syphilitic contagion in the rite of circumcision. *New York Medical Journal* 18: 561-82.

Teale, Mr. 1883. Letter. *British Medical Journal,* 14 April, 720.

Temkin, Owsei. 1973. *Galenism: Rise and decline of a medial philosophy*. Ithaca, NY: Cornell University Press.

Thomas, Robert. 1816. *The modern practice of physic*. 5th ed. London.

Thompson, E. P. 1968. *The making of the English working class*. Rev. ed. Harmondsworth: Pelican Books.

———. 1991. *Customs in common*. New York: Penguin.

Thompson, Henry. 1852. Nitrate of silver in spermatorrhoea, and a new instrument for applying it. *Lancet* 1: 89-90.

Thomson, Matthew. 2001. Neurasthenia in Britain: An overview. In *Cultures of neurasthenia from Beard to the First World War,* ed. Marijke Gijswijt-Hofstra and Roy Porter, 77-96. Amsterdam: Rodopi.

Three treatises on child rearing. 1985. Walter Harris, *A treatise of the acute diseases of infants* (1742); *The nurses' guide: Or the right method of bringing up young children* (1729); and William Cadogan, *An essay upon nursing and the management of children, from their birth to three years of age* (1750). Facsimile reprint. New York: Garland.

Tissot, S.-A. 1974. *Onanism: A treatise on the diseases produced by masturbation*. Trans. by a physician. Facsimile reprint of the 1832 New York ed. In *The secret vice exposed: Some arguments against masturbation.* New York: Arno. (*Onanism* orig. pub. in English in 1758.)

Tosh, John. 1991. Domesticity and manliness in the Victorian middle class: The family of Edward White Benson. In *Manful assertions: Masculinities in Britain since 1800,* ed. Michael Roper and John Tosh. London: Routledge.

———. 1999. *A man's place: Masculinity and the middle-class home in Victorian England*. New Haven: Yale University Press.

Towers, Bernard. 1968. The impact of Darwin's *Origin of species* on medicine and biology. In *Medicine and science in the 1860s,* ed. F. N. L. Poynter. London: Wellcome Institute for the History of Medicine.

Townsend, Joanne. 1999. Private diseases in public discourse: Venereal disease in Victorian society, culture and imagination. PhD diss., University of Melbourne.

Treves, Frederick, ed. 1895. *A system of surgery*. 2 vols. London: Cassell.

Trumbach, Randolph. 1998. *Sex and the gender revolution*. Vol. 1, *Heterosexuality and the third gender in Enlightenment London*. Chicago: University of Chicago Press.

Tuke, D. Hack, ed. 1892. *A dictionary of psychological medicine*. London: Churchill.

Van Howe, Robert S. 1998. Circumcision and infectious diseases revisited. *Pediatric Infectious Diseases Journal* 17: 1-6.

———. 1999. Does circumcision influence sexually transmitted diseases? A literature review. *BJU International* 83 (suppl. 1) (January): 52-62.

Venette, Nicolas de. 1712. *The mysteries of conjugal love reveal'd*. Done into English by a gentleman. 3rd ed. London. Reprint, Paris: Charles Carrington, 1906.

Vitkus, Daniel. 2000. *Three Turk plays from early modern England*. New York: Columbia University Press.

———. 2001. *Piracy, slavery, and redemption: Barbary captivity narratives from early modern England*. New York: Columbia University Press.

Wagner, Peter. 1983. The veil of medicine and morality: Some pornographic aspects of *Onania*. *British Journal for Eighteenth Century Studies* 6:179–84.

———. 1988. *Eros revived: Erotica of the Enlightenment in England and America*. London: Secker and Warburg.

Walkowitz, Judith R. 1980. *Prostitution and Victorian society: Women, class, and the state*. Cambridge: Cambridge University Press.

Wallerstein, Edward. 1980. *Circumcision: An American health fallacy*. New York: Springer.

Walter [pseud.]. 1888–92. *My secret life*. 3 vols. London: Arrow Books.

Wan, Julian. 2002. Gomco circumcision clamp: An enduring and unexpected success. *Urology* 59:790–94.

Watson, Patrick Heron. 1860. Recent works on venereal disease. *Edinburgh Medical Journal* 6:635–50, 911–35.

Watters, Greg, and Stephen Carroll. 2003. Just like dad: Maternal attitudes to neonatal circumcision in an Anglo-Celtic settler society. Paper given at the Urological Society of Australasia, Annual Scientific Meeting, Queenstown, New Zealand. March.

Wear, Andrew. 1993. The history of personal hygiene. In *Companion encyclopaedia to the history of medicine*, ed. W. F. Bynum and Roy Porter, 1283–1308. London: Routledge.

Webster, Richard. 1995. *Why Freud was wrong: Sin, science, and psychoanalysis*. London: Fontana.

Weeks, Jeffrey. 1981. *Sex, politics, and society: The regulation of sexuality since 1800*. London: Longmans.

Wehrbein, H. L. 1935. Therapy in gonorrhoea: An historical review. *Annals of Medical History*, n.s., 7.

Weiss, Gerald N. 1997. Prophylactic neonatal surgery and infectious diseases. *Pediatric Infectious Diseases Journal* 16:727–34.

Weisse, H. V. 1904. The religion of the schoolboy. *Contemporary Review* 85:697–706.

West, Charles. 1866. Letter. *Lancet*, 17 November, 560.

———. 1874. *Lectures on the diseases of infancy and childhood*. 6th ed. London: Longmans.

———. 1879. *Lectures on the diseases of women*. 4th ed. Revised by J. Matthews Duncan. London: Churchill.

Whiddon, Daniel. 1953. The Widdicombe file: Should baby be circumcised? *Lancet* 262 (15 August): 337–38.

Whitfield, D. W. 1927. An alternative to circumcision in phimosis. *British Medical Journal*, 29 January, 187.

Williams, A. H. 1935. Letter. *British Medical Journal*, 26 October, 822.

Wilson, Leonard. 1990. The historical decline of tuberculosis in Europe and America: Its causes and significance. *Journal of the History of Medicine and Allied Sciences* 45:366–96.

Wilson, Marris. 1856–57. Contributions to the physiology, pathology, and treatment of spermatorrhoea. *Lancet* (1856): 215–17, 300–302, 482–84, 643–44; (1857): 376–77.

Winter, Alison. 1997. *Mesmerised: Powers of mind in Victorian Britain*. Chicago: University of Chicago Press.

Wirth, J. L. 1980. Current circumcision practices in Canada. *Pediatrics* 66:705–8.

Wohl, Anthony S. 1983. *Endangered lives: Public health in Victorian Britain*. London: Constable.

Wolbarst, Abraham. 1914. Universal circumcision as a sanitary measure. *Journal of the American Medical Association* 62:92–97.

Wolper, Roy. 1982. Circumcision as polemic in the Jew Bill of 1753: The cutter cut. *Eighteenth-Century Life* 7: 28–36.

Worboys, Michael. 2000. *Spreading germs: Disease theories and medical practice in Britain, 1865–1900*. Cambridge: Cambridge University Press.

——. 2004. Unsexing gonorrhoea: Bacteriologists, gynaecologists, and suffragists in Britain, 1860–1920. *Social History of Medicine* 17: 41–59.

Worsley, T. C. 1967. *Flannelled fool: A slice of life in the thirties*. London: Alan Ross.

Wright, J. E. 1967. Non-therapeutic circumcision. *Medical Journal of Australia*, 27 May, 1083–86.

Yellen, Hiram S. 1935. Bloodless circumcision of the newborn. *American Journal of Obstetrics and Gynecology* 30 (July): 146–47.

Yellowlees, D. 1876. Masturbation. *Journal of Mental Science* 22: 336–37.

——. 1892. Masturbation. In *A dictionary of psychological medicine*, ed. D. Hack Tuke, 784–86. London: Churchill.

Youngson, A. J. 1979. *The scientific revolution in Victorian medicine*. Canberra: Australian National University Press.

INDEX

Acton, William: on age of male maturity, 86; cauterization with silver nitrate treatment for spermatorrhea, 134, 176, 179, 181; on congenital phimosis, 220; on continence, 38, 54, 77, 124, 128, 134, 269; on the foreskin, 118, 121, 129, 132-33, 146, 181-82, 328n35; genital hygiene, 131-32, 247, 328n37; glans as site of sexual pleasure, 122; on masturbation, 126, 128, 134, 211, 270-71; medical education of, 123; moral convictions vs. scientific knowledge, 133; on physician's authority, 106, 108; on preventive circumcision, 132-33; *Principles of Human Physiology* (Carpenter), 102; on prostitution, 134, 266-67, 268-69; on semen retention, 11, 12, 57, 126, 127, 179; on sexual activity, 12, 74, 87, 125-26, 134; on spermatorrhea, 134, 173, 176, 177, 179-80, 181-82; on venereal diseases, 79, 110-11, 175, 176, 273, 275
Ainsworth, R., 233, 234, 305
Allen, James, 256-58
antisensualism movement, 54, 56-57, 74, 75, 81, 83-84, 307
Aristotle, 23-24, 34, 40-41, 120, 122, 303, 313
Arnold, Thomas, 193, 195
Arthur, Richard, 90
Asher, Rabbi, 205
Atwell, Samuel, 143-44
Auden, W. H., 297, 299-300
Australia, circumcision in, 314-15
autointoxication theory, 113, 249, 250

Baker Brown, Isaac. *See* Brown, Isaac Baker
Baldwin, Peter, 74-75, 83, 269-70, 275, 336n5, 336n25
Bantock, Granville, 155, 156
Barbarity of Circumcision (Snow), 172, 303
Barnes, Dr., on Baker Brown, 153-54, 160
Beale, Lionel, 190-91
Beard, George, 103, 104
bed-wetting, 139-40, 225, 287
Beggars Benison, 29
Beisel, Nicola, 82, 290
Benjamin, Zoe, 232
Benn, Miriam, 327n21
Bernheim, Dr., 253
Bertwhistle, A. P., 292-93
Beugnies, Dr., on effects of circumcision, 205-6
bilharziasis (schistosomiasis), 256-58, 256-59
Binns, Joseph, 261
birth control. *See* contraception
birth rate, 43, 76, 77, 82, 246
Blackwell, Elizabeth, 301
Bland-Sutton, John: on circumcision, 116, 169, 229, 246, 286-87, 294-95; on the foreskin, 169, 170, 228; obstetric procedures of, 228, 334n50; on phimosis, 228-29
Boerhaave, Hermann, 52
Booth, Charles, 245
Booysen, Cecile, 233
Borneman, Ernest, 333n91
Bouce, Paul-Gabriel, 57
Bristow, Edward, 82, 193

Bristowe, John, 112, 275
British Medical Journal: on circumcision, 115, 172, 202-4, 227, 233-34, 285-86, 288, 300, 303-5, 308-14; on clitoridectomy, 147, 152, 153, 154, 160; Contagious Disease Act endorsed by, 267-68; on Darwinism, 113; glans-foreskin structure in fetus, 228; Ernest Hart and, 241, 267-68; moral tone of, 127; on phimosis as imaginary disease, 233; on physician's authority, 159; on venereal disease, 265, 267
Brooke, Rupert, 81
Brown, Isaac Baker: on clitoridectomy, 104, 142, 144, 151-53, 155-56; critical reviews of, 15, 147, 148, 151-55, 162-63; expulsion from Obstetrical Society, 155-56, 159; informed consent for operations, 153, 156, 158; London Surgical Home, 145, 146; medical background of, 145, 158, 160; nervous disease theory, 144-45, 146
Brown, John, 38, 101, 103
Brown, S. G. A., 253-54
Brown-Sequard, Charles-Edward, 104, 145-46
Bryant, Thomas, 223
Buchan, William, 37, 175, 218, 279
Budd, William, 239
Bulwer, John, 24, 25, 313
Burton, Richard, 4, 32, 144, 206
Butler, Josephine, 268, 269
Bynum, W. F., 10, 112
Byrd, William, 28

Cadell, Francis, 201, 237, 260, 277
Cameron, Charles, 240
Canada, circumcision in, 316-17, 339n16
cancer of the penis, 7, 221, 233, 251, 254-47, 333n22
Cannon, John, 27-28
Cantlie, James, 187-88
Capel, Richard, 47
Carlile, Richard (*Every Woman's Book*), 12
Carpenter, William: rider controlling the horse metaphor, 78-79, 102
Carpenter, William/W. B.: erectile tissue, 120; on foreskin's value, 169-70; on glans' sensitivity, 122, 170; hydraulic concept of finite bodily forces, 127; moral philosophy and medicine, 112; on moral virtues of purity, 127; on mortality from excessive genital manipulation, 128; *Principles of Human Physiology*, 101-2

castration, 10, 52, 53, 60-61, 140, 148, 197, 198
Catholic Church, 4, 32, 34
cauterization treatment: death from, 182-83; homosexuality, 181; prostatic section of the urethra, 66-67; for seminal emissions, 176, 184; silver nitrate use in, 134, 176, 179, 181; for spermatorrhea, 66-67, 176, 179, 180, 182, 186-87; urethral, 123, 134, 175, 176-77, 186-87
Chadwick, Edwin, 98, 101
Chambers, Thomas, 55, 178, 182-83
Chapman, John, 265
chemical theory of disease, 239
Chesser, Eustace, 307
Child, G. B., 175
child-care manuals, 202-3, 217, 232, 271, 307, 314
children: age of puberty, 56, 86-88; child-care manuals, 202-3, 217, 232, 271, 307, 314; peer networks of sex information, 24, 29-30, 90-92, 191, 195, 207; public schools, 193-95, 201, 207, 288; sexuality of, 53, 56, 86, 89, 129-30, 203, 325n71, 328n37; surgery for, 116; surveillance of, 56, 60, 64, 86, 90-91, 131, 203. *See also* masturbation; prepubescent males
circumcision: aesthetics of, 4, 42; bed-wetting prevention and, 139-40, 225, 287; case studies, 224-25; clitoridectomy compared to, 144, 148, 149, 161-62, 196-97, 235; complications and mortality of, 9, 294-95, 312; decline of, 308-13; epilepsy and, 148, 225; germ theory and, 239, 246-47; hygiene, 7, 41-42, 68-69, 171, 231, 236, 274-75, 356n5; males and, 230, 296-300; masturbation and, 6-8, 68, 121, 138-39, 158, 185, 192-93, 200-214 (210t), 224-25, 271, 300; methods of, 114-15, 225-26, 291-94, 338n32; nerve force theory, 87, 185, 225; outside Great Britain, 114, 281, 314-17, 337n95, 339n16; paralysis treated with, 68-69, 103, 220-21; parental consent for, 85-86, 287-88, 296-98; penile cancer, 254-56; phimosis and, 67, 132, 178, 204, 220, 222-23, 232, 328n35; postoperative care, 226-27, 285, 287-88; preventive circumcision, 116-17, 132-33, 137, 162, 263-64; in quack medicine, 286; rise of, 317-19; sexual pleasure and, 34, 45, 161, 205, 213, 275, 277, 330n70; social class and, 82, 193, 285-86, 288-90, 314-15; spermatorrhea, 121, 177-78, 185, 188; syphilis and, 223, 261-

62t, 272, 276-79, 280-83, 302, 328n35, 356n5; trauma of, 227, 234-35, 287-88, 291, 293-300, 302; tuberculosis prevention and, 253-54; vaccination compared to, 99, 271, 286, 318. *See also* Brown, Isaac Baker; foreskin; Jewish circumcision; masturbation; Muslim circumcision

Circumcision: Its Advantages and How to Perform It (Clifford), 202

Clark, Andrew, 103

Cleland, John, 42

clergyman's throat, 180, 254, 331n51

Clifford, M., 202, 277-78, 294

clitoridectomy: British medical profession's reputation and, 154, 155-56; childbearing after, 148-49, 154, 161; circumcision compared to, 144, 148, 149, 161-62, 196-97, 235; epilepsy, 147-48; hysteria, 7, 145, 146, 147, 148; informed consent for, 153, 156, 159-60; insanity, 143, 160; as mutilation, 144, 151, 158, 159; women's sexuality after, 148, 154, 156-57, 161. *See also* Brown, Isaac Baker

Cold, Chris, 167-68

Comfort, Alex, 13, 289

Comstock, Anthony, 290

condoms, 84, 263, 274, 275-76, 282, 283, 336n5

Condorcet, Marquis de, 76-77

congenital phimosis: case studies of, 223-25; circumcision and, 204, 220, 222-23; diagnosis of, 121; epilepsy, 140; J. Cooper Forster on, 135-36, 204, 220; germ theory and, 220, 225; hygiene, 220, 222; as medical error, 234; nerve force theory, 220-21, 225; paralysis, 221; reality of, 135, 234; urination, 135-36, 140, 219-20; use of term, 219-20. *See also* phimosis

Connolly, D. I., 232-33, 252

Contagious Disease Act: endorsements of, 123, 264, 267-68; immorality, 268-69; medical profession and, 107-8; regulation of prostitution, 83, 266-69; repeal of, 75, 272-73

continence: as abstinence, 77, 124, 269; foreskin, 276; legislation for, 272; masturbation, 124; physical exercise, 126, 127, 131, 135, 178, 194-95; religious views on, 124-26; sex education, 88

contraception: attempted abstinence as, 81-82; foreskin and, 325n45; as immoral, 75, 77, 85; information on, 12, 23, 76; overpopulation, 76; sexual relationships and, 13, 64, 308

Cook, Hera, 74, 75-76, 82, 252-53, 307, 325n71

Cooper, Astley, 219

Coote, Holmes, 154-55, 273

Cooter, Roger, 116

Copland, James, 119, 137-38, 146, 192, 242

Corfield, W. H., 240, 241

Corner, Edred M., 203, 229-30

Courtenay, F. B., 173-74, 182, 187

Crozier, Ivan, 134, 173, 175, 327n21, 333n85

Cullen, James, 101

Cullen, William, 38

culture of abstinence. *See* antisensualism movement

Curling, T. B., 116, 119, 137, 177, 204

Curtis, Henry, 246

da Carpi, Jacopo Berengario, 24-25, 119, 121

Dally, Ann, 17-18

Daniel, Peter, 250-51

Daniell, W. F., 143, 148

Darwinism, 61, 78-79, 111, 113, 170-71, 331n13

Davenport, John, 205

Davenport-Hines, Richard, 106, 299

Davidson, Alexander, 193, 224, 243

Davis, Dick, 297

Dawson, Richard, 173, 178, 182-83

Dictionary of Medicine (Quain), 104, 187, 188, 241

Dictionary of Practical Medicine (Copeland), 157-58

Digby, Ann, 116

Dionis, Pierre, 26, 217-18

Dixon, Edward, 220

Dock, Lavinia, 271, 274

Douglas, Mary, 100

Doyle, Arthur Conan, 111

Driberg, Tom, 299, 300

Drysdale, George: on circumcision, 262-63, 281; on contraception, 13, 263, 274, 276; on sexual activity, 29, 55, 77, 125; on spermatorrhea, 179, 180

Dubois, Dr., 144

Duncan, Matthews, 334n50

Eagle, Chester, 213

Edinburgh Medical Journal, 292

Ellis, Havelock: on circumcision, 232, 294; homology of clitoris to penis, 122; on masturbation, 62, 211-12, 232, 306, 333n85; on sex education, 91-92, 108, 110; on Symonds' homoeroticism, 181

epidemics, 11, 95-96, 100, 107, 112, 328n35